T0137246

Suicide by Self-Immolation

César A. Alfonso • Prabha S. Chandra
Thomas G. Schulze

Editors

Suicide by Self-Immolation

Biopsychosocial and Transcultural Aspects

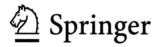 Springer

Editors
César A. Alfonso
Department of Psychiatry
Columbia University Medical Center
New York, NY
USA

Prabha S. Chandra
Department of Psychiatry
National Institute of Mental Health
Bengaluru
India

Thomas G. Schulze
IPPG
Klinikum der Universität München
Munich
Germany

ISBN 978-3-030-62615-0   ISBN 978-3-030-62613-6   (eBook)
https://doi.org/10.1007/978-3-030-62613-6

This Springer imprint is published by the registered company Springer Nature Switzerland AG
The registered company address is: Gewerbestrasse 11, 6330 Cham, Switzerland

Foreword

This book gives rare access to the subject of suicide by self-immolation in all its complexity and challenge. It brings together the topics of suicide and the mental health of women and girls. This convergence is quite uncommon in itself. Death by suicide is most often considered predominantly a male problem, consistent with epidemiological patterns in some parts of the world. The influence on each of these topics of the social and cultural environments and the psychological and biological functions of individuals is another prominent theme.

This lethal means of suicide primarily affects women in low- and middle-income countries. Its occurrence is deeply influenced by the cultural traditions and social realities with which the women live. It is endemic in several parts of the world in which disadvantage and adversities are also common, adversities related to poverty, pandemic, conflict, natural disasters and exposure to interpersonal violence and abuse of human rights. It is also a way of death for men, as recognised more widely even though less common.

Rich transcultural and historical accounts of the phenomenon open the book and are threaded through the commentaries that follow on this form of death in Iran, Afghanistan, India, Indonesia and Papua, Sub-Saharan Africa, Tibetan communities, the Arab world and in high-income countries. Death by self-immolation is rooted in ancient historical traditions in certain parts of the world. Yet it is enabled by modern forms of flammable liquids and perpetuated in contemporary communities and conditions. Even though the death by burning of a venerable religious figure in Vietnam in 1963 is a modern point of reference to altruistic sacrifice as described in the book, it is far from representative of the present-day phenomenon of self-immolation.

The gendered analysis of the causation and prevention of suicide by burning is one of the book's features. For both women and men, death in this way is sometimes related to poverty or oppression and sometimes to persecution and protest. Its transcultural meaning is examined in the opening chapter and in those that follow from several parts of the world. The biological, psychodynamic, phenomenological, social science and spiritual bases of suicide are considered after that, and the need for multidisciplinary work and psychiatric support in the care of people who have survived. The dangers of dichotomous thinking become apparent. Whether it is thinking about social or biological causes of suicide or individual or collective approaches to prevention, narrow perspectives curtail the needed responses. Patterns of suicide among men and women and boys and girls are different across regions, countries and settings. In all settings, the intermix of personal, family, community, cultural and social factors finally influences suicidal behaviour and death.

Suicide by self-immolation may be considered in one sense a strange and atypical form of suicide. It is poorly represented in the world's scientific literature and rarely discussed in gatherings of experts on suicide prevention. It is atypical compared with most scientific accounts of suicide—from high-income countries—in that most of those who die are women using a violent means. As described here, however, suicide by self-immolation exemplifies the need for local and gendered analysis in designing approaches to prevention of suicide. The participation of local people is crucial in consulting on needs and approaches and in the implementation and evaluation of interventions. This gendered, local and participatory approach to prevention needs support and greater development: to relieve the suffering of women and men directly affected; illuminate the prevention of suicide more broadly and increase the understanding of how the mental health of women is inter-twined with their own health and functioning and that of their families and communities.

I congratulate the editors for conceiving this book. They have brought together an extraordinary group of talented and experienced authors. They have worked with them to cast light on an under-recognised phenomenon of cultural, psychiatric and scientific significance. I am proud to see the role of the World Psychiatric Association in the genesis and publication of the book. I recommend it to those in communities and among clinicians, scholars and policymakers who wish to work together to prevent death by self-immolation, to investigate and evaluate the interventions and to understand this phenomenon more fully. Reading it will also reward those interested in the broader questions of suicide prevention and the mental health of women and girls worldwide.

Helen Herrman
President of the World Psychiatric
Association (2017–2020)
Geneva, Switzerland

Director of the WHO Collaborating
Centre in Mental Health
Melbourne, Australia

Contents

Transcultural Aspects of Suicide by Self-Immolation

César A. Alfonso and Prabha S. Chandra

> *"… the pain of not enjoying any basic human rights is far greater than the pain of self-immolation"*
>
> *(Excerpt from suicide note recorded by Tibetans Sonam and Choepak Kyap)*
>
> *"Violence in the lives of Afghanistan's women comes from everywhere: from her father or brother, from her husband, from her father-in-law, from her mother-in-law and sister-in-law"*
>
> *(Dr. Shafiqa Eanin, plastic surgeon in the Herat Burn Hospital, Afghanistan, interviewed by the New York Times)*

1 Introduction

In this book we define self-immolation as the act of burning as a means of suicide by deliberately pouring and igniting kerosene, gasoline or other liquid accelerants on one's body. A self-immolation suicide attempt is lethal 50–90% of the time [1, 2]

C. A. Alfonso (✉)
Columbia University Medical Center, New York, NY, USA

Universitas Indonesia, Jakarta, Indonesia

National University of Malaysia, Kuala Lumpur, Malaysia

World Psychiatric Association Psychotherapy Section, Geneva, Switzerland
e-mail: cesaralfonso@mac.com, caa2105@cumc.columbia.edu

P. S. Chandra
National Institute of Mental Health and Neurosciences, Bangalore, India

International Association of Women's Mental Health, Bangalore, India
e-mail: prabhasch@gmail.com, chandra@nimhans.ac.in

© The Author(s), under exclusive license to Springer Nature Switzerland AG 2021
C. A. Alfonso et al. (eds.), *Suicide by Self-Immolation*,
https://doi.org/10.1007/978-3-030-62613-6_1

and the few who survive populate burn units with agony and high morbidity. Self-immolation survivors return unprotected upon medical discharge from burn centers to the same chaotic home and social environments that generated extreme distress, impulsivity and suicidality. Self-immolators are scarred for life, both factually and symbolically, stigmatized in ways that add psychological insult to bodily injury. Self-immolation invariably follows oppression and characteristically represents an attempt to speak out against and ultimately escape intolerable psychosocial conditions, cultural subjugation and marginalization.

Suicide accounts for close to one million deaths annually worldwide, making it an important cause of death with major public health and prevention implications [3]. It is the leading cause of death in persons 15–24 years of age globally [4]. Since only one third of world countries have adequate vital registration data, suicide death estimates are based largely on modelling methods and suicides may be underreported. According to the World Health Organization (WHO) [3] more than 80% of suicides by self-immolation occur in low-and-middle-income countries (LAMICs). Countries with disproportionate high prevalence of self-immolation include Iran, Iraq, Afghanistan, India, Sri Lanka, Papua-New Guinea, Zimbabwe, and Tibet. Perhaps with the exception of Tibetan regions, self-immolators in LAMICs tend to be young women experiencing extreme forms of abuse and oppression [1, 5].

In high-income countries self-immolation usually occurs as a rare symbolic display of political protest among men (who may not have a psychiatric diagnosis) or associated with severe psychopathology [2, 5]. Psychiatric diagnoses associated with self-immolation in high-income countries include psychotic disorders, substance use disorders, major depression, posttraumatic stress disorder and adjustment disorders [2, 5, 6]. Recent unemployment has also been identified as a risk factor in self-immolators, especially in those with adjustment disorders, in high-income countries [5, 6].

In low- and-middle-income countries self-immolation is highly prevalent, primarily affects women, and may be one of the most common suicide methods in regions of Central and South Asia and parts of Africa [2, 5–7]. While in high-income countries self-immolation constitutes 0.6–1% of all suicides, in some LAMICs it comprises 40–70% of suicides [1, 2, 6]. In LAMICs, trauma and stressor-related disorders are the most common psychiatric diagnoses associated with self-immolation suicides, although many persons who self-immolate in LAMICs do not have a psychiatric diagnosis [2, 6].

This chapter will review psychosocial determinants of self-immolation, identify pertinent psychodynamic, ethnographic and sociocultural elements, and provide an overview of common factors and culturally specific antecedents that may be relevant for the design and implementation of suicide prevention strategies.

2 Historical, Religious and Sociopolitical Antecedents of Self-Immolation

Self-immolation accounts exist in historical and religious texts dating back millennia. Self-immolations occur worldwide in the context of most religious traditions. Historical emphasis has been given to immolations in Hindu and Buddhist societies, although important historical accounts of Daoist and Christian self-immolations similarly influenced other regions of the world.

Sati in India is the practice describing widow self-immolation by ritualistically ascending on to the funeral pyre of the deceased husband [8]. It is named after the Hindu goddess of marital felicity and longevity. Widow self-immolation in India dates back to the fourth century BCE but did not become widespread until the seventh century AD. Mention of Sati is present in the Sanskrit Mahabharata and in Tamil Sangam literature. Sati served the purpose of perpetuating karmic marital union and optimized chances for a husband's heavenly rebirth. Sati practices spread throughout the centuries and to all socioeconomic strata inside and outside of India to Indonesia, China, Myanmar and the Philippines [9]. Sati was abolished in the nineteenth century in India after strong opposition by Hindu reformers and Christian evangelists. In the late twentieth century a Sati Prevention Act passed to prohibit the glorification of Sati self-immolations. Nevertheless, self-immolation role models and stories remain part of the cultural armamentarium of the collective psyche of millions of women in the Indian subcontinent. Bhugra [10] refers to Sati as a cultural form of suicide and exhorts awareness of the cultural idioms that widowhood reflects in Indian culture when devising prevention strategies and programs. Social pressures in Indian society may compound acute grief, which may lead to depersonalization and carrying out culturally endorsed self-immolations, since the psychological experiences and attitudes towards widowhood include stigma, oppression, guilt and a sense of failure [10].

Indian and Mahayana Buddhist ancient texts report accounts of self-immolation so as to achieve enlightenment and altruistically sacrifice oneself for the benefit of others. Over centuries self-immolation in China took on a political purpose as well [11]. Non-Buddhist Chinese descriptions of self-immolations include the self-immolation of King Tang, founder of the Shang Dynasty, who burned himself as a sacrifice to his people to alleviate a devastating drought. Many notable Daoist self-immolations of rulers and high-ranking officers for procuring rain followed in subsequent centuries throughout China [12].

Maltreatment of Christians during the era of Roman Emperors Diocletian and Maximian resulted in subjugation, persecutory practices, desecration of churches, imprisonment and executions. Many executions occurred by burning Christians alive. A memorable standoff between the Christian priest Glycerius and the Roman Emperor, in the year 304, resulted in what is now known as the 20,000 Martyrs of Nicomedia event, where parishioners were either burned alive for not renouncing their faith, or willingly self-immolated as an act of protest [13, 14]. Over a thousand years later, in seventeenth-century Russia, factions of the Orthodox Church protested government-ordered religious reforms. Friction between Church and State peaked and thousands of Kapitonist Old Believers set themselves on fire in an infernal mass baptismal suicide to affirm religious fervor denouncing the Russian Czar as the Antichrist [13].

The self-immolation of five Falun Gong supporters in Tiananmen Square in Beijing in 2001 on the Eve of Chinese New Year celebrations catalyzed Chinese propaganda and persecution of Falun Dafa practices but also brought international attention to the group. Although there is lack of clarity as to what motivated the Falun

Gong self-immolations, there is no doubt that it communicated a powerful message all over the world by creating awareness of the intolerance of the Chinese government towards the spiritual-religious activities of this group, practices which are rooted in Buddhist, Daoist and Confucian traditions and followed by millions [15].

3 Psychosocial Determinants of Self-Immolation

There is no unique psychological profile of persons who self-immolate. Some commonalities may exist, especially in culture-specific ways. Psychosocial determinants of self-immolation in LAMICs are summarized in Table 1.

Suicide by self-immolation may be more common in recent immigrants who have not yet acculturated to their host countries. This has been observed, for example, in immigrants from India who relocated to Australia, UK or the Caribbean [22, 23].

Although identifying risk factors may help prevent suicide, a multidimensional ethnographic approach provides a more nuanced and culturally informed understanding of motivation and meaning of suicidal behaviors than the classic psychiatric approach that focuses on individual biomedical and interpersonal psychosocial factors. Is suicide an unvarying or a culturally specific phenomenon? This is a question that anthropologists ponder, and perhaps an exploration of complementary perspectives through cross-fertilization of overlapping research in the fields of psychology, psychiatry, sociology and anthropology may help in the design of more effective suicide prevention programs.

Table 1 Psychosocial determinants of self-immolation in LAMICs (low- and middle-income countries)	• Forced marriages [16–18]
	• Violence in the household [16, 18, 19]
	• War-torn countries and regions [16, 18]
	• Young age (ages 19–21) [16, 18–20]
	• Female [16–18, 20]
	• Conflict with spouse [16, 18–20]
	• Conflict with in-laws [16, 18, 19]
	• Conjugal fights [16, 18–20]
	• Romantic disappointment [19, 20]
	• Poverty [16, 18–21]
	• Dowry disputes [22]
	• Hunger [16, 18]
	• Overcrowding when families merge [16–18]
	• Impulsivity [19, 20]
	• Illiteracy and low education [18–20]
	• Affective states of hopelessness and helplessness [18–20]
	• Adjustment, depressive and trauma related disorders [18–20]

4 Psychodynamic and Socioenvironmental Formulations of Self-Immolation

Psychodynamic formulations are beneficial in order to understand motivation and choice and inform cultural and socioenvironmental formulations. Psychodynamic formulations should not be generic and must include the specific circumstances and life trajectory of the individual, including the cultural context [24].

The psychodynamics of self-immolation remain elusive and complex. People who self-immolate engage in an act of self-sacrifice, historically glorified in many cultures and associated with martyrdom. Imitation is an important dynamic when considering suicide by contagion. Media reports of suicides are often followed by copy-cat suicides, also known as the Werther effect or imitative suicidal behavior [25]. Recent research demonstrates that young women in both LAMICs and high-income countries are particularly vulnerable to imitative suicidal behavior [26]. In cultures in which cremation is the rite of passage for the dead there may be a propensity towards self-immolation as a way to precipitate death. Conversely, in cultures where cremation is prohibited or taboo, self-immolation may serve the purpose of protest and rebellion against what is normative and socially sanctioned. At times, self-immolation could be understood as a demonstrative act to seek revenge by creating guilt, or as an illusory form of self-defense, especially when being victimized by intimate partner violence.

Durkheim [27], and later Dollard [28] proposed a link between frustration and aggression in the genesis of suicide, a formulation that echoes Freud and Abraham's [29, 30] psychodynamic understanding of suicide as internalized anger that is violently acted out in states of depression and despair. While biomedical paradigms regard suicide as a defect, deficit, failure of adaptation or pathological, *sociologists regard suicide as rooted in a society that fails to protect the individual from the vicissitudes of life* [31]. The sociological paradigm may be more appropriate and relevant when designing public health self-immolation suicide prevention interventions in LAMICs.

Suicide gives a voice to the oppressed, and suicide as protest may be an opportunity to symbolically rebel against the aggressors and escape distress. Disenfranchised minorities, members of alienated religious groups, and vulnerable individuals victimized by senseless intimate partner violence may choose to communicate protest, fight back and speak up through the act of suicide. Self-immolation is a particular choice that allegorically links religion, mythology and popular culture in a dramatic and powerfully theatrical manner. By burning one's skin, an essential organ that protects and separates the individual from the environment, boundaries between self and others cease to exist and a powerful message is communicated to family survivors, perpetrators and communities at large.

5   The Skin, Haptics, Proxemics, Attachment and Epigenetics

The skin is the body's largest organ, serving as a protective barrier between external and internal worlds. The average adult has 2 m^2 of skin weighing up to 3.5 kg. Its multiple biological functions include insulation, immune and hormonal regulation, vitamin synthesis, temperature regulation, and somatosensory perception and communication. Haptics is defined as communication and perception that occur via the sense of touch [32]. Psychologically, the skin is closely linked to self-esteem and sexual and relationship health. Individuals from all cultures value their appearance, protect and nurture their skin, and maintain interpersonal health largely through the sense of touch and haptics.

The sense of touch, including proprioception and haptic perception, is mediated peripherally by complex and interactive neuroreceptors signaling upon stimulation via neural pathways the somatosensory brain cortex. Most touch receptors are contained within the skin. These include Pacinian corpuscles (sensing high frequency vibration signals, joint positional and rapid pressure changes), Meissner corpuscles (sensing light touch, vibration and minute stretch), Ruffini corpuscles (sensing positional movement), Merkel cells (responding to deep pressure to sense shapes), and free nerve endings, which are the most numerous receptors (involved in the perception of pain, pressure, temperature and stretch) [33]. The complexity of this biological system is also reflected in the intricacy of cultural norms regarding touching as a way of communicating. Although social touching varies in its expression across and within cultures, it is indispensable to express emotional closeness and modulate relationships through contact and boundaries. Haptic communication stimulates the production of growth hormone in infants [34] and mediates emotional attachments later in life with measurable changes in circulating neuropeptides such as oxytocin and vasopressin [35].

Cultural anthropologists developed the concept of *proxemics* to understand the interrelationship of the human use of space with behavior and social interactions [36]. Attachment theorists emphasize the importance of early life experiences in determining interpersonal security later in life [37–40]. The sensitive period of attachment bonding and security comprises the pre-school years, largely when children are nonverbal. It would follow that nonverbal communication is of essence in establishing security in infants and young children and providing a sense of safety and connectedness thereafter. Nonverbal behaviors include haptics (touch) and mimicry, and mirroring through praxis and vocalizations. The biometric study of proxemic behaviors in anthropology examines various dimensions of interpersonal distance surrounding an individual at any given point in time, including intimate, personal, social and public distance. In proxemic theory [41] there are subdivisions of space surrounding the body. These include, from proximal to distal: body, home, interactional and public territory. Navigating these spaces with psychological comfort greatly depends on emotional memories encoded after primal dyadic interactions. Those who were cared for and protected in a consistent, attentive and nurturing way will venture out with comfort into the interactional and public spaces later in life.

Attachment security is maintained intergenerationally [40] and traumatic life experiences affect our biology and cause epigenetic changes [42]. Adversity becomes programmed molecularly, leaving behind biological memories that persistently alter genome function and increase susceptibility to illnesses [42]. Epigenetics refers to the alteration of gene activity without changes in DNA sequences. Epigenetic processes occur mainly through DNA methylation and acetylation [43]. The interactions between acute trauma, enduring stressors, emotions, hormonal and peptide surges, up and down regulation of receptors and neurotransmission cause epigenetic changes in the brain with associated changes in endocrine and immune systems and inflammatory response [44]. Epigenetic processes are heritable by offspring and may be associated with the intergenerational transmission of trauma. Epigenetic changes may partially determine increased suicide risk [45] as a consequence of gene-by environment interactions.

Intimate partner violence constitutes a transgression of psychological boundaries that causes bodily injury and threatens the person's basic sense of safety. Being physically attacked and emotionally tortured by those who are meant to love us unconditionally causes a near state of psychological disintegration. When defense mechanisms such as dissociation and isolation of affect fail to protect the individual who is being abused, destroying the skin by burning becomes an extension of the psychological destruction of the protective boundary that separates and protects the self from others. Self-immolation is common in regions of the world where women marry young and are displaced from their family units onto a new hostile surrogate family in an overcrowded environment, with a husband who is physically abusive, and in-laws who are physically and emotionally abusive, especially when the husband is mostly absent earning a living or fighting a war. This set of circumstances compounds poverty, terror, alienation, helplessness, powerlessness, and hopelessness.

6   Culture Specific Aspects of Self-Immolation

Self-immolation suicides are often viewed as acts of protest aiming at redemption, freedom from oppression and realization of basic human rights. Protest suicides occur within a matrix of cultural-historical embeddedness [46]. Self-immolation suicides are prevalent in ancient cultures where fire has iconographic and mythological prominence with transformational qualities [46]. When religious oppression and cultural impositions occur as part of the ethnographic framework, self-immolation becomes a meaningful tool, communicating a public message to the social units, attracting notice and influencing public opinion [46, 47]. Such is the case of the dramatic self-immolation of Vietnamese and Tibetan monks [1, 48], peace activists protesting war and armed conflicts [49], and most recently the suicides during the Arab Spring [50]. Religious and social motivations at times determine the choice to self-immolate, as in the case of sacrifice to preserve a sense of honor, protest against reform, demand reforms, and affirm one's beliefs in spite of persecution, discrimination and alienation [49].

6.1   The Role of Gender and Violence Against Women

Most self-immolations in the world occur among women living in an environment of poverty, overcrowding, and subjected to repeated intimate partner violence and other forms of domestic violence. Access to means is a known risk factor for all suicides. In oppressive patriarchal cultures where women live in poverty and their actions restricted to the immediacy of the household, self-immolation may result as there is easy access to kerosene or other volatile substances in kitchens. Women, when not allowed to go out to obtain or buy pills or pesticides, may resort to using readily available volatile substances to end their lives.

In India self-immolations often involve dowry disputes [22], although some are acts of academic and political protest [49]. In Iran, women with lower education and socioeconomic status and of Kurdish ethnicity seem to be at higher risk [51]. In Afghanistan the prevalence of self-immolation is perhaps the highest in the world. Fifty-seven percent of Afghan women marry before 16 years of age, 29% are forced into marriage to settle tribal conflicts, 84% are illiterate, and the average woman gives birth to eight children. High rates of intimate partner violence and domestic violence by in-laws and husband's other wives compound overcrowding, poverty and result in the self-immolation of vulnerable young women in Afghanistan [52]. In regions such as the Herat province of Afghanistan, the prevalence of suicide by self-immolation is alarmingly high. In spite of recent legislative changes in the country aimed at improving human rights, social change lags behind, self-immolation suicides persist, and efforts have failed to protect vulnerable young women at risk [52].

7   Recommendations and Prevention

The WHO suicide prevention guidelines [3] are comprehensive and can be tailored to target populations at risk. Suicide prevention intermediations can be further subdivided into *universal, selective, indicated* and *postvention* interventions (see Table 2).

Prevention of suicide by self-immolation needs to take into consideration the cultural milieu of vulnerable groups and individuals. All suicidal persons at risk would benefit from improving current mental health services. Health and social services should include sensitive evaluations for partner violence and have provisions for support when detected. Providing capacity-building opportunities in low- and middle-income countries is of essence to prevent suicide by self-immolation.

Table 2 WHO Suicide Prevention Intermediation Guidelines (2014)

Type of intervention	Target	Examples
Universal	*Population at large*	Increasing access to health care
		Promoting mental health
		Decreasing use of harmful substances
		Promoting responsible media reporting
		Restricting access to means
		Implementing mental health policies
Selective	*Vulnerable groups* (e.g. Trauma survivors, affected by disaster, refugees and migrants, suicide survivors)	Suicide helplines
		Training community gatekeepers
		Training religious leaders
		Training clinicians
		Encouraging protective factors
		Encouraging adaptive coping
		Legislation to protect vulnerable groups
		Legislation to preserve social ties
Indicated	*Vulnerable individuals*	Community support to reduce stigma
		Follow-up upon discharge
		Training healthcare workers
		Improving diagnosis of mental disorders
		Assessment and management of suicidality
Postvention	Bereaved families and friends	Outreach to family and friends
		Grief counseling for families
		Grief counseling for friends
		School-based postventions
		Bereavement support groups for survivors

Recognition of psychopathology and screening for mental-health problems are pivotal, as well as understanding the nuances of interpersonal relationships among women at risk of self-immolation.

Women-oriented mental health programs could improve access to care and provide psychosocial support to susceptible individuals living in fragile and volatile environments. Peer support groups are a useful method of creating spaces for women to share distress and learn ways of coping. Funding and empowering NGOs that support human rights of women, passing legislation that protects women, and enforcing egalitarian laws to facilitate a cultural shift away from discriminatory attitudes are all necessary. In addition, there needs to be a strong move in these countries to focus on men's mental health, substance use and their methods of conflict resolution and handling emotions. Traditional forms of masculinity encourage patriarchy and the subjugation of women and these need to be questioned. Men and boys need to be taught more adaptive ways of family life and handling relationships.

Upstream suicide prevention approaches include addressing risk and protective factors early in life and may be of particular importance to prevent suicide by self-immolation in LAMICs [3]. Childhood adversity and trauma correlate with poor health outcomes and suicide [53]. Connectedness, reduction of alienation, and eliminating a person's sense of expendability are suicide protective [54, 55]. Upstream prevention interventions may include home visits, mentoring and buddy programs, optimizing adolescent health by improving access to care, and encouraging help-seeking via training of gatekeepers.

Promoting gender equality legislation and working towards eliminating forced marriages, especially of the very young, should be strongly pursued. Media guidelines are important to properly educate the public about mental illness and engaging in responsible reporting of suicides. Communities play a key role in suicide prevention, particularly in cultural enclaves at risk for self-immolation. Prevention efforts must take place beyond the individuals at risk and target vulnerable groups and survivors.

Regions of the world with high prevalence of self-immolation should systematical assess their national suicide prevention strategies. A national strategy must involve the following ten essential components: *surveillance, means restrictions, responsible media reporting, access to treatment, training and education, crisis intervention, postvention, stigma reduction, oversight coordination* of efforts by NGOs and governmental organizations, and *measuring outcomes* [3].

8 Conclusions

Suicide by self-immolation is a grave and unaddressed public health problem in LAMICs and cultural enclaves worldwide. It has historical, sociopolitical and religious antecedents dating back millennia in Judeo-Christian, Hindu, Buddhist and Daoist traditions. Transcultural factors of relevance include suicides as acts of protest aiming at redemption, freedom from oppression and realization of basic human rights. The psychosocial context of self-immolation, particularly in LAMICs, includes family dynamics where intimate partner violence, forced marriages, and interpersonal conflicts compound exposure to war related life events, poverty, forced migration and ethnic conflicts. Sociologists' view of suicide as rooted in a society that fails to protect the individual from the vicissitudes of life may inform suicide prevention interventions by mental health clinicians. Selective and indicated suicide prevention strategies are needed in areas of the world with a high prevalence of self-immolations. These include, in addition to optimizing access to mental health treatment, developing regional and national suicide prevention strategies and promoting legislations that take into account specific transcultural needs of vulnerable individuals and marginalized groups.

References

1. Laloë V. Patterns of deliberate self-burning in various parts of the world: a review. Burns. 2004;30(3):207–15.
2. Suhrabi Z, Delpisheh A, Taghinejad H. Tragedy of women's self-immolation in Iran and developing communities: a review. Int J Burn Trauma. 2012;2(2):93–104.
3. WHO. Preventing suicide: a global imperative. Geneva: World Health Organization; 2014. https://apps.who.int/iris/bitstream/handle/10665/131056/9789241564779_eng.pdf;jsessioni d=4DB114A485E61068593DDC2ACC1BEB4F?sequence=1. Accessed 7 Feb 2020.
4. Fazel S, Runeson B. Suicide. N Engl J Med. 2020;382:266–74. https://doi.org/10.1056/NEJMra1902944.
5. Zamani SN, Bagheri M, Nejad MA. Investigation of the demographic characteristics and mental health in self-immolation attempters. Int J High-Risk Behav Addict. 2013;2(2):77–81.
6. Poeschla B. Self-immolation: socioeconomic, cultural and psychiatric patterns. Burns: J Int Soc Burn Inj. 2011;37(6):1049–57. https://doi.org/10.1016/j.burns.2011.02.011.
7. Sheth H, Dziewulski P, Settle JAD. Self-inflicted burns: a common way of suicide in the Asian population. A 10-year retrospective study. J Burns. 1994;20(4):334–5.
8. Brick SD, Kitts M. Matyrdom, self-sacrifice and self-immolation: religious perspectives. Oxford: Oxford University Press; 2018.
9. Hawley JS. Sati, the blessing and the curse: the burning of wives in India. New York, Oxford: Oxford University Press; 1964.
10. Bhugra D. Sati: a type of nonpsychiatric suicide. Crisis. 2005;26(2):73–7.
11. Benn JA. Burning for the Buddha: self-immolation in Chinese Buddhism. Hawaii: University of Hawaii Press; 2007. p. 9–10.
12. Yu J. Reflections on self-immolation in Chinese Buddhist and Daoist traditions. In: Kitts M, editor. Martyrdom, self-sacrifice and self-immolation. New York: Oxford University Press; 2018. p. 264–79.
13. Verini J. A terrible act of reason: when did self-immolation become the paramount form of protest? *The New Yorker*. May 16, 2012.
14. Walsh MJ. A new dictionary of saints: east and west. Collegeville, MN: Liturgical Press; 2007. p. 401.
15. Pan, P.P. Human fire ignites Chinese mystery. *The Washington Post*. February 4, 2001.
16. Aziz N. What self-immolation means to Afghan women. Peace Rev: J Soc Justice. 2011;23:45–51.
17. Hasrat-Nazami W. Afghan women escape marriage through suicide. In: World, Society. Berlin: Deutsche Welle; 2013.
18. Hauslohner A. Afghanistan: when women set themselves on fire. *Time*. Wednesday July 7, 2010.
19. Ahmadi A, Mohammadi R, Schwebel DC, Yeganeh N, Soroush A, Bazargan-Hejazi S. Familial risk factors for self-immolation: a case-control study. J Women's Health (Larchmt). 2009;18(7):1025–31.
20. Saadati M, Azami-Aghdash S, Heydari M, Derakhshani N, Rezapour R. Self-immolation in Iran: systematic review and meta-analysis. Bull Emerg Trauma. 2019;7(1):1–8. https://doi.org/10.29252/beat-070101.
21. Rehkopf DH, Buka SL. The association between suicide and the socio-economic characteristics of geographical areas: a systematic review. Psychol Med. 2006;36:145–57.
22. Chen Y, Wu KC, Yousuf S, Yip PSF. Suicide in Asia: opportunities and challenges. Epidemiol Rev. 2011;34(1):129–44.
23. Raleigh VS, Balarajan R. Suicide and self-burning among Indians and West Indians in England and Wales. Br J Psychiatry. 1992;161:365–8.
24. Alfonso CA. A psychodynamic approach to complex psychiatric disorders. In: Alfonso CA, Friedman RC, Downey JI, editors. Advances in psychodynamic psychiatry. New York, London: Guilford Press; 2019.

25. Niederkrotenthaler T, Fu KW, Yip PSF, et al. Changes in suicide rates following media reports on celebrity suicide: a metanalysis. J Epidemiol Community Health. 2012;66:1037–42.
26. Hahn Yi JH, Hyun-Jin B, Kim N. Age and sex subgroups vulnerable to copycat suicide: evaluation of nationwide data in South Korea. Nat Res Sci Rep. 2019;9:17253. https://doi.org/10.1038/s41598-019-53833-8.
27. Durkheim E. The division of labour in society. Simpson G, translator. London: Collier Macmillan Publishers; 1893. p. 1933.
28. Dollard J, Doob LW, Miller NE, Mowrer OH, Sears RR. Frustration and aggression. New Haven: Yale University Press; 1939.
29. Freud S. Mourning and melancholia. In: Standard edition of the complete psychological works of Sigmund Freud. Strachey J, translator, vol. 14. London: Hogarth Press; 1917. p. 237–60.
30. Abraham K. Notes on the psychoanalytical investigation and treatment of manic-depressive insanity and allied conditions. In: Selected papers on psychoanalysis. Byran D and Strachey A, translators. New York: Basic Books, 1960; 1911. p. 137–56.
31. Durkheim E. A study in sociology. Suicide J.A., Spauding JA, Simpson G, translators. London: Routledge; 1951; [1897]
32. Proksch E, Brandner JM, Jensen JM. The skin: an indispensable barrier. Exp Dermatol. 2008;17(12):1063–72.
33. Boron WF, Boulpaep EL. Medical physiology. Philadelphia: Saunders; 2003. p. 352–8.
34. Field T, Schanberg SM, Scafidi F, et al. Effects of tactile/kinesthetic stimulation on preterm neonates. Pediatrics. 1986;77:654–8.
35. Chambers J. The neurobiology of attachment: from infancy to clinical outcomes. In: Alfonso CA, Friedman RC, Downey JI, editors. Advances in psychodynamic psychiatry. New York, London: Guilford Press; 2019.
36. Hall ET. A system for the notation of proxemic behavior. Am Anthropol. 1963;65(5):1003–26.
37. Bowlby J. Attachment and loss (Volume III). New York: Basic Books; 1980.
38. Cassidy J, Schaffer PR. Handbook of attachment: theory, research and clinical applications. New York: Guilford Press; 2008.
39. Wallin D. Attachment in psychotherapy. New York: Guilford Press; 2007.
40. Main M, Hesse E. Parents' unresolved traumatic experiences are related to infant disorganized attachment status. In: Greenberg MT, Cicchetti D, Commings EM, editors. Attachment in the preschool years: theory, research and intervention. Chicago: University of Chicago Press; 1990.
41. Moore N. Nonverbal communication: studies and applications. New York: Oxford University Press; 2010.
42. Dunn EC, Soare TW, Zhu Y, Simpkin AJ, Suderman MJ, Klengel T, Smith ADAC, Ressler KJ, Relton CL. Sensitive periods for the effect of childhood adversity on DNA methylation: results from a prospective, longitudinal study. Biol Psychiatry. 2019;85:838–49.
43. Szyf M, Bick J. DNA methylation: a mechanism for embedding early life experiences in the genome. Child Dev. 2013;84(1):49–57. https://doi.org/10.1111/j.1467-8624.2012.01793.x.
44. van Heeringen K, Mann JJ. The neurobiology of suicide. Lancet Psychiatry. 2014;1:63–72.
45. Adam EK, Sheldon-Keller AE, West M. Attachment organization and history of suicidal behavior in clinical adolescents. J Consult Clin Psychol. 1996;64:264–72.
46. Andriolo K. The twice killed: imagining protest suicide. Am Anthropol. 2006;108(1):100–13.
47. Biggs M. Dying without killing: self-immolations, 1963–2002. In: Gambetta D, editor. Making sense of suicide missions. Oxford: Oxford University Press; 2005. p. 173–208.
48. Barnett R. Political self-immolation in Tibet: causes and influences. Revue d'Etudes Tibétaines. 2012;25:41–64.
49. Donaldson DB. The self-immolators. 2013. http://thespeakernewsjournal.com/wp-content/uploads/2013/06/The-Self-Immolators.pdf. Accessed 7 Feb 2020.
50. Staples J, Widger T. Situating suicide as an anthropological problem: ethnographic approaches to understanding self-harm and self-inflicted death. Cult Med Psychiatry. 2012;36:183–203.
51. Rezaeian M. Epidemiology of self-immolation. Burns. 2013;31(1):36–42.

52. Raj A, Gomez C, Silverman JG. Driven to a fiery death—the tragedy of self-immolation in Afghanistan. N Engl J Med. 2008;358(21):2201–3.
53. Chesney E, Goodwin GM, Fazel S. Risks of all-cause and suicide mortality in mental disorders: a meta-review. World Psychiatry. 2014;13:153–60.
54. Cottrell DJ, Wright-Hughes A, Collinson M, et al. Effectiveness of systemic family therapy versus treatment as usual for young people after self-harm: a pragmatic, phase 3, multicentre, randomized controlled trial. Lancet Psychiatry. 2018;5:203–16.
55. Dunster-Page C, Haddock G, Wainwright L, Berry K. The relationship between therapeutic alliance and patient's suicidal thoughts, self-harming behaviours and suicide attempts: a systematic review. J Affect Disord. 2017;223:165–74.

Suicide by Self-Immolation: Historical Overview

Jeremie Sinzelle

> *If all that changes slowly may be explained by life, all that changes quickly is explained by fire. Fire is the ultra-living element. It is intimate and it is universal...*
>
> Gaston Bachelard
>
> *The Psychoanalysis of Fire, 1938*

1 Introduction

Among all medical fields, psychiatry is probably the closest to social sciences and humanities. Initially called alienism, psychiatry addresses mental disease, psychological suffering of individuals, and its treatment. For one of its pioneers, Philippe Pinel, the challenge to its practice was basically medical-philosophical. This may lead us to the reflection that many topics in psychiatry can benefit from the lights of sociology and history. The topic of this volume, self-immolation, is particularly emblematic of the different views developed through medical and psychiatric approaches, on a common subject, which can contribute to innovative prevention efforts of this dramatic act.

Self-immolation entered psychiatry by the mid-nineteenth century. In the twentieth century, technical progress and the general use of gasoline and matches, compounded by the growing mediatization of all topics and events, led to an increase of self-immolations that peaked after the burning sacrifice of the venerable Thich Quang Duc in Saigon in 1963 during the Buddhist Crisis in South Vietnam.

J. Sinzelle (✉)
Private Practice Psychiatrist, Paris, France

World Psychiatric Association (WPA), Section on History of Psychiatry, Geneva, Switzerland
e-mail: docteursinzelle@gmail.com

© The Author(s), under exclusive license to Springer Nature   15
Switzerland AG 2021
C. A. Alfonso et al. (eds.), *Suicide by Self-Immolation*,
https://doi.org/10.1007/978-3-030-62613-6_2

Even if most self-immolations of men are often described and mediatized as a political message, especially in high-income countries, the main problematic nowadays is located in Central and South Asia where these suicides are more frequent, silent, and affect mostly women. Most patients managed in burn recovery units suffer from a wide range of psychiatric disorders.

The WHO report *"Preventing Suicide, A Global Imperative"* [1], issued in 2014, notes that:

> ... *the social practices of certain religions have also encouraged self-immolation by fire among specific groups such as South Asian women who have lost their husbands. Therefore, while religion and spiritual beliefs may offer some protection against suicide, this depends on specific cultural and contextual practices and interpretations.* [1]

Rezaeian highlights cultural and sub-regional epidemiological variance of self-immolations. With an over-representation of Central and South Asians, the most vulnerable individuals seem to be married young women with low levels of education who experience marital discord and violence in the household. [2] The psychosocial dimensions of self-immolation are of paramount importance in understanding motivations and devising prevention strategies.

2   The Historic Symbolism of Fire

In the foreword of his work on *"The Psychoanalysis of Fire"* [3], the French philosopher Gaston Bachelard, who was a physicist in his early career, states that modern chemistry books rarely mention the phenomenon of fire: *"fire is no longer a reality for science"*. Fire has however fascinated and inspired humans since the most ancient days, fostering an *"initial charm"* that could be everlasting. Controlling fire, one of the first innovations of humankind for over one million years, is both intriguing and challenging. An objective approach to deconstruct the meaningfulness of fire is difficult. Bachelard refers to this as *"the psychological problem posed by our convictions about fire"*. Our oral and written traditions offer a plethora of allegorical allusions to the power of the fire. Relevant to this chapter is that destructive fire also has a purifying role in most religions.

In biblical traditions, Moloch (or Molekh) was a Canaanite deity that appeared when children were to be sacrificed through war or fire. His name, based on the three-consonant M-L-K, means *"King"* in Semitic languages. He is depicted as a giant with permanent fire emanating from within from being fed human lives. He was worshipped in the Kingdom of Ammon and in Carthago, as Baal-Hammon. Josias (648 BC–609 BC) forbade the cult in the Kingdom of Israel, showing that attempts to eradicate sacrifices through fire have existed for about two and a half millennia [4].

The main figure in the ancient Kurdish religion shares almost the same name. In Yazidi religion, it is believed that when God (Xwedê) created the world he shaped seven angels. The first of them and his deputy on Earth was Melek Tawus, depicted as a peacock. An illumination of fire from God created Melek Tawus, who then created the world from a single egg. He should enlighten humans and reveal their divine nature. Kurdish populations are one of the most affected by self-immolation [5]. In the same regions, fire to this day plays an important role in Zoroastrian religion, and similar rituals are integrated in the cult of Agni, the Vedic fire god of Hinduism.

Virgil, (79 BC–19 BC), in his exaltation book on nature and agriculture, presents fire as a means to attain purification:

It's often been beneficial to fire the stubble fields,
and burn the dry stalks in the crackling flames,
whether the earth gains hidden strength and rich food from it,
or every poison is baked out of it by the fire ... [6]

Diodorus, Virgil's contemporary who traveled through Persia to the Indian subcontinent, offered detailed accounts of self-immolation.

3   Immolation as a Traditional Indo-European Custom

Diodorus the Sicilian (90 BC–30 BC) left us an account of the travels of Alexander the Great through Persia. He noted that some Indian mercenaries joined Alexander's troops. One of them, Calanus, decided to end his happy, healthy and fulfilled life and asked Alexander to order his men to erect a funeral pyre to be lit as he stood over it. Alexander tried to dissuade him, but Calanus was determined and died on the very same day. There is no mention of possible religious motives and in retrospect it is unclear if we can qualify the event as a religious self-sacrifice or self-immolation suicide:

... and there Calanus (according to the rules and dictates of his own opinion) with great courage ascended the pile, and both he and it were consumed together. Some who were present judged this act to be an effect of madness, others nothing but a piece of vain glory, though some there were who admired his noble spirit and contempt of death; and the king caused him to be honourably buried. [7]

There is another depiction of self-immolation by Diodorus, reporting on the death and funeral rites of Ceteus, an Indian commander within Alexander's Army. Ceteus had two wives, who competed to be burnt over his dead body on the pyre. Eventually the older woman was chosen to be *"honored"* by the custom. The detailed description is astounding:

For there was one Ceteus, who commanded them that came out of India, and fought with great resolution, but died in this battle; he left two wives behind him, who followed him all along during the campaign: one he had but lately married, the other had been his wife for some years before; and both loved their husband exceedingly. It had been an ancient custom in India for men and women to marry with their own mutual liking, without consulting the advice of their parents ... another law therefore was made - That wives should be burnt together with their dead husbands, except they were with child, or had born children... The spectators were affected, some with pity, another with admiration, and extraordinary commendation of her resolution. However, there are some who condemn this law as cruel and inhuman. [7]

The most famous depiction of a cremation ritual comes from the direct observations of Ibn-FaÐlān in 921 AD. As an Ambassador of the Caliph Al-Muqtadir of Bagdad, Ibn-FaÐlān's mission was to reach Almish, the King of Volga Bulgars, and try to convince him to change from the Hanafi to the Baghdadi Shafei school of thought. Ibn-FaÐlān found himself with a group of Rūsiyyah and described their funeral immolation customs. One of the tribal chiefs died, and one of his slaves was to be cremated with him:

> *I was told that when their chieftains die, the least they do is to cremate them... They placed him in his grave and erected a canopy over it for ten days... When their chieftain dies, his family ask his slaves... "Who among you will die with him?" and some of them reply, "I shall"... The crone called the "Angel of Death" placed a rope around her neck in such a way that the ends crossed one another and handed it to two of the men to pull on it ... until she died... Then the deceased's next of kin approached and took hold of a piece of wood and set fire to it... He ignited the wood that had been set up under the ship after they had placed the slave-girl whom they had killed beside her master. Then the people came forward with sticks and firewood. Each one carried a stick the end of which he had set fire to and which he threw on top of the wood. The wood caught fire, and then the ship, the pavilion, the man, the slave-girl and all it contained. A dreadful wind arose, and the flames leapt higher and blazed fiercely.*

Although Ibn FaÐlān describes witnessing an unfamiliar funeral ritual, we cannot say it corresponds to a self-incineration per se. As immolation in *stricto sensu* is not necessarily through fire, we can say the slave offered herself in sacrifice and volunteered for immolation to be cremated next to the defunct. We should also point out that the ethnic affiliation of the group remains unclear to specialists: it was a group called Rūsiyyah, but from several origins sharing the same rituals (predominantly Varangians-Vikings, with a strong Slavic influence, and Finnic components) locates it in the Russian state that was just being constituted (Kievan Rus'). Although Ibn FaÐlān had an interpreter it is unclear what was language they spoke [8].

It is not known if the Ancient Greeks, before the Mycenaean era, carried out human sacrifices and rituals through fire like other Indo-Europeans [9]. Crooke noticed a possible common origin behind the phonetic similarity between one of the titles of Agni, the Hindu god of fire- Pramantha, and the Greek Titan Prometheus, who was petrified in punishment after giving fire to humanity for civilization. The homonymous Pramantha/Prometheus association may be coincidental. Archaeological findings demonstrate that human sacrifices almost certainly occurred in Minoan Crete [10] but we lack evidence for Continental Greece.

Embedded in the collective unconscious of European culture is the burning of heretics, which corresponds to a religious ritual given the fact that at the time judges were clergymen, such as the judgement of Joan of Arc's by Pierre Cauchon, bishop of Beauvais [11].

Alireza Ahmadi reminds us that, before the political combat of Raja Ram Mohan Roy in the 1820s, *"sati"* (self-immolation by a woman over the funeral pyre of her husband) and *"jauhar"* (mass suicides by self-immolation among Rajput women to avoid molestation by soldiers invading their land) traditions were practiced for a long time [12].

In 1872, Jules Verne in his famous book *"Around the world in 80 days"*, introduced the character of a woman, Mrs. Aouda, an Indian widow. She was married very young to an older man and when he died a *sati* ceremony was prepared for the young widow. Mr. Phileas Fogg ordered his butler to rescue her from the burning pyre. This romantic love story captured in the book matches the prevailing subversive fantasy of a wealthy colonial European salvaging young women from nefarious circumstances [13]. The practice of *sati* raises questions on the representation of the fate and human rights of Indian women. Is *sati* a voluntary or forced act? Chapter 5 addresses *sati* in a multidimensional context.

In 1983, Gayatri Chakravorty Spivak opened up a new chapter of post-colonial studies with her article *"Can the subaltern speak?"* [14]. With vast knowledge of European philosophy, her starting point was a philosophical Marxist point of view and the use of a terminology that allows her to describe how post-colonized people, and now populations of low-and-middle-income-countries, differ from the people from high-income countries [15]. The expertise of Professor Spivak on the works of Jacques Derrida [16] allows her to incorporate Foucault's Marxist activism to focus on issues deeply buried within her mind. Her example of a family secret, her great-aunt dying by suicide to hide her involvement in the independence movement, reveals the existence of a privileged protected area of speech among women within the family unit. Can this protected circle be accessible to medicine? Is psychiatry ready to hear what self-immolators say?

4   Emergence of Psychiatry and Early Works on Suicide

Classical French alienism progressively developed conceptions on suicide and offered descriptions of suicide by burning. One of the first monographs on suicide was the doctoral thesis of Chevrey, in 1816, from the Paris Medical Faculty. The title of his work is precisely *"Medical Essay on Suicide, considered, in any case, as the result of mental alienation"*. In the section *"Opinions we've had so far about suicide"*, he states: *"The brahmin still knows in Indostan how to exalt the imagination of women to the point of making them rush to the pyre which consumes the corpse of their husbands"* [17]. His knowledge of *sati* did not exceed this short sentence, but it is noteworthy to state that shortly before Raja Ram Mohan Roy began his activism, the plea of Indian women was not unknown.

In 1822, Jean-Pierre Falret, a psychiatrist very involved in the social movement for a welfare state, commented on the suicide by burning practice of *sati* and the contradictions of colonial power:

> *Everybody knows the barbaric custom where women burn themselves on a pyre after the death of their husbands. So! The French, the Dutch, the Danes have wished to abolish this horrible superstition through severe regulations. What happened? The regulations have been eluded, by performing the sacrifices in regions outside the districts that were dominated by these peoples. The British were not happier. Lord Binning and Mr. Bathurst assure that after the bill had been published on this subject by the English government, the number*

of people who set themselves on fire was all the more considerable. Last year, 2366 people had thus sacrificed themselves on pyres; and in this number, it included only the sacrifices made publicly, being unable in any way to specify the number of women who had burned themselves voluntarily in their private houses. Among the victims of superstition, we saw some who were not yet fourteen, twelve, ten, and even one who was only eight years old... [18]

Esquirol, the disciple of Pinel, expressed in 1838 interesting remarks on how hidden pathologies are difficult to ascertain and assess. He reminded us of the subjectivity of suicide:

All that I have said hitherto, together with the facts which I have related, prove that suicide offers all the characteristics of mental alienation, of which it is, in reality, a symptom: that we must not look for a single and peculiar sign of suicide, since we observe it under circumstances the most opposite, and since it is symptomatic or secondary, either in acute or febrile delirium, or in chronic delirium. Finally, the opening of the dead bodies of suicides has shed little light on the subject [19]

Esquirol was aware that knowledge in psychiatry is predominantly clinical, and that the pathogenesis of mental disorders is not to be found on the surface, but much deeper within the mind.

Brierre de Boismont reported in 1856 a case presented by Bricheteau at the Medical Academy, referred by Dr. Madin from Verdun. It was one of the first detailed descriptions of agony after severe burns caused by suicide by self-immolation:

Case report of voluntary combustion of an insane, during a delusional outburst.

Mr. P, 36 years old, was so affected by the loss of his beloved wife that he fell into a deep melancholia, with sight and auditory hallucinations. This delusional state was only intermittent and did not prevent Mr. P from fulfilling his public office. After quite a long quiet period he thought of remarrying; his difficulties to get married brought him back his delusions; hallucinations came more and more often, and of a more frightening nature. Dr. Madin was called to him and found him handed over the strangest delirious misconceptions: among other things, he thought he had received the mission to burn bad books and other items that were supposedly contrary to common decency. His growing propensity for burning brought M.r P to light his house with flaming torches. His delusion was not continuous and showed interruptions where he was keen on laughing of his pranks.

On January 18th, 1836, at two hours at night, Mr. Madin was called to Mr. P who had voluntarily given himself up to the flames, for expiation of his sins he was ashamed of. He had erected a pyre in the fireplace of the kitchen and placed himself on it, after setting it on fire. Smoke from combustion had already warned the neighbors of this tragic event; a huge quantity of fat mixed with blood had flowed up to two meters from the hearth.Dr. Madin was surprised to find the patient calm and smiling amidst a horrible smoke that barely allowed him to breathe. Mr. P was openly delighted to join his deceased wife, after atonement of his deeds on his own stake, following God's orders. The patient had legs, thighs and his posterior entirely burnt, his bones were whitened and calcined, his genitals were charred, and his hands reduced to shapeless blackish stumps; the rest of the body was intact. Ten minutes after being wrapped in a huge waxed sheet, his voice which was strong and resounding suddenly weakened; a thready pulse; death was imminent. Dr. Madin has suddenly removed his stethoscope, and didn't see that the popliteal artery, corroded by fire, had resulted in a fatal hemorrhage. [20]

By the end of the nineteenth century sociologists in Europe began to study the determinants of suicide. After the rejection of his thesis on *"Principles of Sociology"* in 1878, Thomas Masaryk (future first president of independent Czechoslovakia), brilliantly defended another thesis on *"Suicide and the Meaning of Civilization"* in 1879 (issued in German in 1881). He was the first to publish a philosophical monograph on this topic, and from it the new study of suicide from a sociological perspective developed [21]. Almost 20 years later, in 1897, Emile Durkheim published statistical results to corroborate observations, and proposed a new classification and a modernized vision of suicide (see Chap. 13 in this book for a more detailed description of the contributions of Durkheim). His practical views had a huge influence across allied disciplines. Both Masaryk and Durkheim demonstrated, with their works on suicide, the importance of identifying sociological risk factors for suicide as predisposing, enabling or protective. [22].

5   Suicide by Burning and Fear of an Epidemic

Honoré de Balzac's 1831 novel, *The Unknown Masterpiece* (*Le chef d'oeuvre inconnu*) integrates a suicide by burning at the end of the narrative:

> ... he said to them, "Adieu, my little friends." The tone of this farewell chilled the two painters with fear. On the morrow Porbus, alarmed, went again to visit Frenhofer, and found that he had died during the night, after having burned his paintings. [end of the novel] [23]

A painter, Master Frenhofer, after searching in vain for the perfect depiction of a feminine model and having seen the disappointment of his disciples, decided to burn his unfinished masterpiece and all of his paintings. He erected a pyre in his atelier and suicided. The fire was seen as an annihilation of his life and all of his creations. No political message was intended by the character, who sought no broader audience from his act. During the nineteenth century, suicide by burning was uncommon and difficult to execute, due to the large amounts of wood required and careful planning. One hundred years later, Picasso illustrated with etchings a reprint of Balzac's book [24]. Picasso moved his own atelier to the very location of the novel, where he painted his masterpiece 'Guernica' in 1937.

In 1951, Lewis published a monograph on *"Pathological firesetting (pyromania)"* [25]. Suicide by burning is depicted as *"vengeance fires"* by *"semi-social outcasts"* with *"self-destructive drives"* worsened by excessive drinking. Proposed antecedent were schizophrenia or depression, and an *"unpredicted explosion"* could lead the offender to paranoid projection with an impulsive desire of aggression. Hate towards the partner in conflict could punctually reverse as a desire for suicide. The *"suicidal ceremony"* could symbolically represent an attempt to repent.

In 1952, Battle and Marshall, from the London St. Thomas Hospital, published an early paper on self-immolation, stressing the necessary cooperation between their two fields of expertise, plastic surgery and psychiatry, in the management of these patients [26]. They described a case of a 30-year-old woman who, during a puerperal depression and after two failed attempts of coal-gas poisoning, set her nightdress on fire. She expressed a profound delusional guilt and underwent electro-convulsive therapy and skin engraftment operations. Euthymia was obtained after a month of treatment and dressings successfully removed 7 weeks after self-immolation.

With industrialization and especially the motorization of vehicles, the growing use of petrol and refined gasoline and kerosene products with high flammability became widely available. Physicians developed experience in the treatment of acci-dental burns, but suicide by burning remained uncommon with low prevalence dur-ing the first half of the twentieth century.

In 1966, in a Welsh congress of forensic medicine, James presented a case report on self-immolations [27]. One case was of a 60-year-old woman who covered her-self in paraffin and lit herself in her bath. She had her body unevenly burnt to the extent that her torso was detached, transpierced the wooden floor and burned to bones in the basement. Another was a 37-year-old separated man who doused him-self with a gallon of petrol while sitting in a remote wasteland. Only his skin was charred, and his clothes were not completely burnt but the hypovolemic shock due to burns was sufficient to cause death.

The possibility of instant self-harm through gasoline raised concern among phy-sicians and incited prevention measures, but the modern society of the 1960s brought about other unexpected dangers. The impact of media coverage was revolu-tionized with the availability of radio and television, with a target audience that could expand to reach almost all mankind [28].

Psychiatrists began to surmise that suicide could be subject to epidemics within distinct groups of people [29]. Various formulations of suicidal behavior in groups were put forward, such as the hypothesis that *"whenever there are covertly-shared pluralistic emotions and desires in a group—for whatever reason—that group will unwittingly strive to adopt, at least temporarily, any suitable idea"* [30]. The pos-sibility exists that the combination of characterologically predisposed or vulnerable persons and specific superimposed stresses could lead to an *"infectiousness of acting-out"* within a community [31].

The emergence of mass media led the authorities to reflect on the potential new vulnerability of patients facing new figures and images in their daily life as if these were part of their personal experience. As early as 1911, the American Academy of Medicine addressed the influence that written media could have on provoking sui-cide. The main concern was to protect patients suffering from *"psychosis"* from loss of *"self-control"* given their vulnerability to suggestion. The warning to the press to refrain from publishing details of suicides remained unheard, due to the apparent impossibility to hinder freedom of speech, and suggestions to deliver important counterinformation and contribute to having medical education reach the general public were not properly followed [32].

Their proposition was to be put in practice much later: in 1945–1949, and espe-cially in 1963–1969. The results were not favorable: the numbers of attempts were not significantly reduced, and even greater numbers were observed in some places:

the fear of the influence of the media over suicidal behavior was not properly veri-
fied. For Motto [33], there would probably be a *"very slight role of imitation on
suicidal behavior"*, agreeing with Durkheim by stating that it would be more prob-
able that these persons reached *"a state which is the true cause of the act and which
probably would have produced its natural effect even had imitation not intervened"*
[34]. Chapter 17 in this book addresses in detail safe reporting of suicide and the
issue of contagion.

6 Self-Immolation as a Burning Message

The term *"suicide by burning"* fell into disfavor and replaced by *"self-immolation."*
Immolation comes from Latin *"immolare"* and means *"offer to a deity by sacrifice"*. Although literally it does not imply that fire is needed, since 1963, it refers
exclusively to burning as an act of self-inflicting death.

The Cold War raged since the end of the Second World War. After the departure
of the Japanese troops, due to the surrender of the Empire and the victorious
Resistance of a national movement backed by the Allies, the project of an independence for the populations in South East Asia seemed within reach. But in Indochina,
although they lost control of the territory during the war, the French tried to re-
establish a colonial power in 1945. In 1954, after an armed conflict, independence
was obtained for Laos, Cambodia, and two Vietnamese republics. In North Vietnam,
the main support shifted from China to the USSR. In South Vietnam, the French
presence was replaced by an American influence and United States military intervention as the war broke out between the two republics.

6.1 The Immolation of Thích Quảng Đức in 1963

In 1963, the authoritarian power of South Vietnam's President Ngô Đình Diệm felt
threatened by the movement of Buddhist monks, and he forbade the traditional fes-
tivities to celebrate Gautama Buddha's birthday. Demonstrations took place and the
army killed nine civilians in Hué. The *"Buddhist Crisis"* mobilized the monks to
decide that radical political action was necessary to shed light on the repression. The
press was alerted that an imminent action would take place. After a collegial decision taken by the Buddhist Clergymen, the Venerable Thích Quảng Đức (66 years
old, born Lâm Văn Tức) volunteered to self-immolate in a public square. He wrote
the following statement, to be revealed after his death:

> *Before closing my eyes and moving towards the vision of the Buddha, I respectfully plead to
> President Ngô Đình Diệm to take a mind of compassion towards the people of the nation
> and implement religious equality to maintain the strength of the homeland eternally. I call
> the venerables, reverends, members of the sangha and the lay Buddhists to organize in soli-
> darity to make sacrifices to protect Buddhism.*

On June 11th, 1963, a procession of around 300 monks wearing the traditional robe and accompanied by lay people walked slowly through the streets of Saigon carrying flags with slogans, behind a small car, a blue Austin Westminster Sedan (now in a museum in Hué). A few blocks from the Presidential Palace, in front of the Cambodian embassy, the procession stopped on a square, surrounded by the police. Thích Quảng Đức sat on the ground praying, on a ritual cushion, in a traditional lotus position (*padmāsana*). Another monk poured the gasoline from a container taken from the car, recited a short prayer to Buddha, and lit a match in the gasoline puddle. Thích Quảng Đức stayed still while his body was burning. The assistant prayed and bowed before him, and some policemen obliged doing the same. Slogans were proclaimed through a microphone: *"A Buddhist priest burns himself to death. A Buddhist priest becomes a martyr."* After 10 min, his consumed body was taken by the monks in sacred sheets and brought to a Pagoda. Two American journalists attended the scene and were later awarded Pulitzer Prizes: Malcolm Browne of *Associated Press* who took a picture of the self-immolation (see Fig. 2 in Chap. 8 photograph reprinted with permission), and David Halberstam of *The New York Times* who described the scene for the press [35].

Thích Quảng Đức is now considered a Buddhist Saint, a *"Bodhisattva"*, and for believers his message overcomes violence, pain, death, and fire, as if his sacrifice through fire made him reach enlightenment. The event became known in all countries, shedding a new light to the troubled situation in Vietnam [36], and eliciting sympathy for the Vietnamese throughout the world. Apart from the mediatic reactions influencing public opinion worldwide, the political outcomes of this action were numerous, in particular the assassination of the President Diệm by a military plot 5 months later (after 7 self-immolations of venerable monks during these 5 months).

7 Self-Immolations Since 1963

After 1963, a semantic shift occurred and self-immolation became the preferred term to describe suicide by burning, revealing a symbolic reenactment of the sacrifice of Thích Quảng Đức. The comparable events that took place in Czechoslovakia in 1969 after the student Jan Palach self-immolated in front of the Faculty of Philosophy (12 self-immolations followed in Central Europe under the Soviet rule) raised awareness of injustices and weakened the power of the Soviet Union in Prague, starting a series of events that culminated with the Velvet Revolution and peaceful transition of government in 1989.

Bourgeois linked the Saigon and Prague events [37], recounting self-immolations occurring for various political reasons in Tokyo, Florence, Seoul, Munich, Madras, Algiers, Oviedo, Khartoum, Moscow, Helsinki, Vienna, Tarragona, Washington, New York, and Montevideo, among other places… Whereas this modus operandi was unusual before 1963 (with only 5 published cases), between June 1963 and May 1969, the number increased to 105 published cases.

Bourgeois noted the peculiar link of certain victims with the Vietnam experience, especially a young French war veteran, but less understandable were suicides of persons without apparent risk factors. He identified a cluster of ten self-immolations in January 1970 in France, including three high school pupils and a medical student, 1 year after Palach's suicide in Prague [38]. Stunned by the emergence of a new modus operandi, he stated:

> *How much the suicide of bonzes changed in its meaning and function... It has lost its Buddhist religious meaning and has become a mere political action... Self-cremations ... have become the signature of commitment and an act of political struggle... This technological world is a world made of massive, continuous and raw data: all channels of information ... instantly spread and broadcast the news and the most sensational pictures. In our "Civilization of the Image", each of us bask in a multitude of urging and violent pictures ... images that bypass our Imaginary and our conscient and unconscious phantasms.... [38]*

Bourgeois took note that suicides by self-immolation are part of the modern world, even if they are rooted in our deep and ancient cultures, and reflect an explosive literal aspiration for light and positiveness:

> *Political suicide reflects suicidal rage... It is a splitting of drives: being destroyed but attacking the enemy and leaving him panic, shame and hopeless remorse, drawing on him a universal dismay... What a temptation for these solitary, violent and suggestible unfortunates to die out after a short moment of fierce enlightenment! [38]*

These very conceptions were discussed by Bostic [39] in 1973, who inspired Andreasen and Noyes to study the psychopathological status of the victims [40]. They acknowledged the problem of the availability and the hazardous nature of gasoline and identified the existence of psychotic processes in most self-immolations. Increased survival of self-immolators in high-income countries was due to attempts of self-immolations occurring in institutions, where gasoline is not available and the fire rapidly put out, and to the improvement of dermatological care in specialized burn recovery units. In 1974, the International Society for Burn Injuries in the United Kingdom founded the scientific journal *Burns*, which was to focus on the topic of medical care of burn injuries.

Crosby and colleagues [41] examined the social phenomenon of protest suicides suggesting that the terms self-immolation and self-incineration should not be interchangeable as immolation conveys altruistic sacrifice and protest while incineration is a general descriptor. Their review of the literature points out the occurrence in ancient cultures in Europe and Asia, but also Africa (Fang culture) and Native American (Mohave culture). They reviewed all cases (N = 131) of self-incineration reported in the *London Times* and *New York Times* during the period of 1790–1971. Of these, 29% occurred before 1963 (a 172-year period), and 71% between 1963–1972 (95 cases). They found that *"none of the self-incinerations reported during the period 1790–1962 was described as political protest"*, and two thirds after 1963 were protest suicides. To be viewed as a political protest, the authors propose immolations should meet all three criteria: a prior statement explaining the protest exists, the act occurred in a public place, there should be no underlying mental illness. They state that there are *"clusters suggestive of epidemics"* amidst many *"isolated events"*; *"epidemics are likely to occur when times were unsettled, emotions inflamed and when no appropriate outlet exists for the expression of commonly shared emotions."*

Crosby and colleagues consider that iterative Buddhist self-incinerations are made possible by the:

> conducive atmosphere of open conflict and emotional tension (focused on) *a dramatic and powerful expression of a widely shared emotion (on) a population of individuals whose religious devotion, personal commitment, and unquestioning obedience perhaps made them particularly susceptible to suggestion from their leaders who may have encouraged the sacrifices for political purposes.* [41]

Furthermore, some *"covertly suicidal persons"* could have suicidal tendencies to meet a general cause: motivation could be interior, but mode to take action could be exterior and influenced by mediatic discourses. Self-incinerations without political motivation could then be almost entirely represented by individuals suffering from depression or schizophrenia. Crosby and colleagues observed that a *"reduction in the incidence of self-incineration has been coincident with an apparent increase in the use of aggressive methods of protest—dramatic acts of terrorism such as hijackings, bombings, hostage-taking, and political assassination"* that may force political change [41].

The suicide contagion effect induced by the media is referred to as the *Werther Effect* [42]. Despite numerous biases, a study indicated that mimicry in action, even actions of self-harm, could be favorized amidst young people prone to identification and being influenced. A review article by Barnett and Spitzer [43] draws attention to imitative tendencies for self-burns that is often overlooked and in the very young.

Biggs review of self-immolations during the last four decades of the twentieth century [44] shows that the larger scale of the problem is overwhelmingly located in Asia. Nevertheless, reliable statistics are not easy to compile without bias due to the controversial status of self-immolation [45]. The epidemiology of self-immolation at present highlights the vulnerability of women in regions of the world where the protection of their human rights is suboptimal [2], but also points out regions of persistent socio-political tension with political impasse and no freedom of speech, such as Tunisia since the Jasmine Revolution subsequent to the self-immolation of Mohammed Bouazizi [46].

8 Self-Immolation and Contemporary Medical Challenges

Albeit all of these historical considerations that help healthcare providers consider the ever-changing clinical and sociological dimensions of self-immolation, cooperation with psychiatrists may benefit prevention and therapeutic aspects of care. Consider, for example, the following challenges:

- In Egypt, 91% of self-immolations are in women, with a mortality rate 73%, most suffering from depressive disorders (see Chap. 9 in this book) [47].
- In Iran, in the Kermanshah province, Ahmadi expressed the need for a national strategy for the prevention of suicide by self-immolation advocating for abandoning kerosene stoves and shifting to domestic gas or electricity (see Chap. 3 in this book) [12, 48].
- In Nigeria, the burn recovery unit of the Sokoto region is one of the few places that studied the determinants of self-immolation in Africa, identifying that persons with underlying psychiatric disorders are less adherent to burn care treatments (see Chap. 7 in this book) [49].
- In Nepal, 29% of burn admissions in 2015 were intentional [50]. Among the 293 self-immolations 82% were women. Additionally, many patients were hospitalized with burns as a result of being assaulted. Of those assaulted, 58% were women. It is possible that there is a cross-over between these categories as a result of inaccurate reporting, and that there is an underestimation of women who face violence. This highlights the need for legislation to protect against gender bias and implementation of violence prevention programs [50].
- In the Herat province of Afghanistan, almost all (93%) persons who suicide by self-immolations are women (93%), and most experience forced marriages (64%) and family violence (57%) (see Chap. 4 in this book).

9 Conclusion

Even if the extent of self-immolation became widespread after 1963 and could have been favored by technical advances (gasoline, kerosene, matches, lighters, media coverage and dissemination), the origins of the act are to be found in the deep forgotten past of cultures and may linger in the collective unconscious worldwide. As most victims seem to be affected by psychiatric disorders such as depressive disorders and stressor related disorders, political motivation by itself does not seem to be the most relevant aspect in terms of public health interventions.

We may state, however, that the marginalization of women is a political issue, and this problematic cannot be absent from the dialogue during psychiatric assessments and prevention efforts. Psychiatric treatments are limited in underserved areas of the world. If a psychiatric intervention is possible, posing the question *"What do self-immolators say?"* could help clinicians develop necessary insights to devise preventive measures. Psychiatrists must be ready to hear what the answers to this question may reveal from our societies, not only framed within medical, surgical, psychiatric, and public health paradigms, but also exploring sociological and political dimensions.

When Gayatri Chakravorty Spivak formulated and published *Can the subaltern speak?* she stressed the development of the individual subject, internal speech, and constructing a new narrative to give voice to the experience of persons in low-and-middle-income-countries. Prevention efforts to protect those at risk for self-immolation must include, in addition to access to clinical services, legislation and societal efforts to help effect a cultural shift that empowers vulnerable persons and reduces violence.

References

1. Saxena S, Krug E, Chestnov O, Fleischmann A, Howlader S, Vijayakumar L, Butchart A. Preventing suicide, a global imperative. Geneva: WHO Report; 2014.
2. Rezaeian M. Epidemiology of self-immolation. Burns. 2013;39(1):184–6.
3. Bachelard G. The psychoanalysis of fire. Routledge: Kegan; 1964.
4. Bible. Leviticus 18:21, 20:2–5, Kings 23:10, Jeremiah 32:35, and Acts 7:43.
5. Açıkyıldız B. The Yezidis: the history of a community, culture and religion. London: IB Tauris; 2014.
6. Virgil (Publius Vergilius Maro). Georgics. Book 1. Verses 84–93.
7. Siculus D. The Historical Library. J Davis, *Military Chronicle Office*. 1814. Vol. I; Book XVII, Chap. X: 246 & Vol. II; Book XIX, Chap II:345–7.
8. Montgomery JE. Ibn FaÐlān and the Rūsiyyah. J Arab Islam Stud. 2000;3:1–25.
9. Crooke W. The popular religion and folk-lore of Northern India. Edinburgh: Archibald Constable & Co; 1896. p. 193. Vol I: 263. Vol II
10. Hughes DD. Human sacrifice in Ancient Greece. London: Routledge; 1991.
11. Pernoud R, Clin MV. Joan of Arc, her story. New York: St Martin's Griffin; 1999.
12. Ahmadi A. Suicide by self-immolation: comprehensive overview, experiences and suggestions. J Burn Care Res. 2007;28(1):30–41.
13. Verne J. Around the World in eighty days. Houghton: Osgood and Company; 1873. p. 96–8.
14. Spivak GC. Can the subaltern speak? In Marxism and the interpretation of culture. Basingstoke: Macmillan Education; 1888. p. 271–313.
15. Spivak GC. A critique of postcolonial reason: toward a history of the vanishing present. Berkeley: Harvard University Press; 1999.
16. Derrida J. Of grammatology. Baltimore: Johns Hopkins University Press; 1976. Translated from French into English by Spivak GC
17. Chevrey J. Essai médical sur le suicide, considéré, dans tous les cas, comme le résultat d'une aliénation mentale. Didot Jeune. 1816: 6.
18. Falret JP. De l'hypocondrie et du suicide, vol. 275. Paris: Croullebois; 1822.
19. Esquirol JED. Mental maladies, a treatise on insanity, vol. 301. Philadelphia: Lea and Blanchard; 1845.
20. Brierre de Boismont A. Du suicide et de la folie suicide. Paris: Baillère; 1856. p. 416–7.
21. Masaryk TG. Suicide and the meaning of civilisation. In: The Heritage of Sociology. Chicago: Chicago University Press; 1970.
22. Durkheim E. Suicide: a study in Sociology. New York: Free Press; 1897.
23. Balzac H. de. The unknown masterpiece. London: Dent; 1896.
24. Balzac H. de. Le Chef d'Oeuvre Inconnu. Eaux fortes originales et dessins gravés sur bois de Pablo Picasso. Paris: Ambroise Vollard; 1931.
25. Lewis NDC, Yarnell H. Pathological fire setting (pyromania). Nervous and Mental Disease Monographs (No. 82). New York. 1951.
26. Battle RJV, Marshall HES. Attempted suicide by burning. Br Med J. 1952;2:1397–8.
27. James WRL. Suicide by burning. Medicine, Science and the Law. Br Acad Foren Sci. 1966;6:48.
28. Schiffer MB. The portable radio in American life. Arizona: University of Arizona Press; 1991.

29. Weiss JMA. Suicide: an epidemiologic analysis. Psychiatry Q. 1954;28:225–52.
30. Taylor Kraupl F, Hunter RCA. Observations of a hysterical epidemic in a hospital ward. Psychiatry Q. 1958;32:821–39.
31. Hankoff LD. An epidemic of attempted suicide. Compr Psychiatry. 1961;2:294–8.
32. Hemenway HB. Report of the Committee on Publishing Details of Suicides in the Public Press—to what extent are suicide and other crimes against the person due to suggestion from the press? Bull Am Acad Med. 1911;12(5):253–63.
33. Motto JA. Suicide and suggestibility—the role of the press. Am J Psychiatr. 1967;124:252–6.
34. Durkheim E. Suicide, vol. 141. Glencoe, IL: The Free Press; 1951.
35. Halberstam D. The making of a quagmire. New York: Random House; 1965.
36. Prochnau WW. Once upon a distant war: David Halberstam, Neil Sheehan, Peter Arnett—young war correspondents and their early Vietnam battles. New York: Vintage Books; 1996.
37. Bourgeois M. Suicides par le feu à la manière des bonzes [Suicides by fire in the bonze manner]. Ann Med Psychol. 1969;2:116–27.
38. Bourgeois M. Les suicides par le feu. Annales Médico-Psychologiques. 1988;147:87–98.
39. Bostic RA. Self-immolation: a survey of the last decade (1963–1973). Life Threaten Behav. 1973;3:66–74.
40. Andreasen NC, Noyes R. Suicide attempted by self-immolation. Am J Psychiatr. 1975;132(5):554–6.
41. Crosby K, Rhee JO, Holland J. Suicide by fire: a contemporary method of political protest. Int J Soc Psychiat Sage. 1977;23:60–9.
42. Schmidtke A, Häfner H. The Werther Effect after television films: new evidence for an old hypothesis. Psychol Med. 1988;18:665–76.
43. Barnett W, Spitzer M. Pathological fire-setting 1951–1991: a review. Med Sci Law. 1994;34(1):4–20.
44. Biggs M. Dying without Killing: self-immolations, 1963–2002. Making sense of suicide missions. Diego Gambetta: Oxford University Press; 2005.
45. Sanghavi P, Bhalla K, Das V. Fire related deaths in India in 2001: a retrospective analysis of data. The Lancet. 2009: 373:1282–8. quoted by Labie D. Le feu, cause multiforme de décès en Inde. Méd Sci. 2010;24:98–9.
46. Barrett MP, Nikkah D, Gilbert P, Dheansa B. Social campaigns are needed to stop any form of self-immolation. Burns. 2014;40:361.
47. Mabrouk AR, Mahmoud Omar AN, Massoud K, Magdy Sherif M, El-Sayed N. Suicide by burns: a tragic end. Burns. 1999;25:337–9.
48. WHO. Self-directed violence. Geneva: World Health Organisation; 2002.
49. Legbo JN, Ntia IO, Opara WE, Obembe A. Severe burn trauma from deliberate self-harm: the Sokoto experience. Niger Postgrad Med J. 2008;15(3):164–7.
50. Lama BB, Duke JM, Sharma NP, Thapa B, Dahal P, Bariya ND, Marston W, Wallace HJ. Intentional burns in Nepal: a comparative study. Burns. 2015;41(6):1306–14.

Self-Immolation in Iran

Seyed Kazem Malakouti and Amir Hossein Jalali Nadushan

1 Introduction

Self-immolation is one of the most common methods of suicide in Iran. Self-immolation accounts for a high percentage of suicide deaths because of its high fatality rate, even in provinces where individuals favor other means of suicide. A study by Haji-Wandy and colleagues (2009) showed that in the southern province of Bushehr, while only 6% of all suicide attempts were by self-immolation, it was the cause of 71% of suicide deaths, followed by hanging causing 69% of suicide deaths [1]. Women in Iran attempt suicide by self-immolation more often than men. A study conducted by the Forensic Medicine Organization in one of the northern cities of the country in the province of Mazandaran showed that 58% of suicide attempts by women were by self-immolation [2]. In terms of lethality, a study found that the chances of death from self-immolation is 12 times higher than when poisoned by pesticides [3]. In general, 27% of suicides in Iran occur by means of self-immolation [4].

In most countries that belong to the World Health Organization/Eastern Mediterranean Region (WHO/EMR), with relatively similar ethnographic and cultural characteristics, self-immolation is one of the commonly chosen suicide methods. Suicide risk is heightened in EMR countries in the presence of

S. K. Malakouti (✉)
Mental Health Research Center, Department of Gerontology and Geriatric Psychiatry, School of Behavioral Sciences and Mental Health, Iran University of Medical Sciences,
Tehran, Iran
e-mail: Malakouti.k@iums.ac.ir

A. H. J. Nadushan
Mental Health Research Center, Department of Psychiatry, School of Medicine,
Iran University of Medical Sciences, Tehran, Iran
e-mail: jalali.am@iums.ac.ir

dispossession, disenfranchisement, poverty, humiliation, forced marriages, and intimate partner violence [5–7]. A review and meta-analysis study in the EMR region showed that the three main methods of suicide were hanging, drug poisoning and self-immolation, accounting for 39.7%, 20.3% and 17.4% of total suicides, respectively [8].

Despite ethnographic and cultural similarities in the region, differences exist among EMR countries and within Iranian provinces that could determine choosing self-immolation as a means of suicide. Iran, with a population of close to 84 million people in 2020, has a cultural diversity that accommodates a multiplicity of ethnic groups, including the Persian, Azeri, Kurd, Arab, Lur, Baloch, Qashqai, Turkmen, Gilaki, Mazandarani, Talysh and other ethnic minorities, with diverse religions, languages and traditions. The epidemiological pattern of self-immolation throughout Iran varies and is not constant over time. In the western and northwestern regions of the country the prevalence of self-immolation is changing in recent years. In the northwestern region of the country, East Azerbaijan province, there was an increasing trend of self-immolations from 1998 (1.48 per 100,000) to 2003 (7.7 per 100,000) [9]. Conversely, in the Ilam province, which is one of the western and border provinces of the country, a decreasing trend occurred from 2010 to 2014 [8] and instead, poisoning with pesticides and drugs increased. Figure 1 depicts the provinces of Iran and Fig. 2 the population breakdown of the country.

Plausible reasons for the decline of self-immolations in some regions of Iran over the last decade include social change empowering vulnerable individuals, declining access to combustible materials decreasing access to means, and an increase in divorce rates providing release from oppressive and violent marriages. In this chapter we review the literature describing predisposing and precipitating factors for self-immolation. We discuss study findings from Iran that assess demographic characteristics, motivations, precipitating stressors, psychological features, psychiatric diagnoses, and socio-economic conditions associated with self-immolation that have implications for suicide prevention.

2 Demographic Characteristics of Self-Immolators in Iran

2.1 Age

In the self-immolation studies reviewed, the age range of the majority of subjects was 15–30 years. The mean age of self-immolators is 30.5 years for men and w 26.3 years for women [7, 9–12]. In people over the age of 30, the risk of self-immolation is 30% lower (relative risk = 0.7) [12]. Nevertheless, the average age of those who self-immolate increased significantly between 2000 and 2016 [13]. Increasing age of marriage in the last decades could account for this but other factors may also play a role.

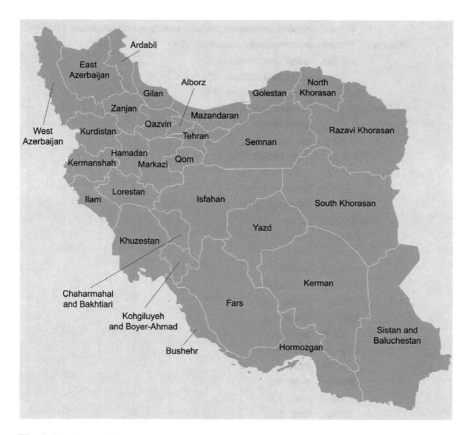

Fig. 1 Provinces of Iran

2.2 Gender

Seventy to eighty-seven percent of persons who self-immolate in Iran are women. Women are 2.5–13 times more likely to self-immolate than men, but this ratio varies from province to province. In the western region of provinces with lower Human Development Index (HDI), self-immolation rates are higher [5, 6, 9–15]. A consistent finding is that self-immolation is higher among women in the western part of the country compared to other regions. This gender difference may correlate with HDI, and our belief is that this correlation may imply causation. We will describe HDI indicators and the meaningfulness of this correlation in more detail in Sect. 3.

2.3 Urban and Rural Areas

Sixty to seventy-seven percent of patients who self-immolate live in urban city areas [11, 16–19]. In one study, the risk of self-immolation in urban areas had an odds ratio of 1.6 compared to rural areas [12]. In contrast, another report found that

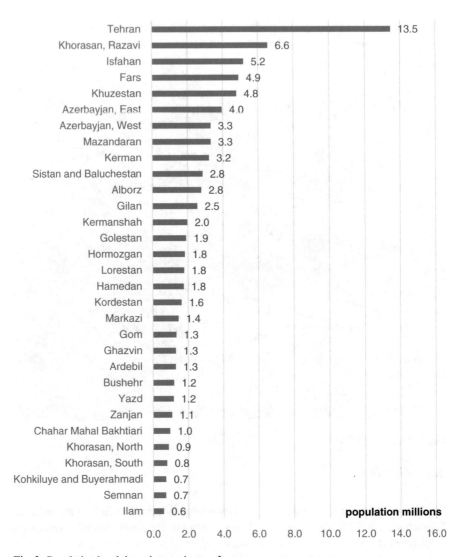

Fig. 2 Population breakdown by provinces—Iran

80–83% of self-immolators lived in rural areas [19, 20]. The prevalence of self-immolation in urban or rural areas does not seem to follow a fixed causative trend.

2.4 Marital Status and Occupation

In Iran, 47.5–63% of self-immolators are married [17–19, 21]. Meanwhile, approximately 6% of self-immolators are pregnant women [15]. The mean age of pregnant patients who self-immolate is 24.2 years [15, 22, 23].

When a precipitating factor is marital discord, the average length of marriage of self-immolators is 4.5 years. When pre-existing mental disorders are a predisposing factor, self-immolators on an average are married for nearly 13 years [24]. This suggests that self-immolation in a majority of patients is more likely to occur in the first few years after marriage, when emotional problems and conflicts peak before adaptive coping skills develop [24]. Moreover, 70–89% of women who self-immolate are homemakers [11, 16, 20, 21], while 50% of men who self-immolate are unemployed [11, 20].

2.5   Education

Self-immolation in Iran occurs more often in persons with lower levels of education. Those who are illiterate constitute 25% of self-immolators [20], while 57% have less than 12 years of schooling [21]. Diploma-level education reduces the risk of self-immolation by 15% (relative risk = 0.85) [12].

2.6   Mortality Rate

The mortality rate of self-immolation in Iran is in the range of 64–92% [9, 15, 17, 18, 20, 21]. The total body surface area (TBSA) affected by burns significantly correlates with severity of intent to suicide (70% for high intent vs. 28% for low intent). TBSA greater than 40% in combination with high intent increases the risk of death [14]. There seems to be a significant relationship between high TBSA affected by burns, low education and higher mortality rate [15]. Regarding to the season of year, the prevalence of self-immolation in Iran is higher in the spring (36.5%) [18].

In general, survival from self-immolation is low, and most deaths occur in the first few days after hospitalization [17]. In fact, people with burns in a TBSA greater than 70% are 17 times more likely to die than those with burns in a TBSA of up to 30%. Hospitalization in burn centers and immediate action without delay is a necessity to ensure survival [25].

2.7   Comparison with Other Suicide Means

A comparison of the demographic characteristics of self-immolators with those who attempt suicide by drug poisoning shows a significant difference between the two groups (see Table 1). [26]. The demographic profile of self-immolators characteristically includes more young women with lower levels of education, who stay at home as homemakers, and are newly married. Intimate partner violence is evident in both groups.

Table 1 Demographic features of suicides by self-immolation and drug self-poisoning [26]

		Self-immolation			Self-poisoning			Across self-immolation and self-poisoning
		Case n = 54 (%)	Control n = 92 (%)	X²(2)	Case n = 88 (%)	Control n = 92 (%)	χ2 (P)	χ2 (P)
Gender	Male	13(24.1)	30(32.6)	1.19 (NS)	44 (50)	41 (51.2)	0.026	9.36 (0.003)
	Female	41 (75.9)	62 (67.4)		44 (50)	39 (48.8)		
Marital status	Single	17 (31.5)	34 (37)	0.45 (NS)	50 (56.8)	51 (63.7)	2.057	8.62 (0.01)
	Married	31 (57.4)	49 (53.3)		32 (36.4)	27 (33.8)		
	Other				6 (6.8)	2 (2.5)		
Employment	Unemployed	15 (27.8)	5 (5.4)	3 (0.000)	12 (13.6)	8 (10)	3	37.78 (P < 0.001)
	Employed	6 (11.1)	34 (37)		58 (65.9)	58 (72.5)		
	Homemaker	30 (55.6)	27 (29.3)		10 (11.4)	5 (6.3)		
	Student	3 (5.6)	26 (28.3)		8 (9.1)	9 (11.3)		
Educational level	<12 years schooling	35 (64.8)	20 (21.7)	32.74	28 (31.8)	19 (23.8)		14.77
	12 years Schooling	12 (22.2)	20 (21.7)	(P < 0.001)	39 (44.3)	35 (43.8)		
	>12 years Schooling	7 (13%)	52 (56.5)		21 (23.9)	26 (32.5)	2.095	(P < 0.001)
Suicidal ideation during past year	Yes	29 (53.7)	14 (15.2)	24.25	46 (52.3)	4 (5)	44.79	0.027 (NS)
	No	25 (46.3)	78 (84.8%)	(P < 0.001)	42 (47.7)	76 (95)	(P < 0.001)	
Domestic violence	Yes	28 (51.9)	26 (28.3)	8.12	53 (60.2)	20(25)	21.16	0.95 (NS)
	No	26 (48.1%)	66 (71.7)	−0.004	35 (39.8)	60 (75)	(P < 0.001)	
Harmful use of alcohol	Yes	4 (7.4)	9 (9.8)	0.237 (NS)	39 (44.3)	14 (17.5)	13.95	21.59 (P < 0.001)
	No	50 (92.6)			49 (55.7)	66 (82.5)	(P < 0.001)	
Harmful use of drugs	Yes	10 (18.5)	6 (6.5)	5.019	9 (10.2)	10 (12.5)	0.216	1.98 (NS)
	No	44 (81.5)	86 (93.5)	(P = 0.03)	79 (89.8)	70 (87.5)		

3 Stressors

Almost always, self-immolation is preceded by psychosocial stressors that act as enabling situational and precipitating factors. The most common are family disputes and conflicts, occurring in up to 56% of persons who self-immolate. Triggering conflicts include heated arguments between older parents and younger adults over academic performance or disapproval of romantic choices, marital conflicts rooted in jealousy or spouse's addiction, and financial problems triggering tension. Studies show that husbands have alcohol or drug dependence 19.5–32% of the time, financial problems 11.7–12.5%, and romantic turmoil is present in 47.4% of instances prior to self-immolation. In married cohorts, conflict with spouse and spouse's addiction, and in single individuals, conflict with parents and parental addiction significantly correlates with self-immolation [10, 15, 22, 25, 27]. When compared to a control group, marital conflict is 7.8 times higher and conflict with other family members ten times greater in those who self-immolate [28]. It seems that women with the demographic characteristics described in Sect. 2, when faced with family stressors, especially when in direct conflict with their spouse or spouse's family, bear the necessary psychological pressure to suicide. A 2009 study by Saadati and colleagues [27] delineates commonly occurring and co-existing enabling and predisposing stressors associated with self-immolation, which co-exist with psychiatric disorders. These are summarized in Fig. 3.

In one study, 84% of self-immolators had a family history or personally knew individuals who self-immolated [29]. Cultural factors modeling suicidal behaviors or intergenerational transmission of trauma may be responsible for these familial suicides. The Werther effect or suicide by contagion phenomenon is of high

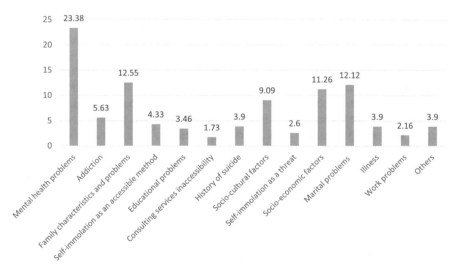

Fig. 3 Prevalence of co-existing enabling and predisposing stressors triggering self-immolation [27]

importance in self-immolations, as the dramatic nature of these suicides remains embedded in the psyche of witnesses or persons with lived experience.

Social and economic stressors such as poverty and unemployment are important risk factors for suicide at the macro-societal level. An examination of the growth and development index and its relationship with self-immolation shows that in provinces in Iran with lower growth and development as indicated by lower HDI had a higher incidence of self-immolation [30]. The HDI is a composite score that takes into account indicators such as life expectancy, educational attainment and GNI per capita as a logarithm of income. These measurements produce an index that captures a country's development based on health, well-being and quality of life. Although the HDI value for Iran is 0.798, placing it in the high human development category (http://hdr.undp.org/sites/default/files/Country-Profiles/IRN.pdf) differences exist within provinces indicating internal inequality. Inequality significantly correlates with suicide by self-immolation. This correlation is relevant throughout the country but most noticeable in the province of Ilam [30].

4 Motivations for Self-Immolation

Motivation is an inner psychological process by which a person urges to engage in or withdraw from activities. By exploring the motivations of people who self-immolate, researchers could better conceptualize suicide prevention interventions. We reviewed several qualitative studies of Iranian cohorts that examine the motivations of vulnerable individuals to choose self-immolation as a means of suicide instead of other methods. Clinicians usually ask suicidal persons: What are the problems? Why suicide? What motivated you to take action by setting yourself on fire? Answers to these questions may guide prevention interventions and help suicidal individuals express distress with words rather than actions and approach problem-solving collaboratively.

In order to address what motivates self-immolation, researchers conducted qualitative studies based on content analysis and grounded theory to elucidate causes and processes that are conducive to this form of suicide. The following summary includes the most important motivational factors gathered from study results of Iranian subjects, primarily women, who self-immolate in response to a variety of triggers [27, 29, 31, 32]:

- Sexism, misogyny, and the disadvantaged position of women within the family unit.
- Exaggerated sense of power and dominance of men that polarizies masculinity towards bigotry, which fuels domestic violence.
- Conflict between new and traditional values in family relationships. In the last decades, remarkable changes in social values transpired, especially among young women who accept globalized standards, creating intergenerational conflict and critical attitudes.

- Showing courage as a way to protest the misery of everyday life. Suicide serves as an act of bravery that provokes a sense of guilt in surviving family members.
- Repeated physical, emotional and psychological abuse by a family member, mainly by husband, but also perpetrated by others, including the father and in-laws.
- Incompatible family facets or extreme stringency within the family.
- Dispossession, poverty and unemployment of spouse.
- Creating an environment of terror with frequent threats of violence by husband against wife.
- Suicide is culturally sanctioned, considered fashionable behavior when inspired by relatives who self-immolated. In some regions of Iran, the general perception of self-immolation is that it is an act of bravery and a last solution for intractable and never-ending problems.
- Fire symbolically serves a cleansing effect to atone for sinful behaviors, especially if there is a discussion of betrayal within the family. In most religions, fire is an element associated with the potential to expunge sins of those tormented by guilt and shame.

5 Psychological Characteristics of Self-Immolations

Some studies examined the psychological profiles and psychiatric diagnoses of persons who suicide by self-immolation. These are the underlying predisposing psychological features of individuals who self-immolate:

- Affective states of helplessness, anger, sadness, anxiety, guilt, and shame.
- Feeling disappointed, disheartened, giving up and ending bad luck by self-immolation.
- Experiencing strange and unusual mental states before self-immolation, which could be characterized as dissociation, a fugue state or an amnestic trance that challenges reality testing. A patient described her state of mind as follows:

  I was in a state of disintegration at the time... I didn't understand or feel environmental stimuli well... I felt that events were happening so fast, and I am not able to remember what I did before setting myself on fire... I cannot remember details of the event.

- Impulsivity. Sixty to seventy percent of subjects who self-immolate endorsed impulsive behavior [11, 19]. While recovering in burn centers, some stated that the act was not planned at all.

6 Psychiatric Diagnoses of Self-Immolators

A risk factor for suicide is the presence of mental disorders. The prevalence of mental disorders in self-immolators is in the range of 33.8–55.6% [11, 18, 26, 33]. In studies conducted in Iran, different methods used to evaluate mental disorders provide dissimilar and sometimes contradictory results. The psychiatric literature includes reports of three methods used to assess psychiatric diagnoses: *self-report*, *unstructured clinical interviews* by psychologists or psychiatrists, and *structured/ semi-structured interviews*.

Using *self-report* methodology, the most common diagnoses in women who self-immolate were adjustment disorder and major depression, while in men major depression and harmful use of drugs ranked higher [16]. Depressive disorders are present in 22–65% of subjects and substance use disorders in 17–26% of persons who self-immolate [18, 20, 34]. Examining intention to die, 67–70% of those who self-immolated regretted their actions, especially those with lower TBSA burn rates [35, 36].

In *unstructured clinical interviews* findings included adjustment disorder in 67% (all women), 7.5–10% substance use disorders (all men), 7–20% dysthymic disorder, 3–40% major depression, and 3% anorexia nervosa. Personality disorders reported included 18.3% of individuals with obsessive-compulsive personality disorder, 11.2% with borderline personality disorder, and 3% with antisocial personality disorder. Seventy-five percent of male self-immolators had alcohol dependence or substance use disorders and 77% of women self-immolators had adjustment disorders. Adjustment disorders increase the risk of self-immolation by a factor of 13 [11, 19].

Studies using *structured or semi-structured diagnostic interviews* should be more reliable. One such study using the Composite International Diagnostic Interview (CIDI) reported the prevalence of adjustment disorders in self-immolators to be 42%, nicotine-dependence 16.7%, and any type of depressive disorder 20% [21]. A study using the Structured Clinical Interview for DSM Disorders (SCID) in self-immolators reported a 1-year prevalence of major depression as 26% (56% when drug intoxication was comorbid), and bipolar disorder 7.4% (17% when drug intoxication was comorbid). Major depression in self-immolators increases the risk of recurrence of suicidal behavior by a factor of 5 (by a factor of ten when drug intoxication was comorbid) [26].

Chronic physical illnesses, which are known to be independent risk factors for suicide in general, may increase the risk of suicide by self-immolation as well. In one study 30% of persons had at least one chronic physical illness, and surprisingly 17.6% reported epilepsy [21].

7 Socio-Cultural Factors and Self-Immolation

Qualitative studies on culture and family background of Iranian women who self-immolate extracted the following factors, which exert inordinate psychological pressure and cause disinhibition and distress [37–39]:

- A traditional marriage structure in which the father and older brother are the main decision-makers. Also, moving in with family after marriage is customary and the newlyweds are forced to live with the spouse's family, compromising autonomy of the younger adults.

- Divorce being considered taboo and highly stigmatized. Many families still believe that one should remained married until death, regardless of circumstances.
- In ordinary conversations the threat to self-immolate often comes up in heated arguments during family conflicts. The dreadfulness of words such as "suicide" and "self-immolation" dissipates, and violent suicidal behavior becomes culturally endorsed.
- A persistent war in the western border provinces, with a high prevalence of depression and posttraumatic stress disorder from repeated exposure to violence in these areas provide grounds for aggressive and impulsive behaviors [37, 38].
- Up to 70% of persons who self-immolate in Iran have a low socio-economic status [39, 41, 42].

8   Conclusion

The biopsychosocial approach to suicide prevention examines individual/psychological, social/economic, cultural/family and environmental factors associated with suicide. The factors delineated in this chapter, which can enable, predispose and precipitate self-immolation suicides, may be classified into four interconnected dimensions. Figure 4 illustrates these multidimensional considerations.

A summary of extensive research conducted in Iran over the last decades examining determinants of suicide by self-immolation can be summarized as follows:

1. Young, married women who are homemakers, with low educational levels are at higher risk for self-immolation. Predominant characteristics of those at risk include disappointment and disenfranchisement, being a victim of intimate partner violence or other violence in the household, having impulsive behavior, and affective states of hopelessness, anger, sadness, guilt and shame.
2. Family characteristics of self-immolators include sexism, misogyny, a dominant patriarchal culture, an over-controlling family, inability to align new acquired values with long-standing traditional family values and turning anger against the self as a way to assert oneself and protest against injustices and maltreatment.
3. Persistent stressors in the form of repeated conflict with one's spouse and parents, and the accumulation of stress reaching threshold may trigger self-immolation. A vulnerable person who is disenfranchised and alienated may engage in impulsive self-immolation. Self-immolation is both a learned behavioral response and a culturally encouraged custom of some regions of the country. Psychological distress and weaknesses in family and social support provide context for self-immolation to occur.
4. In the social, cultural and economic dimensions, factors such as prolonged war in border areas, acceptance of "self-immolation" as one of the social realities of the region, casual expressions of "self-immolation" in ordinary conversations without a sense of dread, and low Human Development Index in certain prov-

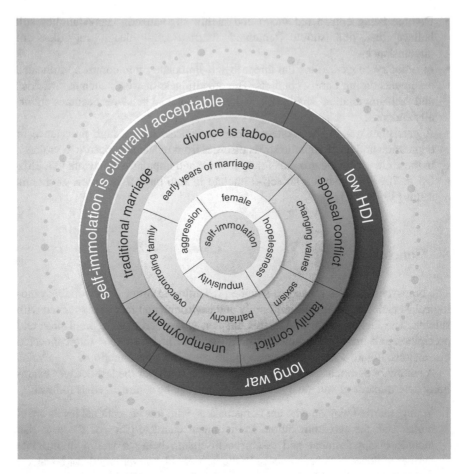

Fig. 4 Enabling, predisposing and precipitating factors associated with suicide by self-immolation in Iran

inces of Iran are all macro-societal and cultural factors associated with self-immolation suicides.

Suicide prevention strategies based on these parameters may include:

1. Restricting access to means, reducing self-immolations by restricting the now ubiquitous flammable liquids.
2. Providing mental health counseling, psychotherapy and screening for mental disorders, targeting interventions to empower women and decrease violence in men [28, 40].
3. Helping to change societal attitudes and the public perception of self-immolation, via responsible reporting of suicides, educational and wellbeing campaigns, and legislation that protects the human rights of women [29].

References

1. Hajivandi A, Akbarizadeh FJM. Epidemiology of suicide in province of Bushehr in 2009. J Heal Syst Res. 2013;9(12):52–61.
2. Pourhossein M, Mir Mohammdi SMAA. Evaluation of demography & methods of successful suicide in corpses referred to Sari Legal Medicine Center during 2009–2010. Iran J Forensic Med. 2016;21(3):199–205.
3. Havassi N, Khorshidi A, Khorshidi A, Jafari AHF. Evaluating the predictors of suicide deaths. J Maz Univ Med Sci. 2017;27(147):217–27.
4. Ahmadi A, Mohammadi R, Stavrinos D, Almasi A, Schwebel DC. Self-immolation in Iran. J Burn Care Res. 2008;29(3):451–60.
5. McDonald M. *Young women in rural Uzbekistan seek escape by self-immolation.* Knight Ridder Newspapers. 2004. http://www.axisoflogic.com/artman/publish/Article_7020.shtml.
6. Aziz N. What self-immolation means to Afghan women. Peace Rev A J Soc Justice. 2011;23(1):45–51.
7. Amin PM, Mirlashari JNA. A cry for help and protest: self-immolation in young Kurdish Iraqi women-a qualitative study. Int J Commun Based Nurs Midwif. 2018;6(1):56–64.
8. Morovatdar N, Moradi-Lakeh M, Malakouti SK, Nojomi M. Most common methods of suicide in Eastern Mediterranean Region of WHO: a systematic review and meta-analysis. Arch Suicide Res. 2013;17(4):335–44.
9. Dastgiri S, Kalankesh LR, Pourafkary N, Vahidi RG, Mahmoodzadeh F. Incidence, survival pattern and prognosis of self-immolation: a case study in Iran. J Public Health (Bangkok). 2006;14(1):2–6.
10. Panaghi L. Prevalence of self-inflicted burn and the related factors in Iran: a systematic review. Iran J Psychiatry. 2007;2(4):174–80.
11. Shaker J, Tatari F, Sadeghi K, Elahe Mohamadi KV. Suicide by self-immolation, a cross sectional study in Kermanshah-Iran. Iran J Psychiatry Behav Sci. 2007;1(2):11–5. https://www.sid.ir/en/journal/ViewPaper.aspx?id=132502.
12. Rostami M, Jalilian A, Rezaei-Zangeneh RSA. Factors associated with the choice of suicide method in Kermanshah Province. Iran Ann Saudi Med. 2016;36(1):7–16.
13. Parvareh M, Hajizadeh M, Rezaei S, Nouri B, Moradi G, Esmail NN. Epidemiology and socio-demographic risk factors of self-immolation: a systematic review and meta-analysis. Burns. 2018;44(4):767–75. https://doi.org/10.1016/j.burns.2017.08.013.
14. Mohammadi AA, Danesh N, Sabet B, Amini M, Jalaeian H. Self-inflicted burn injuries in southwest Iran. J Burn Care Res. 2008;29(5):778–83.
15. Mehrpour O, Javadinia SA, Malic C, Dastgiri S, Ahmadi A. A survey of characteristics of self-immolation in the East of Iran. Acta Med Iran. 2012;50(5):328–34.
16. Ahmadi A, Mohammadi R, Almasi A, Amini-Saman J, Sadeghi-Bazargani H, Bazargan-Hejazi S, et al. A case-control study of psychosocial risk and protective factors of self-immolation in Iran. Burns. 2015;41(2):386–93.
17. Dastgiri S, Kalankesh LR, Pourafkary N. Epidemiology of self-immolation in the North-West of Iran. Eur J Gen Med. 2005;2(1):14–9.
18. Hosseini S, Yazdanpanah F, Ghannadzadegan H, Fazli M. Evaluation of Self-Immolation Suicide attempt in Sari City (north of Iran) between 2011 to 2014. Int J Med Investig. 2016;5(2):65–8.
19. Ahmadi A, Mohammadi R, Schwebel DC, Yeganeh N, Hassanzadeh M, Bazargan-Hejazi S. Psychiatric disorders (Axis I and Axis II) and self-immolation: a case-control study from Iran. J Forensic Sci. 2010;55(2):447–50.
20. Ghalambor A, Zarei J, Peypolzadeh M. Assessing individual and social characteristics as risk factors in self-immolation (in pesian). Jundishapur Sci Med J. 2010;4(16):95–102. https://www.sid.ir/fa/journal/ViewPaper.aspx?ID=203045.

21. Zarghami M, Khalilian A. Deliberate self-burning in Mazandaran. Iran Burns. 2002;28(2):115–9.
22. Farrokh-Eslamlou HR, Khorasani-Zavareh D, Oshnouei SMS. Epidemiology of burns injury among women in reproductive age in the West Azerbaijan Province of Iran: a three year case-study. Saf Promot Inj Prev. 2014;2(1):31–8.
23. Maghsoudi H, Samnia R, Garadaghi A, Kianvar H. Burns in pregnancy. Burns. 2006;32(2):246–50.
24. Fazli M. Demographic factors affecting the motivations of suicide by self-burnin (hospitalized in Burn Unit of Zare hospital Sari-Iran). Q J Educ Psychol. 2015;6(21):60–72.
25. Moradinazar M, Amini S, Baneshi M, Najafi F, Abbasi N, Ataee M. Survival probability in self immolation attempters: a prospective observational cohort study. Ulus Travma Acil Cerrahi Derg. 2016;22(1):23–8.
26. Malakouti SK, Taban M, Nojomi M, Eftekhar Ardebili M, Mohammadi Farsani H, Ghiasi Z, Khazaie H, Zarghami M, Karimi MAK. Comorbid psychiatric diagnosis in suicide attempters using self-immolation and self-poisoning: a case-control and multisite study. J Suicide Prev. 2019;1(1):25–32.
27. Saadati M, Azami-Aghdash S, Heydari M, Derakhshani NRR. Self-Immolation in Iran: systematic review and meta-analysis. Bull Emerg Trauma. 2019;7(1):1–8.
28. Ahmadi A, Mohammadi R, Schwebel DC, Yeganeh N, Soroush A, Bazargan-Hejazi S. Familial risk factors for self-immolation: a case-control study. J Women's Health. 2009;18(7):1025–31.
29. Safari-Faramani R, Khanjani N, Najafi F. Self-immolation causes and preventive strategies from the viewpoint of healthcare providers: a qualitative study. Sci J Sch Public Heal Inst Public Heal Res. 2014;12(3):37–51.
30. Veisani Y, Khazaei S. Inequality in self-immolation incidence according to HDI in Iran. Burns. 2018;44(3):726–8.
31. Yoosofilabani J, Mirzaei H. The study of factors affecting of self-burning among women. J Heal Syst Res. 2013;9(7):672–81.
32. Yoosefilebni J, Mansourian M, Hossain Taghdisi M, Khosravi B, Ziapour A, Demir Özdenk G. A study of Kurdish women's tragic self-immolation in Iran: a qualitative study. Burns. 2019;45(7):1715–22. https://doi.org/10.1016/j.burns.2019.05.012.
33. Shakeri J, Mohamadi E, Valinia K, Hakim SM. Self-immolation in Kermanshah City, Iran; a serious suicide intention? Int Arch Heal Sci. 2016;3(3):139–43.
34. Azami, Y, Yavari, A, Pournazari M. Social factors influencing the tendency of young women to self-immolation (Case study: cities Paveh & Javanrud). Q J Kermanshah Police Sci. 2014;1393:17–31.
35. Ahmadi A. Suicide by self-immolation: comprehensive overview, experiences and suggestions. J Burn Care Res. 2007;28(1):30–41.
36. Alaghehbandan R, Lari AR, Joghataei MT, Islami A, Motavalian A. A prospective population-based study of suicidal behavior by burns in the province of Ilam, Iran. Burns. 2011;37(1):164–9. https://doi.org/10.1016/j.burns.2010.04.010.
37. Rezaie L, Hosseini SA, Khankeh HR, Rassafiani M, Shakeri J, Khazaie H. Exploration of how culture influences on attempting suicide by self-immolation among women. Tehran Univ Med J TUMS Publ. 2016;73(11):832–5. http://tumj.tums.ac.ir/article-1-7197-en.html. Accessed 11 Feb 2020.
38. Khankeh HR, Hosseini SA, Rezaie L, Shakeri J, Schwebel DC. A model to explain suicide by self-immolation among Iranian women: a grounded theory study. Burns. 2015;41(7):1562–71. https://doi.org/10.1016/j.burns.2015.03.015.
39. Rastegar Lari A, Alaghehbandan R. Epidemiological study of self-inflicted burns in Tehran. Iran J Burn Care Rehabil. 2003;24(1):15–20.
40. Karim H. What factors play a role in preventing self-immolation? Results from a case-control study in Iran. J Inj Violence Res. 2015;7(2):59–63.

41. Safiri K, Rezaienasab Z. A qualitative study of women self-immolation phenomenon in Ilam city (in Persian). Q J Woman Soc. 2016;7(1):123–41.
42. Taban M, Malakouti SK, Ranjbar H, Eftekhar Ardebili M, Motavalian SA, Zarghami M, et al. Making a symbolic gesture: a qualitative examination of self-immolation in Iran. Qual Quant. 2019;53(4):2117–30. https://doi.org/10.1007/s11135-019-00859-9.

Self-Immolation in Afghanistan

Thambu Maniam, Sayed Sabour Ahmad Mansouri, Sayed Azimi, Mohammad Farris Iman Leong Bin Abdullah, Frozan Esmati, Hatta Sidi, and César A. Alfonso

T. Maniam
Universiti Kebangsaan Malaysia Medical Centre, Kuala Lumpur, Malaysia
e-mail: tmaniam@yahoo.com

S. S. A. Mansouri
Sayed Sabour Psychiatric Clinic, Kabul, Afghanistan
e-mail: sabouram@gmail.com

S. Azimi
Mental Health Unit, Ministry of Public Health, Kabul, Afghanistan
e-mail: sayedazimi@hotmail.com

M. F. I. L. B. Abdullah
Lifestyle Science Cluster, Advanced Medical and Dental Institute, Universiti Sains Malaysia, Pulau Pinang, Malaysia
e-mail: farris@usm.my

F. Esmati
New Zealand Psychologist Board, ACC Sensitive Claims Registered, Wellington, New Zealand
e-mail: fesmati@worldbank.org

H. Sidi (✉)
Faculty of Medicine, Department of Psychiatry, Universiti Kebangsaan Malaysia Medical Centre, Kuala Lumpur, Malaysia
e-mail: hattasidi@hotmail.com

C. A. Alfonso
Universiti Kebangsaan Malaysia Medical Centre, Kuala Lumpur, Malaysia

Columbia University Medical Center, New York, NY, USA

Universitas Indonesia, Jakarta, Indonesia

World Psychiatric Association Psychotherapy Section, Geneva, Switzerland
e-mail: cesaralfonso@mac.com

C. A. Alfonso et al. (eds.), *Suicide by Self-Immolation*,
https://doi.org/10.1007/978-3-030-62613-6_4

47

1 Introduction

Suicide by self-immolation is highly prevalent in low-income countries. In Afghanistan, especially in the Herat region bordering Turkmenistan and Iran, it attracted international attention during and after the Taliban rule, occurring primarily among violently victimized women living in oppressive conditions [1, 2]. A 2010 article in *Time* magazine describes self-immolation as a "practice that has long existed as a method by which Afghan women try to escape their sorrows", identifying forced marriages and violence in the household as common precursors [2]. Medica Mondiale, a German NGO protecting human rights of women and children, conducted a survey in 2006 in burn units in Afghanistan, finding an alarming number of cases, almost all young women [1]. To date, there are no systematic studies and few publications exist examining the psychosocial and psychiatric correlates of suicide by self-immolation in Afghanistan. Reliable epidemiological studies and commentaries addressing the mental health of Afghans are scant in the medical and social sciences literature.

The authors of this chapter collaborated in a research project studying a cohort of psychiatric outpatients in 2012–2013 in the Herat Mental Health Clinic, with the aim of identifying psychosocial factors associated with suicidal behaviors and self-immolation ideation. In addition to presenting the results of the study to determine psychosocial predisposing factors, we will provide a review of historical and cultural antecedents of suicide by self-immolation in Afghanistan.

2 Country Profile and History of Afghanistan

Afghanistan comprises what was once referred to as the Ariana and Khorasan territories. It is now a much smaller landlocked country in central Asia with a total area of 652,225 square kilometers and a population of around 25 million people, of which 77% live in rural areas. Neighboring countries include Pakistan, Iran, Turkmenistan, Uzbekistan, Tajikistan and China. The adult literacy rate in Afghanistan is 31% (43% for males and 20% for females). Afghanistan is a low-income country with a GDP per capita of US$352 [3].

According to the Ministry of Public Health of Afghanistan [4] general government expenditure on health is 5.5% of total disbursements covering around 33.2% of health costs, with two-thirds of total health expenditures paid out-of-pocket. In terms of human resources, as of 2008, Afghanistan had 0.2 physicians and 0.5 nurses per 100,000 population. Although the health status of the population improved since 2001 [5], statistics from the WHO collected between 2003 and 2006 show that total life expectancy at birth is 46 years (47 for males and 45 for females), infant mortality rate is 129 per 1000 live births, under age five mortality rate is 191 per 1000 live births, and 39% of children are underweight [3].

Important primary sources written by Afghan historians include Gholam Mohammad Ghobar's book, *Afghanistan in the course of history* [6], and Mir

Mohammad Sediq Farhang's *Afghanistan in the last five centuries* [7]. Although evidence exists substantiating human settlements for millennia in what is current day Afghanistan, the first systematized government started with the mass immigration of Indo-Aryans into the region, from where they proliferated to India, Iran and Europe. After gradually renouncing nomadic lifestyle in favor of farming in fertile lands and building, these original Indo-Aryan colonists expanded around the Persian territories.

Afghanistan is a country conquered and rebuilt many times with different iterations and fluid borders. The Greeks conquered it and ruled for many years, Afghanistan being the easternmost region of the Greco-Bactrian Kingdom. It was also incorporated into the Persian Achaemenid and Parthian Empires that encompassed most of Central Asia.

Independent kingdoms of Kabul kings ruled after Muslims entered the country from Herat. Some remnants of the ancient walls still exist atop the mountains near Kabul. They referred to the country's name as Khorasan and an era of prosperity started among the resilient people who accepted Islam. A man from Khorasan called Abu Muslim had a major role in overthrowing the Umayyad dynasty during the Abbasid revolution. The vast Abbasid caliphate from thereon ruled most of Central Asia and Northern Africa during the zenith of the Islamic Golden Age, from approximately 800–1300 AD.

Invasion of Mongols in the thirteenth century devastated the land and decimated Khorasanian cities. Yet, survivors at times led vital regional pockets of strength. The Sarbedaran Rebellion in Herat is a notable example of triumph against invasion. The last middle ages empire of Persia that ruled almost all of what is current day Afghanistan and Iran had its last capital in Herat. Nonetheless, and for several centuries, most of Afghanistan was either controlled by the Mughal Empire of India, isolated local governments, the Uzbek Khanate of Bukhara, and Persian governments based in current Iran.

In the eighteenth century, under the leadership of Ahmad Shah Duranni, battles led to consolidation of the land of most of what constitutes present-day Afghanistan. Duranni established a Pashtun ruled empire that was in control of what is currently Afghanistan as well as most of current Pakistan, in addition to some parts of current Iran and Turkmenistan. Nevertheless, subsequent Afghan kings gradually lost territory to other governments, including to the British East India Company, until the current boundaries of the country remained.

Afghanistan literally means land or place of Afghans. The name became of common usage during the nineteenth century. The first written document with Afghanistan in it is the Anglo-Persian Treaty of 1801 AD. Pashtun rulers led Afghanistan after Ahmad Shah Duranni, except for a short period of a few months at the beginning of the nineteenth century and few years at the end of twentieth century, when non-Pashtuns had control of Kabul and a handful of provinces.

Afghanistan is a country at a geographical crossroads and Afghans constitute an amalgam of different ethnic groups, including Pashtuns, Tajiks (Persians), Hazaras, Turkic tribes such as Turkmen and Uzbecs, Moghols, and Gujjar Indians. Dari (Persian, Farsi) and Pashto are the most widely spoken languages, each with many distinct dialects, followed by Turkic languages. While ethnic diversity of Afghans creates cultural richness, it also serves as a source of conflict and an obstacle to needed ethno-culturally sensitive research design in psychology and social sciences.

3 Honoring Fire in Literature, Religion and Oral Traditions in Afghanistan

Shahnameh (the Book of Kings) [8] is an influential Persian literary masterwork. Abu Mansur Daqiqi wrote the first one thousand verses of the epic poem in his native Afghanistan province of Balkh, where Buddhism, Islam and Zoroastrianism co-existed. After Daqiqi's untimely death, the notorious poet Abukl-Qasem Ferdowsi in Persia completed the masterpiece in the year 1010 after several decades of effort, reaching close to fifty thousand captivating verses in over one thousand pages. The *Shahnameh* recounts the mythical history of Persia from the creation of the world up to the seventh century through the reign of 50 kings. It also serves as an account of the Zoroastrian religion. Zarathustra, the founder of the influential Zoroastrian religion, refers to fire as holy and fire is of utmost importance in Zoroastrian religious rituals. Fire always burns upwards and connotes righteousness. Zoroastrian community worship involves lighting and maintaining eternal fires in temples, and fire connotes purity, energy, illumination, warmth, creation, justice, and protection.

Customary beliefs in Central Asian countries consider interacting with fire as redeeming and freeing. For example, jumping over fire results in good luck and cleanses your sins. It is particularly auspicious to do so before the *Nowruz* holiday during the last Wednesday of the solar year, an ancient tradition that persists as part of the festival of *Charshanbe suri* in present day Iran and Afghanistan.

The allegory of Ibrahim is a legendary account of surviving immolation. Embedded in the collective psyche of the region is the story of Ibrahim surviving his execution, as an example of surviving immolation to prove innocence and being free of sin. The exemplar Ibrahim was an exalted prophet venerated in Judaism, Christianity and Islam religions. In Islamic tradition he is considered a patriarchal archetype and model citizen. When sentenced to be executed by Nimrod of Babylon, Ibrahim was chained and catapulted to his death into a fire. Saved by Allah as he calmly accepted his fate, the fire freed him from the chains, and he walked out from within the blaze serenely and unharmed as testimony of his faith and piousness.

Numerous poems in Afghan literature glorify burning and immolation. Consider the following verses:

پروانه نیستم که به یک شعله جان دهم شمعم که پاک سوزم و جان را فدا کنم

...I am the candle that burns cleanly to the end as I sacrifice my life.

گرچه خاموشم ولی آهم به گردون می رسد دود شمع کشته ام که در انجمن پیچیده ام

Although I am extinguished my sigh reaches the heavens like the dissipating smoke of a blown off candle

4 From Honor Killings to Self-Immolation: A Crisis of Women's Rights in Afghanistan

The practice of honor or shame killings, commonplace in central and south Asia dating back to the time of the invasion of Mongols, continues at alarming rates to this day in certain regional and ethnic enclaves. Such murders include daughters, sisters and wives by their fathers, brothers and husbands, for a variety of reasons that are culturally offensive, including forbidden love that deviates from accepted norms, killings of victims of rape, and slaying women who protest marital discontent. This misogynistic practice persists and results in the death of thousands of women every year, and relevant to our chapter is that *many women choose to self-immolate to avert impending murder*. The relationship between honor killings and forced suicides by self-immolation, although horrific, is understandable in the cultural context of patrilineal societies that restrict women's freedom and ability to express sexuality, and cultural precepts that blame victims in order to justify senseless violence.

A magnanimous historical figure killed in this manner was Rabia Balkhi, a famous and highly educated Afghan poet who rose to international prominence in the tenth century AD. An all-girls' school and a women's hospital in Kabul are named after her. Although historical accounts differ, a commonly accepted story is that Rabia Balkhi died as a result of an honor killing after the perception of a romantic transgression based on the content of her love poems. Her father ordered her brother to kill her to avenge and preserve family honor.

A reading of the *Shahnameh* asserts the misperception of women as inferior or second-class citizens. Persian and Pashto literature commonly attribute manipulation, wrongdoing and lying as inherent to femininity, misguided beliefs that unfortunately persist in current-day Afghanistan. Feminists and iconic women fighting for human rights include the consummate poets Sayyida Makhfi Badakhshi (1876–1992) and the aforementioned Rabia Balkhi. Others, such as Goharshad Begum, deftly worked behind the scenes to positively influence their environments. A women's university in Kabul and a high school in Herat bear Begum's name. Goharshad Begum led a cultural renaissance during the fifteenth century, politically outmaneuvering men in power to become a *de facto* ruler at a time when this was not permissible.

To this day, women's rights remain compromised in Afghanistan. Oftentimes self-immolations occur to escape violence, oppression and threats of death, taking control of one's destiny through suicide before being murdered by a family member.

Nadia Anjuman 2005–1980) نادیا انجمن), a foremost woman Dari poet, died at the age of 25 in Herat. The circumstances of her death remain a mystery. Although reported as a suicide, most believe she was a victim of domestic violence and was beaten to death by her husband, who resented her choice to continue writing after her first book gained regional and international notoriety. Poetic expression by a woman is still commonly considered an intolerable transgression in present day Afghanistan. Anjuman wrote:

Do not question love as it is the inspiration of your pen
My loving words had in mind death.—Nadia Anjuman, *"Strands of Steel"*, in the book
Gul-e-dodi (Dark Red Flower) [9]

As educated leaders in Afghan cities take on the dutiful task of protecting women's rights as human rights, others in healthcare struggle to provide basic mental health services to communities in need and vulnerable individuals at risk for suicide and other multimorbidities.

5   Mental Health Services, Suicide and Mental Disorders in Afghanistan

Mental-health services in Afghanistan remain perilous and inadequate even after the collapse of the Taliban's rule. [10] Limited research exists on the mental health status of the Afghan population. As a war-torn country with overwhelming needs and scarce resources, vulnerable groups such as women and children suffer the most. War-related tension gets displaced into the household with a high incidence of domestic violence [11]. Hundreds of thousands Afghans are likely to be suffering from depression, anxiety and syndromal or subsyndromal incapacitating posttraumatic stress disorder (PTSD) [12].

According to the WHO report of a fact-finding mission in Pakistan, 30% of Afghan refugees seeking medical help presented psychosomatic complaints related to psychological health [13]. A study of mortality rate and causes of death among displaced and non-migratory populations in Kabul found that 33% of deaths among the displaced and 48% of deaths among resident populations, in all age groups, result from gunshot and war-related trauma [14, 15]. There are anecdotal reports suggesting that the number of persons attempting suicide by self-immolation is exceedingly high in the Herat province. Exact statistics are not available but according to a news report from the Herat Burns Unit, more than 80 self-immolation cases are in record for 2008 alone, suggesting that Herat has the highest prevalence of suicide by self-immolation in Afghanistan [16].

Having a mental illness is a risk factor suicidal behavior [17], together with socio-demographic determinants such as living in poverty and war zones, being geographically displaced, of female gender, unmarried, divorced, widowed or separated, and having lower education [18]. To the best of the authors' knowledge there is no systematic research of the mentally ill in Afghanistan. Furthermore, there are frequent media coverage reports of suicidal behavior among Afghan women. Most of these reports suggest a connection between suicide and intimate partner violence, also within the context of forced marriages [19, 20].

The authors, under the leadership of Prof. Maniam Thambu and Dr. Sayed Sabour Ahmad Mansouri, designed a study to explore the psychosocial determinants of suicide among Afghan psychiatric patients by looking at the prevalence and circumstances surrounding suicidal behavior and self-immolation in an outpatient mental health clinic in the Herat province of Afghanistan. Our objective was to identify the associated risk factors for suicidal behavior by self-immolation in the study cohort.

6 Self-Immolation Ideation Among Psychiatric Outpatients in Herat-Research Study

6.1 Methods

We aimed to explore the proportion of persons with suicidal ideation among attendees of the Mental Health Training Centre of Herat, also known as the Herat Mental Health Clinic, and examine the associated psychosocial factors correlating to suicidal behaviour and specifically self-immolation ideation and plans. The clinic serves as a treatment center for the mentally ill in the Herat province and the western region of Afghanistan. It is also a site for practical mental health training for medical and nursing students, medical officers and primary health care staff. The total number of patients seen in this clinic during the study period was 3993 with 1202 new cases. Almost 97% of attendees were from the Herat province, with 53% living in rural areas. The study was conducted from 25th June 2012 until 31st November 2013.

Randomized patients had to fulfil inclusion criteria including age over 14 years and ability to communicate in Persian (also known as Dari, Farsi) or Pashto (also known as Pakto and Pakhto). Patients excluded were those who could not give informed consent for any reason, had severe psychotic symptoms that interfered with the interview process, had profound mental retardation or severe dementia and lacked decisional capacity to consent, or had physical disability such as deafness that could interfere with the interview.

The cross-sectional exploratory study used proportion estimation and regression models to assess the relationship of suicidal behaviors to demographic variables, life events, impulsivity and major mental health conditions. Psychometric instruments used included demographic questions, Brugha's List of Threatening Experiences (LTE) [21] with modifications, Barratt's Impulsiveness Scale (BIS-11) [22], and the Mini International Neuropsychiatric Interview (M.I.N.I) version 6.0.0 [23, 24], and open ended questions to understand the reasons some participants would consider self-immolation as a suicide method. A team of translators translated questionnaires into the two national languages.

The Postgraduate Research Scientific Committee of the Department of Psychiatry of the National University of Malaysia Medical Centre (UKMMC) evaluated and approved the research proposal and the Ethics Committee of UKMMC Ethical Board approved the methods and merits of the study. Co-authors of this chapter are UKMMC professors and served as liaisons for these functions. The Ministry of Public Health of Afghanistan gave verbal approval before conducting the study as well.

6.2   Results

Of the 117 patients included in final data analyses, 70% were female. The most common psychiatric diagnosis was major depressive disorder (70% of patients), followed by obsessive compulsive disorder, generalized anxiety disorder, phobia, post-traumatic stress disorder, bipolar disorder, psychotic disorders, and panic disorder, present in 7–27% of patients. 78% of participants reported suicidal ideation. The 18–29 years age group and a diagnosis of major depressive disorder were associated with current suicidality (Odds ratio, OR = 3 [95% Confidence Interval, CI 1.0–8.6] and OR = 4.3, [95% CI 1.6–11.2]) respectively. We also found that experiencing serious illness, being assaulted by a close relative, and conflict with in-laws, significantly correlated with higher suicidality (OR = 3.5, 95% CI 1.1–11.3 and OR 6.3, 95% CI 1.3–30.4 respectively).

Thirty percent of subjects thought about a method of suicide. Fifty-one percent of subjects who thought about a method thought of poisoning and 38% thought about self-immolation. When exploring reasons for selecting a particular method, it initially appeared that reasons related to impulsive decision making was the main answer to the question "why did you select this method?" Almost all participants (97%) who thought of a suicidal method answered with statements such as "It just came to my mind suddenly". However, upon further exploration, 30% of brought up access to means as a factor, 19% stated endorsed their choice as a learned method, and 11% spoke of simplicity as a factor. Of those who specifically thought of self-immolation, 36% endorsed accessibility as a factor, and 29% endorsed it as a learned method.

Table 1 summarizes demographic variables of persons with self-immolation ideation or plans.

Table 2 summarizes the relationship of adverse life events with self-immolation ideation or plans.

Table 1 Demographic variables of persons with self-immolation ideation or plans		Number	Percentage
	Age (18–29)	9	64
	Gender (female)	13	93
	Education		
	No education	13	93
	Traditional education	1	7
	Living area		
	Herat City	10	71
	Herat Village	4	29
	Marital state (Married)	14	100
	Number of children		
	0	2	14
	≥3	12	76
	Immigration	3	21

Table 2 Relationship between adverse life events and self-immolation ideation or plan

	Number	Percentage
Experiencing serious illness, injury or assault	5	36
Witnessing serious illness, injury or assault of a close relative	7	50
Serious problems with a close friend, neighbor, or relative	8	57
Conflict with spouse	8	57
Forced marriage	9	64

In addition to psychopathology and adverse life events, impulsivity was another common characteristic, with 85% of persons with self-immolation ideation or plan having total impulsivity scores ranging from 61 to 90.

6.3 Discussion

Our study generates clinically relevant data that could help identify and prevent suicidal behavior and understand the determinants of suicide in Afghanistan, in particular when self-immolation is considered as a means of self-harm.

The study showed that major depression is the main associated factor with self-immolation suicidal ideation; younger age (18–29), being female, married, in a forced marriage, uneducated, having >3 children are also associated factors. Increased risk of suicide in the 18–29 year age group is in accordance with the recent trend of increased suicidality among younger people [25]. This is similar to higher prevalence of suicidal ideation found in other countries with adolescents and young adults being more vulnerable to suicide. For example, in a Malaysian general population study those in the 16–24 year age group were found to have significantly higher rates of suicide [26].

Higher impulsivity scores is a determining factor as well. However, the severity of suicidality is substantially and significantly associated with adverse life events. The most important life events associated with high suicidal risk were experiencing serious illness, injury, or an assault by a close relative. Family conflicts with sisters-in-law, husband or mother in-law were also important associated factors. These are known risk factors in other cohorts of suicidal patients as well [27, 28].

Afghans lived through consecutive decades of war and poverty encountering catastrophic life events. The majority of study participants endorsed several threatening adverse life events in addition to conflicts with their spouse, in-laws, and paternal family, and reported distress associated with forced marriages. Human rights organizations and clinicians are mindful of the frequency and severity of family conflicts and domestic violence in Afghanistan [29], recognizing the rampant victimization of women as a result of intimate partner violence. Although new laws passed to protect the human rights of women in Afghanistan, a cultural shift lags behind in this regard.

A study of Afghan refugees in Pakistan reports a high rate of conflicts with in-laws as an important aspect of domestic violence [30]. In our study, conflict with spouse, sister in-law and with all in-laws altogether indicated and association with increased suicide risk. When families merge and with overcrowding, conflicts among members of different family facets compound conjugal tension and exacerbate psychological distress. There is clear emphasis on the recognition of violence against women perpetrated by men [31, 32], but less attention given to conflicts between women in the extended family. To the best of the authors' knowledge, conflicts with in-laws contributing to suicidal behavior is not sufficiently emphasized elsewhere in the suicide prevention literature. Our finding of conflicts with sister in-laws being a significant predisposing factor for suicide is an area that may benefit from further exploration and study in the context of Afghan culture.

Self-immolation is the second most common method of suicide reported as a plan or ideation, after poisoning, in our study participants from Western Afghanistan, placing these individuals at great risk given the lethality of the method. Other investigators identified a high prevalence of suicides by self-immolation in this region of the world [33]. A descriptive study in a burn unit in Bandar Abbas in the more economically developed neighbouring country of Iran found that domestic violence against women, family problems, romantic disappointments and conjugal fights often preceded self-immolation suicide attempts [34]. Similarly, a study in Western Iran showed that almost all women treated in burn units after self-immolation attempts are survivors of intimate partner violence [35].

7   Prevention of Suicide by Self-Immolation in Afghanistan

In view of the high rate of suicidal ideation among the mentally ill in our study population combined with the finding that suicidality goes clinically unnoticed in mental health settings in Afghanistan, it would be sensible to enhance services and provide systematic training on suicide prevention to mental health caregivers. Research shows that suicidal ideation strongly correlates with suicide attempts and eventual death by suicide [36]. We recommend a concerted effort to establish suicide prevention initiatives as well as support and treatment for survivors of suicide.

Improving current mental health services, especially providing capacity-building opportunities, is perhaps the most feasible approach to consider. Recognition and screening of mental-health problems are crucial [37, 38]. In mental health centers similar to the clinic where we conducted our study, or even in primary health centers in Afghanistan, a translation of the M.I.N.I suicidality module may help to detect persons at risk for suicide. This module could be simply administered by a trained nurse or mental health paraprofessional.

Our study increased our understanding of the nuances of inter-personal relationships among women at risk of self-immolation in Herat, Afghanistan.

Women-oriented mental health programs could improve access to care and provide psychosocial support to vulnerable individuals living in fragile and volatile environments [39]. Psychoeducational programs designed for men at risk of violence with the goal to reduce intimate partner violence could also lower suicide rates. Forced marriages, especially of the very young, should be strongly discouraged or prohibited, a difficult task in traditional cultures. As self-immolation is common among non-educated women, it is again strongly recommended to support education programs for women.

Imitation and suicide by contagion appear to be contributory factors in our clinical experience, whereby hearing or witnessing deaths of other women by self-immolation plants a seed that could eventually evolve into replication of actions. When there is a constriction of cognition and suicide becomes a maladaptive coping mechanism as all else fails, socially endorsed forms of self-harm are revisited and perpetuated. Implementing research validated media guidelines that are suicide protective is important to properly educate the public about mental illness and responsible reporting of suicides. [40].

Furthermore, funding and encouraging volunteerism and empowering organizations that support human rights of women, passing legislation that protects women, and enforcing egalitarian laws to facilitate a cultural shift away from discriminatory attitudes are all necessary to catalyze suicide prevention efforts [41].

References

1. Medica Mondiale. https://www.medicamondiale.org/en/nc/latest/evaluation-afghanistan-decidedly-side-by-side-with-women.html. Accessed 6 Jan 2019.
2. Hauslohner A. Afghanistan: when women set themselves on fire. *Time*. Wednesday July 7, 2010.
3. Country Profile-Afghanistan. http://www.emro.who.int/emrinfo/index.asp?Ctry=afg. Accessed 20 Feb 2020.
4. MOPH Afghanistan. The essential package of hospital services for Afghanistan. Kabul: USAID; 2005. p. 1–52.
5. The Lancet editorial. Revitalizing health in Afghanistan. Lancet. 2009;374(9691):664.
6. Mohammad GMG. Afghanistan in the course of history, volume two. Alexandria, VA: Hashmat K Gobar; 2001.
7. Sediq FMM. Afghanistan in the last five centuries. Lahore: Irfan Publications; 2008.
8. Ferdowsi A. Shahnameh: The Persian Book of Kings. New York: Penguin Books; 2007.
9. Anjuman N. The complete poems. Tehran: Iran Open Publishing Group; 2014.
10. World Health Organization. WHO-AIMS report on mental health systems in Afghanistan. Kabul: WHO and Ministry of Public Health; 2006. p. 1–19.
11. van de Put W. Addressing mental health in Afghanistan. Lancet. 2002;360(Suppl):s41–2.
12. Ventevogel P, Azimi S, Jalal S, Kortmann F. Mental health care reform in Afghanistan. J Ayub Med Coll Abbottabad. 2002;14(4):1–3.
13. World Health Organization. The invisible wounds: the mental health crisis in Afghanistan. 6 November 2001.
14. Gessner BD. Mortality rates, causes of death, and health status among displaced and resident populations of Kabul, Afghanistan. JAMA. 1994;272(5):382–5.

15. De Jong E. Mental Health Assessment Ghurian and Zendah Jan districts, Herat Province Afghanistan. Amsterdam/Kabul: Medecins sans Frontieres Holland; 1999.
16. Patience M. Afghan women who turn to immolation. In.: BBC; 2009.
17. World Health Organization. Preventing suicide: a resource for counsellors. Geneva: World Health Organization; 2006.
18. Nock KMGB, Cha CB, Chiu WT, Hwang I, Sampson NA, Hinkov H, Lepine JP, Ono Y, Beautrais A. Sociodemographic risk factors for suicidal behavior: results from the WHO World mental health surveys. In: Nock KMGB, Ono Y, editors. Suicide: global perspectives from the WHO world mental health surveys, vol. 1. Cambridge: Cambridge University Press; 2012. p. 391.
19. Sultani MMHA, Nusrat MH, Zahidi A, Elham S, Hasrat MH. Report on the situation of economic and social rights in Afghanistan-IV. In: Afghanistan Independent Human Rights Commission (AIHRC). Report on the Situation of Economic and Social Rights in Afghanistan. December 2009. https://www.refworld.org/docid/4b3b2df72.html. Accessed 23 Feb 2020.
20. Hasrat-Nazami W. Afghan women escape marriage through suicide. Deutsche Welle. 18 April 2013. https://www.dw.com/en/afghan-women-escape-marriage-through-suicide/a-16750044. Accessed 23 Feb 2020.
21. Brugha TS, Cragg D. The list of threatening experiences: the reliability and validity of a brief life events questionnaire. Acta Psychiatr Scand. 1990;82(1):77–81.
22. Patton JH, Stanford MS, Barratt ES. Factor structure of the Barratt impulsiveness scale. J Clin Psychol. 1995;51(6):768–74.
23. Sheehan DV, Lecrubier Y, Sheehan KH, Amorim P, Janavs J, Weiller E, Hergueta T, Baker R, Dunbar GC. The Mini-International Neuropsychiatric Interview (M.I.N.I.): the development and validation of a structured diagnostic psychiatric interview for DSM-IV and ICD-10. J Clin Psychiatry. 1998;59(Suppl 20):22–33; quiz 34–57.
24. Sheehan DV, Lecrubier Y, Harnett Sheehan K, Janavs J, Weiller E, Keskiner A, Schinka J, Knapp E, Sheehan MF, Dunbar GC. The validity of the Mini International Neuropsychiatric Interview (MINI) according to the SCID-P and its reliability. Eur Psychiat. 1997;12(5):232–41.
25. World Health Organization. Figures and facts about suicide. Geneva: World Health Organization; 1999.
26. Institute for Public Health. Psychiatric morbidity in adults. In: The Third National Health and Morbidity Survey (NHMS III) 2006. vol. 2. Ministry of Health Malaysia; 2008.
27. Seponski DM, Somo CM, Kao S, Lahar CJ, Khann S, Schunert T. Family, health, and poverty factors impacting suicide attempts in Cambodian women. Crisis. 2019;40(2):141–5.
28. Ásgeirsdóttir HG, Valdimarsdóttir UA, Þorsteinsdóttir ÞK, Lund SH, Tomasson G, Nyberg U, Ásgeirsdóttir TL, Hauksdóttir A. The association between different traumatic life events and suicidality. Eur J Psychotraumatol. 2018;9:1.
29. Jewkes R, Corboz J, Gibbs A. Trauma exposure and IPV experienced by Afghan women: analysis of the baseline of a randomised controlled trial. PLoS One. 2018;13(10):e0201974.
30. Hayder AA, Zarin N, Tsui E. Intimate partner violence among Afghan women living in refugee camps in Pakistan. Soc Sci Med. 2007;64(7):1536–47.
31. Raj A, Gomez C, Silverman JG. Driven to a fiery death—the tragedy of self-immolation in Afghanistan. N Engl J Med. 2008;358(21):2201–3.
32. Aziz N. What self-immolation means to Afghan women. Peace Rev: J Soc Just. 2011;23:45–51.
33. Central Statistics Organization (CSO) MoPHM, ICF Inter-national. Afghanistan Demographic and Health Survey 2015. 2016.
34. Zamani SN, Bagheri M, Nejad MA. Investigation of the demographic characteristics and mental health in self-immolation attempters. Int J High-Risk Behav Addict. 2013;2(2):77–81.
35. Ahmadi A, Mohammadi R, Schwebel DC, Yeganeh N, Soroush A, Bazargan-Hejazi S. Familial risk factors for self-immolation: a case-control study. J Women's Health (Larchmt). 2009;18(7):1025–31.
36. Taylor PJ, Hutton P, Wood L. Are people at risk of psychosis also at risk of suicide and self-harm? A systematic review and meta-analysis. Psychol Med. 2015;45(5):911–26.

37. Shekhani SS, Perveen S, Hashmi D-E-S, Akbar K, Bachani S, Khan MM. Suicide and deliberate self-harm in Pakistan: a scoping review. BMC Psychiat. 2018;18:1.
38. Thapaliya S, Sharma P, Upadhyaya K. Suicide and self harm in Nepal. A scoping review. Asian J Psychiatr. 2018;32:20–6.
39. Ventevogel P, van de Put W, Faiz H, van Mierlo B, Siddiqi M, Komproe IH. Improving access to mental health care and psychosocial support within a fragile context: a case study from Afghanistan. PLoS Med. 2012;9(5):e1001225.
40. World Health Organization. Preventing suicide: a global imperative 2014. https://apps.who.int/iris/bitstream/handle/10665/131056/9789241564779_eng.pdf;jsessionid=9478E002BDC3F065E43053273FBEFC9D?sequence=1. Accessed 23 Feb 2020.
41. Anderson S, Genicot G. Suicide and property rights in India. J Dev Econ. 2015;114:64–78.

Self-Immolation in India

Naveen Manohar Pai and Prabha S. Chandra

1 Introduction

Suicide is a major public health problem. While suicide by self-immolation is an unusual occurrence in the developed world, it is more frequent in Asian countries and particularly in India. Unusually high rates of suicide by self-immolation are seen among unschooled, young and married woman in low-and middle-income Asian countries, perhaps due to various cultural and socio-economic motives [1]. While the occurrence of these deaths inside the domestic environment is very high, self-immolation receives very little media coverage compared to other fire-related deaths that occur in the general community. While men continue to have a higher total number of completed suicides, there is a remarkably high rate of suicide among women by means of self-immolation [2]. One must keep in mind unique historical and cultural country-specific aspects in order to understand suicides by self-immolation in India. In this chapter the authors will offer a brief historical review of fire related deaths and events, the role of sociocultural factors, Indian research and current epidemiological trends of suicide by self-immolation, and discuss prevention strategies.

N. M. Pai
National Institute of Mental Health and Neurosciences, Bangalore, India
e-mail: dr.naveen.pai@gmail.com

P. S. Chandra (✉)
National Institute of Mental Health and Neurosciences, Bangalore, India

International Association of Women's Mental Health, Bangalore, India
e-mail: prabhasch@gmail.com, chandra@nimhans.ac.in

© The Author(s), under exclusive license to Springer Nature Switzerland AG 2021
C. A. Alfonso et al. (eds.), *Suicide by Self-Immolation*,
https://doi.org/10.1007/978-3-030-62613-6_5

2 Scriptures, Mythology and History of Self-Immolation in India

Ancient scriptures (*Dharma shastras*), which describe various codes and conduct for individuals in Indian society, are unambiguous in their criticism of suicides. Some of these scriptures endorse suicide when a person is unable to perform his or her duties and describe various ways to end one's life. The great mythological text *Ramayana* provides a glorified description of *Agni Pareeksha* (the fire test) [3]. When Lord Rama finds his wife Sita after the victory over the evil Ravana, he is unable to trust her and questions her sanctity on the hearsay of his factions. Upon hearing these allegations she is outraged and protests her innocence by asking Rama's brother to build a pyre for her. She enters the fire offering herself in sacrifice in order to settle the question of her sanctity. This is one of the instances in Hindu mythology where sacrificing one's own life is associated with adoration of the deed, resulting in the glorification of suicide.

Until recently, existing societal norms were by and large conventional and conservative and individuals in society were to a greater extent influenced by these. As proposed by Durkheim, when such repressive sanctions exist, violation of the sociocultural norms are often met with punishments. Conscious or unconscious glorification of these incidents and stories in the ancient texts might have led to the commonly held belief that self-immolation is a form of altruistic suicide [4].

3 The Practice of *Jauhar* and *Sati: Self-Immolation Unique to Women*

The ritual practice of *Jauhar* falls under the category of mass suicide, a group self-immolation practice carried out by women of certain communities in ancient India to avoid insufferable shame when their menfolk faced defeat. This practice was largely prevalent among the Rajput community of North India. The women of the community would build a huge pyre; they along with their children would jump into it. These women were subsequently worshipped as pure and selfless as it was believed that they expressed heroic devotion towards their husbands and other menfolk. What motivated *Jauhar* was the fear of being raped and abused by captors if husbands died at war, which would cause irreparable harm to the self-respect and dignity of the clan. During these instances of honour suicides a whole tribe of women could become non-existent in a matter of a few hours. The ritual of *Jauhar* symbolizes protest among women against the carnages of subjugators. A popular example was the *Jauhar* performed by Rani Padmini of Chittor (presently the Chittorgarh district of Rajasthan, India) who self-immolated along with thousands of kin women when faced with the invading army of the Delhi Sultanate. *Jauhar* mass suicides of women were commonplace in India from the thirteenth to the seventeenth century and abolished by law in 1829 [5].

The term *Sati* (also known as *suttee*) was given to a woman who was burned on the pyre along with the body of her dead husband. This particular form of ritual self-immolation of widows was not widespread until after the eighth century A. D. The majority of the literature on this custom suggests that it was an important form of culturally sanctioned suicide for widows. It was considered to be an important aspect of one's righteous deed as a woman and wife. Mythology describes *Sati* as another name for the Goddess Parvati, who was the daughter of Daksha and consort of the God Shiva. When her father, Daksha organized a massive *yagna* (ritual with a specific objective), he invited various deities to the proceedings but as a form of offense towards God Shiva he purposefully ignored him. Upon hearing this news, the Goddess Sati felt that she and her husband had been shamed and offered herself in sacrifice in the fire of the *yagna* by self-immolation [3]. A common belief was that by doing such a deed, a woman who performed *Sati* would secure a place in heaven for the family for the next seven generations. In addition, women who performed ritual self-immolation—*Sati* were glorified and worshipped endlessly. An alternate belief held was that through *Sati* husband and wife would reunite in an eternal marriage in heaven [5]. Ambiguities in mythological and religious texts pertaining to the practice of *Sati* could also be re-interpreted in various ways with each passing generation, and such interpretations mutually influenced the prevailing customs and practices, as well as religion.

The traditional construct in India is that a woman's primary responsibility is to tend to the needs of her husband by serving, being faithful, and placating him. After the death of her husband a woman is vulnerable and becomes subject to accusations that question the strength of her marital devotion. Thus, ritual self-immolation, *Sati,* became a way for a woman to prove devotion through self-sacrifice. Some critics report that in the background of the prevailing cultural practices when *Sati* was commonplace, a woman's status after the death of her husband was indeterminate and her right to exercise this particular ritual was considered an essential act of selflessness. After several revolts against this ritual and proposed reforms, it was during the period of British occupation that *Sati* formally ended by passing a legislation against its practice.

Women who died by *Sati* were unlikely to be suffering from any form of severe mental illnesses like depressive disorders or psychosis. Some rudiments of grief and possibly aspects of complicated bereavement leading to depersonalisation might have predisposed such individuals to this form of suicide. Also, factors related to the social and cultural pressure experienced by such individuals should not be excluded as enabling these deaths. Thus, *Sati* remains of historical importance as an unusual example of a cultural form of suicide that is tolerated and encouraged by religious and popular beliefs [6].

4   Epidemiology of Suicide by Self-Immolation in India

The mortality rate due to suicide in India is 16.3 per 100,000 population, which is more than the global average of 10.6/100,000. The suicide rate in India is higher when compared to other South and East Asian countries (regional average of 13.2/100,000) [7]. In India the only official source of information about estimates of burns morbidity and mortality is obtained from the listings of these incidents in police records. The national crime records bureau, which maintains a database on Accidental Deaths and Suicide in India (ADSI), estimates the rate of suicide to be around 10.2/100,000. As per the ADSI report there is a steady increase in hanging and drowning as means of suicide, while suicide by self-immolation has seen a downward trend from 10.7% in early 2000 to 4.4% in 2018 [2].

In low- and middle-income countries suicide rates among men is 1.6 times higher than in women [8]. In contrast, the recently concluded National Mental Health Survey of 2014 in India reports that the overall suicide rate is higher amongst women than men. Women had the highest prevalence in the age group of 40–49 years. Overall prevalence of suicide in women is 1.75 times more than in men, which differs from global reports of suicide in low- and middle-income countries [9]. This is further supported by evidence from other studies which suggests that even though the mortality rates from suicide is characteristically lower in females than males, the prevalence of suicidal behaviour is higher in females, thereby giving rise to the gender paradox of reported suicides [10, 11].

Suicide by self-immolation still continues to be one of the common methods of suicide in India. Indian men are twice as likely as women to die by suicide, but out of all the methods of suicide self-immolation is the only one that claims more women than men. According to the ADSI report of 2018, suicides by fire/self-immolation claimed 3809 female deaths out of 5950 in total [2]. The majority of the suicides by self-immolation were in the age group of 16–30 years. Several studies report that the most commonly used accelerants for self-immolation are kerosene based as these are easily available. The mortality rate following self-immolation in India is close to 60% and the majority of survivors die secondary to complications of burns such as sepsis, cardiogenic and hypovolemic shock, and carbon monoxide poisoning [12].

5   Self-Immolation and Intimate Partner Violence

Suicide by self-immolation of women homemakers in India is closely linked to intimate partner violence. A large number of these suicides occur when couples cohabitate with their extended families (a common occurrence in India). One possible explanation is that traditionally the newlywed woman is expected to immediately adjust to her new family and take up the majority of the burden of household duties. In this regard, she is subjected to emotional abuse and harassment by extended family members when performance expectations are not met. Fatigue, confinement and burnout, without a neutral outlet to express emotion, may result in suicide by self-immolation preceded by affective states of desperation, hopelessness and helplessness. When confined over time mostly to the kitchen space, availability of kerosene makes self-immolation the preferred option.

A retrospective study in a tertiary centre in North India of 152 women homemakers with burn related injuries noted that approximately 21% (n = 32) of deaths were due to suicide by self-immolation. The majority of the study population was in the age group of 15–30 years and suicide by self-immolation before the age of 16 years was an uncommon occurrence. The most common venue for such suicides was the common living area of the house. The extent of burns sustained by the victims suggests that little or no rescue attempts were made to save these women. Only 28% of this study population survived for more than 24 hours following the incident. Kerosene was the most commonly used accelerant, which further potentiated the extent and depth of burn injuries. The investigators found that majority of patients in this cohort were young brides and there was an ongoing dowry dispute in most cases [12].

Human rights activists who are critical of the existing social structure in India describe that Indian women perceive marriage as the only option to secure a future, together with the view that a woman's responsibility is first and foremost to her husband and his family, with tending to their needs being the utmost priority. When women are additionally faced with intimate partner violence, options become limited resulting in a constriction of cognition and the perception that choices are seemingly limited to either staying married or dying. An important finding in Kumar's study is that majority of the female victims of suicide by self-immolation have low educational levels. Hence it is suggested that as the level of education increased among women in India in recent years, this resulted in fall in the incidence of suicides by self-immolation [12]. The investigator critiques that the social system in India fails to provide developmental options to protect disenfranchised women, as marriage seems to be the central focus for women in India.

6 The Influence of Mass Media and Social Media on Suicide by Self-Immolation

Philips coined the term the *Werther* effect [13]. He noted that sensational reporting of suicide leads to an increase in the number of additional suicides in the subsequent months. The degree to which vulnerable individuals identify with the suicide method described by mass media is an important predictor of imitation suicides, also referred to as copycat suicides. The theory of social learning helps us place the phenomenon of copycat suicides in context. There are only a handful of studies that examine the impact of mass media reporting on suicide. One such study was done by Chandra and colleagues on the quality of newspaper reports of suicide published in the city of Bangalore in Southern India. The major findings from this study are numerous instances of sensational reporting of suicides by newspapers with detailed reporting of specific aspects like suicide pacts or mass suicides, photographs of the venues and victims, and excerpts of suicide notes. Also, in some cases, the media glorifies suicide as immediate death without suffering [14]. There are no studies examining the direct effects of mass media reporting on suicides by self-immolation in India, but findings from the study by Chandra and colleagues are worrisome since in a majority of occurrences the media in this region does not portray suicide in a sensitive manner.

There is an increasing body of evidence suggesting that internet and various social media platforms can influence rates of suicide and suicide related behaviour. Social media today has a huge potential for creating virtual communities without physical borders and engaging people who are generally difficult to engage, and has a particular impact on vulnerable adolescents and young adults. Although limited, most of the data in this regard is preliminary and comes from high income countries [15, 16]. Social media platforms may influence vulnerable individuals through formation of extreme communities and online groups that promote beliefs and behaviours that are typically unacceptable, which could include suicide by self-immolation, with forums that provoke communal hatred and emulation of problematic practices. Despite the obvious benefits of isolated individuals gaining support through social media, internet communities may place at risk vulnerable ones with a sense of thwarted belongingness who may be coerced to engage in self-destructive behaviours. Hence, there is an urgent need to monitor, flag, and perhaps regulate content in social media platforms as part of suicide prevention strategies.

The Press Council of India recently adopted guidelines on reporting of suicides in accordance with the WHO suicide prevention report from 2014 [8, 17]. Some of the important highlights of these guidelines include restrictions on sensational reporting of suicides by self-immolation, minimizing the use of photographs and video footage and use of language that either stigmatises or provokes similar incidents.

7   Research on Self-Immolation in India

There are very few of studies looking at the aetiology and pathogenesis of suicide by self-immolation and the majority are accounts from hospitalized survivors and interviews with family members of those who suicide. The exact prevalence and psychosocial factors associated with self-immolation are difficult to study due to under reporting of suicides, questionable methodology and reliability of data. Rezaeian points out that the number of indexed articles in PubMed covering various aspects of self-immolation substantially increased over the past few decades worldwide [18]. However, over the past decade there is a steady decline in research reports on self-immolation in Indian settings, which could be attributed to either the decreasing trend of self-immolation as means of suicide or strong legal stances against these suicides.

The Mandal Commission was formed in 1979 under the direction of the then ruling party of the Republic of India. This particular commission was given the task of identifying the needs of socially and educationally backward classes (SEBC) in order to address their difficulties and help achieve social equality. To bring about social change in society the committee recommended that 27% of employment opportunities in the government sector should be reserved for people from SEBC. This determination created uproar and unrest, particularly in the student community, and a series of self-immolations resulted as part of the protests against the recommendations of the Mandal Commission report.

Mahla and colleagues reported a case series of survivors of self-immolation who protested against the recommendations of the Mandal Commission of 1979. Three of the four (75%) subjects in the study had a diagnosable DSM Axis I psychiatric disorder, a conclusion that needs to be viewed as tentative as the study is limited by small sample size. The study suggests that a socio-political movement acted as a catalytic agent in already predisposed individuals, emphasizing the importance of social factors predisposing to suicide by self-immolation [19].

Kannappiran and colleagues, in an attempt to study the psychological factors associated with self-immolation, compared 31 subjects who attempted suicide by means of self-immolation with 31 subjects in a control group who attempted suicide by other means. They used the Sixteen-Personality Factor Questionnaire to assess personality traits in these groups. The study identified that self-immolators were emotionally less stable, had poor frustration tolerance and were easily annoyed by acts/situations compared to subjects in the control group. The study inferred that self-immolators have very high levels of impulsivity and behave differently from those who are depressed and attempt suicide [20].

Singh and colleagues conducted a cross sectional study of 22 subjects who attempted suicide by self-immolation. All the subjects attempted suicide as a form of protest in the wake of the recommendations from the Mandal Commission of 1979. The study subjects showed high degree of vulnerability, hostility and feelings of alienation from society (anomic suicides). In contrast to the previous study done by Mahla and colleagues, all study subjects showed high level of suicidal intent in the absence of diagnosable Axis I psychiatric disorders [21]. Table 1 summarizes research results of several studies of suicide by self-immolation in India.

8   Self-Immolations in the Post-independence Era

In the post-independence era in India, self-immolation for political, religious or self-sacrificial motives has also been reported, although infrequently. One of the earliest reports included a series of suicides by self-immolation occurring during the anti-Hindi agitations of 1965 [22]. A school teacher in the southern district of India committed suicide by self-immolation, which led to a series of 5 other self-immolations subsequently. There are reports of families of victims with complicated grief for many years subsequently. There are other incidents of similar nature

Table 1 Salient findings of studies on suicide by self-immolation in India

Author & year	Sample size	Type of study	Salient findings	Limitations
Mahla et al. (1992)	4	Case series	• 3 out of 4 subjects had Axis I disorder • Socio-political movement brought forward these suicides in already predisposed individuals	• Small sample size
Kannapiran et al. (1997)	Cases = 31 Control = 31	Cross-sectional, comparative	• Those in study group were emotionally less stable and had poor frustration tolerance • No diagnosable Axis I disorder in those in the study group	• Severely burnt suicide attempters were not included
Singh et al. (1998)	22	Cross-sectional	• Participants showed high degree of ambition, hostility and alienation scores • No diagnosable Axis I disorder	• Severely burnt suicide attempters were not included
Kumar (2003)	32	Retrospective cohort	• Majority of the affected were in the age group of 21–25 years • Sustained more than 50% burns • Most common cause of death was cardiogenic shock	• Sample was limited to only females • Bias of recall

reported thereafter, including the series of self-immolations as a form of protest against the recommendations of the Mandal Commission report of 1979 as mentioned earlier [5]. Protest suicides by self-immolation still continue as Tibetans in India dispute the Chinese rule of Tibet with demands for an independent state [23].

Reports of other isolated incidents include a death of a widow by self-immolation in September of 1987, giving rise to a chain of events leading to social and political protests against the act of *Sati*. Investigations into this event brought about the disparity in versions from the family and general public witnessing what occurred, including a suggestion that the widow was drugged and coerced to self-immolate by her family members. Believers of this traditional practice praised her and made pilgrimage to the pyre in which she perished. These events subsequently led to the formation of The Commission of Sati Prevention Act of 1987. From a psychiatric perspective, *Sati* is triggered by social and cultural factors. Thus, it is important to differentiate a person who is mentally ill from other individuals who are coerced to self-immolate in the setting of societal pressures and expectations [5, 6].

9   How Can We Prevent Self-Immolation Suicides?

Suicide prevention in India targets social and public health objectives more than conventional mental health interventions. Suicide prevention programmes need to be multidimensional, require collaborative care and coordination of various stakeholders including the general population. Implementation of prevention programmes at the national level need to be cost effective, identify pertinent risk factors and address those that are relevant to the needs of the community. Some of the major risk factors identified for suicide by self-immolation are family problems, loss and sense of alienation, lower education levels, female gender and prevailing sociocultural norms endorsing suicidal behaviour. A comprehensive suicide prevention strategy needs to take into account all these risk factors and deliver evidence-based interventions. It should also identify both short- and medium-term plans and allocate available resources efficiently. Regular monitoring and outcome measures are essential for effective future planning. For a population of over one billion, there are close to 9000 psychiatrists in India. The existing mental health services are inadequate to deal with the current burden of mental illness, which is about 10.6 weighted percent [24]. Rapid urbanization, industrialization and the diminishing of traditional support systems result in social turmoil and distress leaving people vulnerable to suicidal behaviour. The scarcity of mental health services to attend to the needs of vulnerable individuals catalysed the emergence of non-governmental organisations (NGOs) in the field of suicide prevention [25]. These NGOs, along with the NGOs that focus on women-oriented programs, could improve access to care and provide psychosocial support to susceptible individuals living in fragile and volatile environments [26]. As the editors mentioned in the introductory chapter of this book, promoting NGOs that support human rights of women, passing legislation that protects women, and enforcing egalitarian laws to facilitate a cultural shift away from discriminatory attitudes are all necessary. In a country like India, there needs to be a strong move that focuses on men's mental health, substance use, violence prevention and non-violent conflict resolution.

There is an urgent need for upstream suicide prevention approaches that include addressing risk and protective factors early in life. Measures taken in this regard that promote connectedness, reduction of alienation, and eliminating a person's sense of expendability are suicide protective. Upstream prevention interventions may include creating peer support groups, optimizing adolescent health by improving access to care, and encouraging help-seeking via training of gatekeepers. Promoting gender equality legislation and working towards eliminating forced marriages, especially of the very young, should be strongly pursued. Communities play a key role in suicide prevention by self-immolation [8]. As mentioned earlier, even mass media could play an important role in the prevention of suicides. All these strategies are effective only when steps are taken to reduce illiteracy and promote education and equality.

The government of India has already taken several steps towards the prevention of suicide by self-immolation. One of the key steps in this regard is 'The Commission of *Sati* (Prevention) Act' of 1987 [27]. The act prevents the observation of any ceremony or procession in relation to *Sati*, prohibits glorification and effects punishment to any person involved in the abatement of such an act. Any person who is involved in coercing or instigating a woman to commit *Sati* is punishable under this act. This act protects the rights of these women and rescues the bereaved widow from this gruesome act of ritual sacrifice.

The Mental Health Care Act of 2017 provides some relief to such vulnerable individuals who attempt suicide by self-immolation. The onus of treatment and rehabilitation of such persons who attempt suicide is transferred to the appropriate state governments who have a duty to provide care to such individuals as they are presumed to be under severe stress, unless proved otherwise [28]. This act has further paved way to protect the rights of the person who attempts suicide and prevents them from being prosecuted under the IPC section 309. It has provisions for families of persons who attempt suicide, in case of emergency, shifting the community resources for effective crisis intervention [29].

Some researchers who work with patients with burn related injuries propose an integrated injury surveillance system for better monitoring of suicides by self-immolation. As a part of this surveillance all essential details are collected from the survivors with burn injuries, their families and all other important witnesses to help understand the victim's environment and identify predisposing and precipitating factors associated with suicide by self-immolation. Such interviews may also help understand and ultimately prevent delays in treatment due to various reasons like fear of facing legal punishments, cost of treatment and other problems accessing health care [30]. A substantial proportion of national resources is required to have such an injury surveillance system in place while there are major public health crises affecting the country, such as infectious diseases, malnutrition, infant and maternal mortality. Supplementing governmental resources with NGO efforts and volunteerism could bridge the prevention and treatment gaps so that suicide by self-immolation receives adequate attention.

10   Conclusion

The existing literature suggests that the prevalence of self-immolation is particularly high in India and countries that share a common border. This pattern of geographical proximity among the affected nations suggests the existence of a geographical belt of self-immolation [1]. Hence these nations should collectively invest in designing culturally sound and appropriate prevention strategies at a national level to fight this important public health problem. Figure 1 demonstrates a collaborative care approach for suicide prevention by self-immolation. There is a high need for cooperation among various national and international agencies which support and promote anti-suicide campaigns. Promoting gender equality and education needs to be an important aspect of such suicide prevention programmes. Some of the major drawbacks of the current system of tracking suicides is non registration

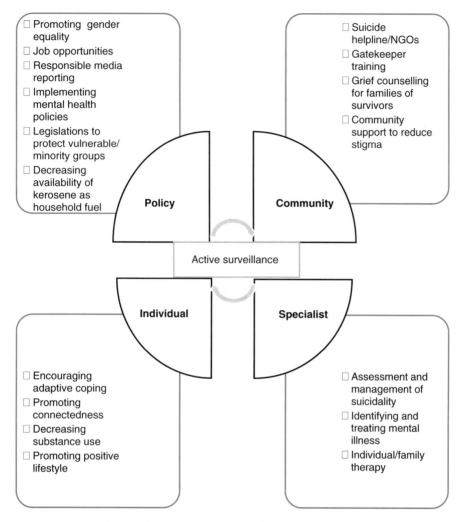

Fig. 1 Prevention of suicide by self-immolation—a collaborative care model

of suicides, fear of public opinions and biases, and inadequate data about the determinants of suicides. A way to overcome such problems is to record all interactions of hospitals, legal systems and others with burns victims and their families as potential sources of data in order to obtain reliable estimates of fire-related deaths. Further distinguishing these incidents from accidents and homicides may help us better understand the magnitude of this problem [30]. A multisector collaborative care approach (as delineated in Fig. 1) that involves not only the health sector but also education, employment, social welfare and judiciary dimensions, along with active surveillance and feedback, may be the key to developing a national self-immolation suicide prevention strategy.

References

1. Rezaeian M. The geographical belt of self-immolation. Burns. 2017;43(5):896–7. https://doi.org/10.1016/j.burns.2017.01.001.
2. Accidental Deaths & Suicides in India. National Crime Records Bureau. 2018. https://ncrb.gov.in/accidental-deaths-suicides-india-2018. Accessed 25 May 2020.
3. Ponnudurai R. Suicide in India—changing trends and challenges ahead. Indian J Psychiatry. 2015;57(4):348–54.
4. Gofman A. Durkheim's theory of social solidarity and social rules. In: The Palgrave handbook of altruism, morality, and social solidarity. New York: Palgrave Macmillan; 2014. p. 45–69.
5. Vijayakumar L. Altruistic suicide in India. Arch Suicide Res. 2004;8(1):73–80.
6. Bhugra D. Sati: a type of nonpsychiatric suicide. Crisis. 2005;26(2):73–7.
7. WHO *Suicide rates per (100,000 population)*. 2020. https://www.who.int/gho/mental_health/suicide_rates_crude/en/. Accessed 25 May 2020.
8. Preventing Suicide. *A global imperative*. 2014. https://www.who.int/mental_health/suicide-prevention/world_report_2014/en/. Accessed 25 May 2020.
9. Amudhan S, Gururaj G, Varghese M, Benegal V, Rao GN, Sheehan DV, et al. A population-based analysis of suicidality and its correlates: findings from the National Mental Health Survey of India, 2015–2016. The Lancet Psychiatry. 2020;7(1):41–51. https://doi.org/10.1016/S2215-0366(19)30404-3.
10. Freeman A, Mergl R, Kohls E, Székely A, Gusmao R, Arensman E, et al. A cross-national study on gender differences in suicide intent. BMC Psychiatry. 2017;17(1):1–11.
11. Canetto SS, Sakinofsky I. The gender paradox in suicide. Suicide Life Threat Behav. 1998;28(1):1–23. http://www.ncbi.nlm.nih.gov/pubmed/9560163
12. Kumar V. Burnt wives—a study of suicides. Burns. 2003;29(1):31–5.
13. Philips DP. The influence of suggestion on suicide: Substantive and theoretical implications of the Werther effect. Am Sociol Rev. 1974;39:340–54.
14. Chandra PS, Doraiswamy P, Padmanabh A, Philip M. Do newspaper reports of suicides comply with standard suicide reporting guidelines? A study from Bangalore, India. Int J Soc Psychiatry. 2014;60(7):687–94.
15. Luxton DD, June JD, Fairall JM. Social media and suicide: a public health perspective. Am J Public Health. 2012;102(Suppl. 2):195–200.
16. Robinson J, Cox G, Bailey E, Hetrick S, Rodrigues M, Fisher S, et al. Social media and suicide prevention: a systematic review. Early Interv Psychiatry. 2016;10(2):103–21.
17. Vijayakumar L. Media matters in suicide-Indian guidelines on suicide reporting. Indian J Psychiatry. 2019;61(6):549–51.
18. Rezaeian M. The trend of indexed papers in PubMed covering different aspects of self-immolation. Acta Med Iran. 2014;52(2):158–62.
19. Mahla VP, Bhargava SC, Dogra R, Shome S. The psychology of self-immolation in. Indian J Psychiatry. 1992;34(2):108–13.
20. Kannapiran T, Haroon AE. Personality profiles of self-immolators. Indian J Psychiatry. 1997;39(I):37–40.
21. Singh SP, Santosh PJ, Avasthi AKI. A psychosocial study of 'self-immolation' in India. Acta Psychiatr Scand. 1998;97:71–5.
22. United in Grief, *50 years after*. https://www.pressreader.com/india/the-new-indian-express/20150121/281556584220318. Accessed 25 May 2020.
23. Tibetan in India dies days after setting himself on fire to protest China. *The New York Times*. https://www.nytimes.com/2016/03/05/world/asia/india-tibet-dorjee-tsering-immolation.html. Accessec 25 May 2020.
24. Garg K, Kumar CN, Chandra PS. Number of psychiatrists in India: Baby steps forward, but a long way to go. Indian J Psychiatry. 2019;61(1):4–5.
25. Vijaykumar L. Suicide and its prevention: The urgent need in India. Indian J Psychiatry. 2007;49(2):81–4.

26. 10 NGOs helping women to fight for their rights in India—GiveIndia's Blog. https://blog. giveindia.org/women/10-ngos-for-women-you-should-support-for-women-rights/. Accessed 25 May 2020.
27. The Commission of Sati Prevention Act and Rules. Ministry of Women & Child Development. *GoI*. https://wcd.nic.in/act/commission-sati-prevention-act-and-rules. Accessed 25 May 2020.
28. The Mental Healthcare Act. 2017. http://egazette.nic.in/WriteReadData/2017/175248.pdf.
29. Math SB, Basavaraju V, Harihara SN, Gowda GS, Manjunatha N, Kumar CN, et al. Mental Healthcare Act 2017—aspiration to action. Indian J Psychiatry. 2019;61(Suppl 4):S660–6.
30. Sanghavi P, Bhalla K, Das V. Fire-related deaths in India in 2001: a retrospective analysis of data. Lancet. 2009;373(9671):1282–8. https://doi.org/10.1016/S0140-6736(09)60235-X.

Self-Immolation in Indonesia and Papua

Rizky Aniza Winanda

1 Introduction

Indonesia is the world's fourth most populous nation with a diverse archipelago of more than 300 ethnic groups and an emerging lower middle-income economy. Despite being the largest economy in Southeast Asia, the vast number of islands and difficult geographic access impose challenges for equal development of remote areas. Even in 2020, there are large discrepancies in almost all sectors of development between the large cities and rural areas. With a population of more than 267 million, nearly 10% still live in poverty and close to 20% hover around the poverty line [1]. This disparity also applies to the health sector, specifically mental health care, where resources and practitioners are limited.

One of the 17,000 islands in Indonesia is Papua, the largest and easternmost island consisting of two provinces of the country's 34 provinces. Unlike the major parts of Indonesia, Papua did not become an official part of the nation until 1969. Formerly known as *Irian Jaya*, it was a Dutch colony until 1961 and then under Indonesian military occupation as well as the United Nations' (UN) temporary administration between 1962 and 1969 [2]. In 1969, the UN General Assembly acknowledged the Act of Free Choice, despite its many controversies, officially recognizing Papua as a part of Indonesia [3]. The complex nature of this island's history caused a large setback in its growth and development. After many years of military oppression, reformation and freedom movements that began in 1998 were met with mixed attitudes from separatist groups and those who wanted to follow in the capital government's development [4]. To this day, the region's search for

R. A. Winanda (✉)
World Psychiatric Association Psychotherapy Section, Geneva, Switzerland

Scholoo Keyen Regional Hospital, West Papua, Indonesia
e-mail: aniza.winanda@gmail.com

© The Author(s), under exclusive license to Springer Nature
Switzerland AG 2021
C. A. Alfonso et al. (eds.), *Suicide by Self-Immolation*,
https://doi.org/10.1007/978-3-030-62613-6_6

identity causes cultural disagreements, political disrupt, a rift between native Papuans and other ethnicities, and hinders progress and economic development [5, 6].

Much of Papua's unique and very different ways of living are considered primordial compared to the advanced city-life of major cities in Indonesia. Besides suffering from intense economic challenges, Papuans struggle with access to proper and equal education, nutrition, electricity, clean water, and advanced technology [7]. In many regions of Papua, many of its inhabitants still live in the forest with little to no clothes, hunting and farming to meet basic daily needs. In contrast, in other parts that began to implement a modern economy, the goal of financial gain has fused with ethnic traditions such as marriage and land grabs [8]. The notion of financial gain also plays a role in fostering gender inequality in Papuan culture [9]. Unlike the largely religion-driven population and marriages in most parts of Indonesia, Papuans follow a custom of financially driven marriage transactions where a man's family must be able to "afford" his wife. Furthermore, it is possible for a man to have many wives and a wife to have many husbands, depending on the woman's family's agreement to the sum of payment provided by the man's family. Apart from wealth, factors such as the ability to conceive, regardless of the child's welfare later on, also play a role in determining the woman's worth as an economic incentive for marriage [10]. It is this tradition that often causes dispute and difficulties in Papuan marriages, with many women becoming depressed within a matrix of oppressive circumstances leading to suicide. Even after suicide affects the family unit, a suicidal woman's family will still seek financial compensation for the woman's near-death or death [11].

Suicide is an increasing concern in Indonesia. Although the World Health Organization official suicide rate for Indonesia is 3.4/100,000 persons, mental health professionals recognize that limited access to care and stigma result in under-reporting of suicides. In their 2018 report, the Indonesian Health Administration stated that as many as 6.1% of Indonesians 15 years old and older experience depressive disorders, with more than 50% admitting to suicidal ideation or self-harm behavior. Suicide is a problem throughout the country affecting all ethnicities, economic groups and regions [12].

With the lowest Human Development Index (HDI) of all 34 Indonesian provinces (see Fig. 1), West Papua and Papua also have high suicide rates with many cases going unsolved and unreported. The difficulty obtaining accurate counts of suicide deaths in Indonesia in general and particularly in Papua is primarily due to the lack of a nationwide suicide death registry system. In addition, suicide is very much taboo in Indonesian as well as Papuan culture, thus leading to many families denying that fact that individuals attempt or die by suicide. The most common reported methods of suicide in Indonesia are hanging (60.9%), ingestion of poisonous agents (18.8%), and medication overdose (8.7%). The other 11.6% comprise various methods often under-reported such as drowning and self-burning [12].

Self-immolation in Indonesia frequently makes news headlines despite rare mention in scientific journals or being recognized in published studies. In the first 4 months of 2020, for example, there has been at least one case of self-immolation

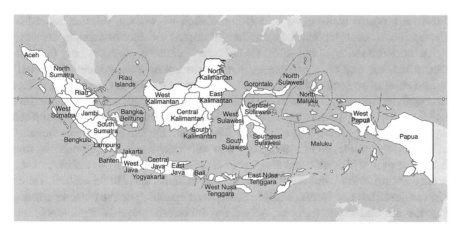

Fig. 1 Provinces of Indonesia

per month in various parts of the country reported in the news. Suicide by self-immolation continues to be a clinical and social problem in Indonesia yet it is clearly under-reported.

This chapter will provide an overview of culturally specific and psychosocial risk factors of self-immolation in Indonesia, focusing on provinces of Papua and West Papua where the author practices as a physician, and describe the challenges of providing adequate care to persons who self-immolate.

2 Under-Reporting of Self-Immolation in Indonesia

In Indonesia, many self-immolation reports trickle down to the popular media. Few cases have been of political protest, the most prominent one being a law student, Sondang Hutagalung, who in 2011, the year following the immolations that fueled the *Arab Spring* in Northern Africa, set himself ablaze in front of the national palace as a protest against corruption and the Indonesian government's neglect of human rights. Although political protest may be a causative factor in some self-immolations in Indonesia, most are due to other stressors. An examination of precipitating factors from media reports and my clinical experience having worked in different parts of the country leads me to conclude that over the last decade the majority of self-immolations occured as a result of depressive and stressor related disorders, financial distress, domestic violence and disenfranchisement of vulnerable individuals.

In Papua, despite the frequent protests that occur throughout the island, including in small and remote villages, there has yet been a single media reported case of self-immolation as part of a political protest. Protests happen almost on a monthly basis and end in road or access to buildings being closed for a certain period until demands are met or a monetary compensation settlement offered. Various media outlets have however reported many cases of self-immolation by women, whether related to depression, relationship/marriage conflicts, domestic violence or financial issues.

A literature search about self-immolation in Indonesia produces only one article, which reviews old Javanese texts and primary historic sources about self-immolation of women in Java and Bali. The article by Helen Creese [13] relates and analyzes historical accounts of suicide by women in Bali and pre-Islamic Java influenced by early settlers from Central Asia. Some of these are notably described by twelfth-century Javanese poets in the *Bharatayuddha* (Javanese *Mahabharata*). It is noted that noble women were known to self-immolate or ascend/descend into a funeral pyre whilst also stabbing themselves with a dagger (*keris/kris*/creese), somewhat differing from the practice of *Sati* in India and Hindu culture. Helen Creese describes two forms of self-immolation, depending on the person performing the act and or its purpose. *Satya,* the Indonesian equivalent of *Sati,* was regarded as an act of loyalty, a display of faithfulness to one's husband, historically recorded several times in scripts from the fifth century and temple reliefs as performed by noble women or wives of army men. The second form of suicide by self-immolation is *Bela,* a common Javanese term that means 'to lay down one's life for another person', whether by fire or not. However, *Bela* was also often used to describe acts of self-immolation performed by concubines, slaves, or other domestics [13].

Consider the following passage that relates a widow's suicide, translated from the fourteenth century epic poem *Sutasoma*:

> The flames of the fire lit up her face,
> as though urging her to follow in death.
> Her *kain* was of fine floral silk;
> Her black and oiled hair hung loose.
> She levelled her *kris* and thrust it into her breast.
> Her blood spurted up but rather than fetid it was fragrant.
> Then bathing her face in blood, steadfastly and bravely paying homage
> She leapt swiftly into the marvelous fire [13].

The practice of *Satya* in Indonesia, which was more common in Bali, was abolished in 1903. Today, self-immolation by women continues but not as an act of loyalty but rather as an act of desperation and escape from subjugation. Despite not being formally recorded, the practice of self-immolation in Papua is a common occurrence as the result of marital conflict. The kitchen of a traditional Papuan home is usually located in the back part of a house and serves not only as a place to cook but also as symbolic of alienation and of the inferior position of women within the family system and society at large. Many Papuan women carry out most of their daily activities and even sleep in the kitchen. After giving birth it is customary to shelter in place and keep the baby in the kitchen during the first month. One reason for this is that the kitchen is deemed to be the warmest and safest part of the house. However, this also becomes the place where a woman seeks refuge and revenge when marital problems arise [14]. As described in several media reports, self-immolations by Papuan women occur by lighting a fire in the kitchen.

In the past two decades, self-immolations in Indonesia as reported by the media usually occur within the home and as a result of intimate partner violence, poverty, depressive disorders or stressor related disorders. Deaths caused by self-immolation are stigmatized by families leading to failure to discuss or disclose details. Even in Papua where self-immolations are settled between families with financial gain after deaths, government or medical institutions are kept in the dark and uninvolved.

The under-reporting of self-immolations in Indonesia in general and Papua in particular make it difficult to adequately estimate the scale of the problem. The taboo of talking about one's death, especially if death is by suicide, inhibits the process of evaluating how the problem can be prevented.

3 Psychosocial Risk Factors of Self-Immolation in Indonesia

No studies exist that analyze the psychological profile of those who self-immolate in Indonesia and Papua. However, a study by Johnson and Sinha of women who self-immolate in the neighboring country of Papua New Guinea reports many similarities to the cases I have encountered in Papua and West Papua, Indonesia. Papua New Guinea shares the Indonesian island of Papua and have many similar cultural characteristics. In their article published in 1993, Johnson and Sinha report that women in Papua New Guinea self-immolate as a result of interpersonal problems, mainly marital disharmony. Only 10% of the reported cases had a psychiatric diagnosis, which is relatively low when compared to self-immolation patients from other parts of the world. Nevertheless, one ought to be cautious to accept this low percentage at face value as stressor-related disorders and sub-syndromal/sub-threshold posttraumatic stress disorders result in great incapacity and are often underdiagnosed unless structured psychiatric interviews are part of the research protocol [15].

Laloë conducted a study in Sri Lanka reporting that 47% of the patients experienced interpersonal problems, mainly in the form of marital discord, as factors enabling self-immolation. Women in particular frequently reported arguments with their husbands immediately prior to self-incineration [16]. Marital disharmony is a common precipitating factor for self-immolation amongst women in Asia, completely deviating from the practice of *Sati* in early Asian history [17]. Self-immolation is often sought as a way out by women experiencing marital problems including financial strife in a marriage [16]. While suicide in Asian history has a place as an expression of loyalty, "the depictions of a patriarchal social order that provide women with no alternatives but marriage or death" [13] may linger in the collective unconscious of disenfranchised women in regions were poverty, violence, gender bias and inequalities abound.

The socioeconomic burden of living in a lower middle-income country in Asia often causes problems in a marriage in which both parties are often required to work in order to meet daily needs. However, many Asian cultural groups still restrict women's roles to domestic duties such as child-rearing and tending to household errands while men work outside the home. Women who have a subordinate position to their husbands are at higher risk of depressive disorders and experiencing complex affective states of perceived burdensomeness and feelings of expendability [9, 14]. Many media outlets in Indonesia report the inability to pay off debt and living in poverty as reasons for a person to suicide. These difficult financial situations compounding marital disharmony may heighten risk of suicide by self-immolation [16].

4   Burn Units and Mental Health Services in Indonesia

Burn wounds are severe injuries due to damage or loss of tissue caused by contact with heat sources that potentially affect organ systems. Injuries to the skin, which serves as a barrier to withhold and protect internal bodily functions, can cause physical morbidity such as fluid loss, breathing difficulties, and require numerous invasive operations while also affecting one's appearance and body image, causing negative feelings [18, 19]. De Sousa and colleagues reported that nearly all burn patients in treatment experience a degree of anxiety, depression, a sense of helplessness, anger, guilt, low self-esteem, and lack of confidence [20].

Apart from negative feelings and associated psychological distress, burn injuries often cause nociceptive and neuropathic pain from the beginning of the injury, throughout treatment, and even for many months following recovery. These factors accumulate to increase stress levels and result in allostatic overload, especially if the injury follows suicide by self-immolation [21]. The management of burn injuries involves a multidisciplinary team consisting of nurses, surgeons, psychiatrists, dieticians, social workers, physiotherapists, occupational therapists, and others; who are able to provide a holistic and comprehensive treatment [20]. Despite many studies reporting the importance of integrated care for burn patients, very few hospitals in Indonesia have the resources to designate a specialized burn unit or center. Only several tertiary hospitals in Indonesia have a burn unit, and there are no designated burn centers in the whole island of Papua.

Several studies report that a high prevalence of burn injuries occur in developing countries such as Indonesia due to the high rates of poverty, low levels of education, and dense population [18]. However, these studies do not specify whether the burn injuries are accidents or acts of self-immolation. To date, there are no published reports that study the association between sociodemographic background and burn injury prevalence in Indonesia.

Not only is the country lacking burn units, but there are also limited human resources such as psychiatrists. As of January 2020, there are approximately 1100 psychiatrists in Indonesia with the majority choosing to practice in large cities. In the Papua province, there are currently eight psychiatrists serving a population of approximately 3.4 million, and two psychiatrists in the West Papua province serving a population of approximately 1.1 million. Adding to the socioeconomic burden is the difficulty to deliver proper care to patients with bun injuries because of a grave scarcity of mental health workers and lack of funding or insurance. In order to reach a larger scope, mental health care in Indonesia, particularly in remote provinces, relies on a public health-informed care delivery model. The lack of integrated care and psychiatric services allows for self-immolation in Papua to be overlooked as a serious matter.

5 Culture Specific Aspects of Self-Immolation in Papua

In Papua alone, there are more than 30 different ethnic groups rich with culture and laws that have withstood time and even modern development [7, 22]. Despite acknowledging the existence of state laws, their implementation and enforcement in Papua is extremely difficult. The same notion applies to traditional practices in marriages and settling disputes between tribes, with others, and within families [4, 7]. There is a vast literature describing traditional Papuan marriages, regional law enforcement practices, and the challenges of bringing Papua into modern practices and globalized standards of development [8].

In a review discussing criminal sanction and blood fines, Martha reports the practice of *otiv-bombari* of the Marind tribe in Papua, where a woman is to sexually serve the chief of the tribe and the husband's elders on the night of her wedding. The practice, besides affirming the diminished place of women within the marriage and society, is meant to provide "experience" in order to please the husband, as well as a mark that she is now "owned" by her husband and his family. Another study by Loppies reports the practice of *Sanepen* among the Biak tribe in which a woman is promised to a certain family and or man prior to the age of 15 years old. While modern age might see these arranged marriages and practices to be primitive and unjust, government officials, medical personnel, law enforcers, as well as religious leaders have been rather unsuccessful in changing or banning these traditions [8]. While the practice of *otiv-bombari* might be considered by outsiders as sexual assault, the tribe sees it as a rite of passage. While the practice of *Sanepen* might be perceived as a violation to human rights and a medical hazard, many see it as an ordinary way of life and guaranteeing a woman's safe future [11].

Despite these marital traditions still being carried out in modern times, many of these women do seek formal education and become informed of the choices they have. Even among the poorly educated, there is a prevailing struggle to become more independent and obtain a higher status in marriage [23, 24]. Women often attempt to do so by farming and selling their products at the local markets. Marriage between Papuan and non-Papuan ethnics are also often plagued with difficulties in aligning cultural differences causing marital disharmony. Extreme differences in communication skills, emotional expression, and expectations following marital unions cause marital disharmony in interracial and exogamous marriages. Differences of opinion and habits managing financial matters also play a role in marital dissatisfaction in interracial marriages in Papua [25, 26].

Gender inequality and power struggles met with financial difficulty many times leads to interpersonal problems that cause women to be unhappy within their marriages and host families. In traditional Papuan culture, divorce is extremely difficult to obtain due to its high cost and potential blood fine, especially when there are children and ownership of land is involved. The decision and discussion to divorce could last for years with many parties including extended family becoming involved in negotiations [14]. Due the complex nature of divorce and dispute settlements, women often seek an easier way to end the marriage, by suicide, and oftentimes by self-immolation.

The symbol of using fire in the kitchen was discussed earlier as to why women in Papua choose to self-immolate as a method for self-harm and or suicide. Women are often objectified in traditional Papuan marriages, which results in common reports of domestic violence with emotional and verbal abuse by husbands as well as in-laws. These women often feel powerless in unhappy and abusive marriages as they also struggle to have a sense of financial independence. When a Papuan woman's suffering ends in a tragic death, her family seeks compensation from her husband's family, sometimes in the form of land but more often in the form of money. The sum is usually large when the woman is known to have been successful in bearing a child. Until this "fine" is paid off, the woman will not be buried. Although self-immolation is very much prevalent in Papua, no study has addressed this serious matter that places monetary value on a person's life and incentivizes suicide deaths [22, 26–28].

6 Recommendations

Many Indonesian governmental and non-governmental organizations have taken steps to lower suicide rate but continue to have difficulty reaching those in remote areas due to an uneven distribution of mental health services and resources. Psychiatric and non-psychiatric organizations have been focusing on increasing suicide awareness, providing suicide helplines and access to mental health care as first-line suicide prevention strategies in Indonesia.

Despite these efforts, services remain limited and prevalence of suicide inadequately recorded. Notwithstanding schools and offices being equipped with capacity-building modules and some form of psychological support, very few people choose to seek mental health help formally or informally. For Indonesia and Papua, there continues to be difficulty in overcoming cultural barriers because of the stigma associated with seeking psychological care. This, along with limited availability of mental health care resources, makes it difficult to prevent suicide both in large cities and remote areas.

Women-protection organizations and programs also exist to empower women, providing psychological aid through peer support. Promoting fair access to education and the importance of financial independence also helps to promote gender equality so that women can strive towards equal status and rights in a marriage and society. Educating the public to increase awareness must also be met in increasing mental health care availability. If telemedicine continues to have difficulty accessing certain vulnerable populations, other methods such as training cadres in the community can be implemented in order to lower the prevalence of suicide by self-immolation [28, 29].

Due to the lack of data on suicide prevalence in general and suicide by self-immolation in particular, it is recommended that Indonesia forms a suicide registry to assess and analyze the scope of the problem and create a proper comprehensive guideline for suicide prevention. Once a national guideline is agreed upon, cultural adjustments can be made tailored to the specific issues in various ethnic groups [29]. It is also important to involve tribe leaders and prominent members of a society to carry out the message of preventing suicide and self-immolation.

7 Conclusions

Suicide by self-immolation in Indonesia and Papua is prevalent despite under-reporting and never being accurately assessed. Since the historical accounts of *Sati/Satya* dating back to the fifth century in Java and Bali, self-immolation among Indonesians continue to make headlines to this day, but never gaining serious attention from sociologists, anthropologists, or mental health researchers, failing to devise and implement prevention strategies. The determinants of self-immolation in Indonesia and Papua today greatly differ from those of *sati/satya*, with a reversal of suicide as a way to express loyalty and idealize marriage to that of escaping poverty, marginalization, violence and marital conflict. Additionally, women in Papua may self-immolate in order to exit abusive marriages in lieu of divorce and to obtain monetary gain from death for the surviving families. The challenges of living in a lower middle-income country also motivates self-immolation in Indonesia. Access to mental health care and burn units in Indonesia and Papua is extremely limited. Many suicides by self-immolation go unreported and unsolved. In order to prevent self-immolation suicides from becoming a greater problem, political leaders and health care officials need to recognize it as public health concern and take steps to prevent it. Culturally specific approaches need to be considered when devising prevention strategies. This may prove to be difficult for a culturally diverse country such as Indonesia, but it is however essential if self-immolation prevention strategies are to succeed.

References

1. Indonesian Bureau of Statistics: poverty rates. 2019. https://www.bps.go.id/pressrelease/2019/07/15/1629/persentase-penduduk-miskin-maret-2019-sebesar-9-41-persen.html.
2. Aditjindro GJ. Cahaya bintang kejora: Papua Barat dalam kajian sejarah, budaya, ekonomi, dan hak asasi manusia. Jakarta: Elsam; 2000.
3. Drooglever P. An act of free choice. Decolonization and the right to self-determination in West Papua. Oxford: One World; 2009.
4. King P. West Papua & Indonesia since Suharto: independence, autonomy, or chaos. Randwick: UNSW Press; 2004.
5. Widjojo M, et al. Papua road map: negotiating the past, improving the present, and securing the future. Jakarta: Buku Obor, LIPI dan TIFA; 2009.
6. Widjojo SM. Nationalist and separatist discourses in cyclical violence in Papua. Asian Journal of Social Sciences. 2006;34(3):410–30.
7. Slama M, Munro J. From 'stone-age' to 'real-time': exploring Papuan temporalities, mobilities, and religiosities. Canberra: ANU Press; 2015.
8. Doirebo ED, Giay B, Yoman SS. Theological declaration of churches in Papua regarding failure of the Indonesian government in governing and developing the indigenous peoples of Papua. 2011. http://www.humanrights.asia/news/forwarded-news/AHRC-FST-014-2011.
9. Rahma AA. Resistensi terhadap ketidakadilan gender di Papua melalui fokalisator dalam novel Tanah Tabu karya Aninda S. Thayf. Tesis Universitas Airlangga. 2011.
10. Kogoya S. Proses pelaksanaan perkawinan hukum adat suku Dani di Distrik Gupura Kabupaten Lanny Jaya Papua ditinjau dari undang-undang nomor 1 tahun 1974. Lex Privatum. 2018;6:28–36.
11. Martha AE. Denda adat dalam penjatuhan pidana (studi kasus kejahatan kekerasan di pengadilan negeri Merauke-Papua). Jurnal Hukum: Ius Quia Iustum, Law Journal of Islamic University of Indonesia; 2004; Number 26 Volume 11: 94–104.
12. Laporan Riset Kesehatan Dasar. Badan Penelitian dan Pengembangan Kesehatan, Kementerian Kesehatan Republik Indonesia. Jakarta: Kementerian Kesehatan Republik Indonesia; 2018. p. 2018.
13. Creese H. Ultimate loyalties: the self-immolation of women in Java and Bali. Bijdragen tot de Taal-, Land- en Volkenkunde Old Javanese Texts and Culture. 2001;157(1):131–66.
14. You Y, et al. Relasi gender patriarki dan dampaknya terhadap perempuan Hubula Suku Dani, Kabupaten Jayawijaya, Papua. Sosiohumaniora-J Ilmu-ilmu Sosial dan Humaniora. 2019;21(1):65–77.
15. Johnson FY, Sinha SN. Deliberate self-harm by means of kerosene fire by women in Papua New Guinea. PNG Med J. 1993;36:16–2.
16. Laloë V, Ganesan M. Self-immolation: a common suicidal behaviour in eastern Sri Lanka. Burns. 2002;28:475–80.
17. Laloë V. Patterns of deliberate self-burning in various parts of the world: a review. Burns. 2004;30(3):207–15.
18. Pujisriyani WA, et al. J Plast Rekonstr. 2012;1
19. Martina NR, Wardhana A. Mortality analysis of adult burn patients. J Plast Rekonstr. 2013;2:497–524.
20. De Sousa A, Sonavane S, Kurvey A. Psychological issues in adult burn patients. Delhi Psychiatr J. 2013;16:24–33.
21. Ahmadi A. Suicide by self-immolation: comprehensive interview, experiences, and suggestions. J Burn Care Res. 2007;28(1):30–41.
22. Deda AJ, Mofu SS. Masyarakat hukum adat dan hak ulayat di provinsi Papua Barat sebagai orang asli Papua ditinjau dari sisi adat dan budaya: sebuah kajian etnografi kekinian. J Administ Publ. 2014;11(2):11–21.
23. Devi A. Sejarah tata cara pernikahan masyarakat Dani Distrik Gupura Kabupaten Lanny Jaya. Universitas Negeri Semarang. 2012;1:1.

24. Nurrokhmah LE. Perbandingan hukum perkawinan berdasarkan hukum adat Biak dan undang-undang nomor 1 tahun 1974. Gema Kampus IISIP YAPIS Biak. 2016;11(2):71–80.
25. Rumbesu FDD. Tradisi perkawinan suku Maniun di desa Anjai distrik Kebar kabupaten Manokwari provinsi Papua Barat. Thesis, Universitas Halu Oleo. 2019.
26. Salabai Y, Nugroho H. Persepsi dan respon orang tua Arfak terhadap pergeseran nilai perkawinan adat suku besar Arfak di Kelurahan Manokwari Barat, Kabupaten Manokwari, Papua Barat. 2010.
27. Utami PN. Optimalisasi pemenuhan hak korban kekerasan terhadap perempuan melalui pusat pelayanan terpadu. J HAM (Hak Asasi Manusia). 2016;7(1):55–67.
28. Latu S. Budaya suku Dani dalam mengimplementasikan program keluarga berencana di kabupaten Jayawijaya provinsi Papua (studi kasus). J Keperawat Tropis Papua. 2018;1(2):58–64.
29. Ahmadi A, Ytterstad B. Prevention of self-immolation by community-based intervention. Burns. 2007;33:1032–40.

Self-Immolation in Sub-Saharan Africa

Matiko Mwita, Olanrewaju Ibigbami, and Anesh Sukhai

1 Introduction

Sub-Saharan Africa is a culturally diverse continental region located south of the Sahara Desert (see Fig. 1), consisting of 48 countries (see Table 1) with a total population of approximately 1.1 billion. Although the United Nations, World Bank and International Monetary Fund listings of countries in this region do not perfectly align, we will refer to Sub-Saharan Africa as all of Africa, including its island nations, except for the North Africa Arab League countries. Chapter 9 in this book addresses the epidemic of self-immolation in North Africa separately.

Suicide by self-immolation is prevalent in developing countries worldwide, accounting for as many as 40–60% of all suicides in some regions [1], primarily affecting women in low-and-middle-income countries, and of clinical and public health relevance in Asia, Africa, and immigrant populations globally [2].

Self-immolation attracts scientific and popular interest, with vast international media coverage and an accumulating literature identifying several transcultural, demographic, psychiatric, and socioeconomic factors that apparently contribute to

M. Mwita (✉)
Department of Psychiatry and Mental Health, Catholic University of Health and Allied Science, Mwanza, Tanzania

Bugando Medical Centre, Mwanza, Tanzania
e-mail: wambula2016@gmail.com

O. Ibigbami
Department of Mental Health, Obafemi Awolowo University, Ile-Ife, Nigeria

Wesley Guild Hospital, OAUTHC, Ilesha, Nigeria
e-mail: oibigbami@oauife.edu.ng

A. Sukhai
Research and Policy Analyst, Cape Town, South Africa
e-mail: anesh.sukhai@gmail.com

© The Author(s), under exclusive license to Springer Nature
Switzerland AG 2021
C. A. Alfonso et al. (eds.), *Suicide by Self-Immolation*,
https://doi.org/10.1007/978-3-030-62613-6_7

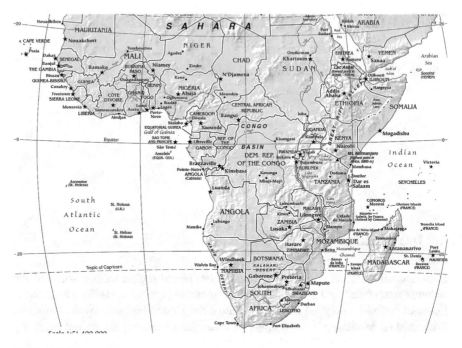

Fig. 1 Sub-Saharan Africa

suicide risk [3, 4]. Despite the fact that self-immolation is considered a major public
health concern and there is a large growing body of research devoted to it, the scarcity of scientific literature on self-immolations in the low- and middle-income countries of Sub-Saharan Africa is problematic. This chapter will review the few scientific
studies that exist and provide clinical guidance.

Both cultural and psychiatric factors are associated with self-immolation [5] and
the behavior is sometimes considered to have religious overtones [6]. In south Asian
cultures self-immolation is a traditional or cultural form of suicide, as in the practice
of *Sati* by Hindu widows who burn themselves in the funeral pyres of their husbands
[7]. Self-immolations in the Tibetan diaspora and those triggering the *Arab Spring*
are politically and altruistically motivated, and often prompted by human rights
violations and accumulating psychosocial distress. Psychosocial and psychiatric
factors identified as predictive of self-immolations in other regions of the world
include poverty, lower level of education, female gender, married status, crowded
home environments, intimate partner abuse and other violence in the household,
posttraumatic and stressor related disorders, harmful use of substances and major
depression [8]. These factors may also play a role in self-immolations in Sub-
Saharan Africa. This chapter will review the epidemiology and transcultural aspects
of self-immolation in Sub-Saharan Africa, identify and provide an overview of common predisposing and protective factors, and propose culturally informed strategies
that might be relevant for the design and implementation of suicide prevention
programs.

Table 1 Countries in Sub-Saharan Africa—Demographic, Social, Health and Economic Indicators[a]

Country	Population (million)	Life expectancy (years)	Secondary school enrollment (%)	GNI per capita	HIV prevalence (ages 15–49) (%)
Angola	31	59.9	50.7	$3370	2.0
Benin	11.5	61.2	59.0	$870	1.0
Botswana	2.3	68.8	80.4	$7750	20.3
Burkina Faso	19.8	60.8	40.7	$670	0.7
Burundi	11.2	60.9	48.5	$280	1.0
Cabo Verde	0.5	72.6	88.2	$3420	0.6
Cameroon	25.2	58.5	60.1	$1440	3.6
Central African Republic	4.7	52.2	17.1	$490	3.6
Chad	1.5	53.7	22.6	$670	1.3
Comoros	0.8	63.9	59.5	$1380	0.1
Congo, Dem. Rep.	84.1	60.0	46.2	$490	0.8
Congo, Rep.	5.2	64.0	52.6	$1640	2.6
Cote D'Ivoire	25.1	57.0	51.0	$1600	2.6
Equatorial Guinea	1.3	58.1	23.5	$6840	7.1
Eritrea	3.2	65.5	47.7	$720	0.7
Eswatini	1.1	58.3	82.4	$3930	27.3
Ethiopia	109.2	65.9	34.9	$790	1.0
Gabon	2.1	65.8	53.1	$6830	3.8
Gambia	2.3	61.4	50.1	$710	1.9
Ghana	29.8	63.5	64.6	$2130	1.7
Guinea	12.4	60.7	39.3	$850	1.4
Guinea-Bissau	1.9	57.7	34.2	$750	3.5
Kenya	51.4	65.9	56.8	$1620	4.7
Lesotho	2.1	52.9	62.0	$1390	23.6
Liberia	4.8	63.3	37.9	$610	0.3
Madagascar	26.3	66.3	36.5	$510	0.3
Malawi	18.1	63.3	40.3	$360	9.2
Mali	19.1	58.5	41.0	$840	1.4
Mauritania	4.4	64.5	36.8	$1160	0.2
Mauritius	1.3	74.5	95.1	$12,050	1.3
Mozambique	29.5	59.3	35.4	$460	12.6
Namibia	2.5	63.0	65.8	$5220	11.8
Niger	22.4	61.6	24.3	$390	0.3
Nigeria	196	54.0	42.0	$1960	1.5
Rwanda	12.3	68.3	40.9	$780	2.5
Sao Tome and Principe	0.21	69.9	89.3	$1890	N/A

(continued)

Table 1   (continued)

Country	Population (million)	Life expectancy (years)	Secondary school enrollment (%)	GNI per capita	HIV prevalence (ages 15–49) (%)
Senegal	15.9	67.4	43.7	$1410	0.4
Seychelles	0.1	74.3	81.4	$15,600	N/A
Sierra Leone	7.6	53.9	41.8	$490	0.5
Somalia	15	56.7	5.9	N/A	0.1
South Africa	57.8	63.5	100	$5750	20.4
South Sudan	11	57.4	11.0	$1130	2.5
Sudan	41.8	64.9	46.6	$1560	0.2
Tanzania	56.3	64.5	29.4	$1020	4.6
Togo	7.9	60.5	61.8	$660	2.3
Uganda	42.7	62.5	24.6	$6205	5.7
Zambia	17.4	63.0	N/A	$1430	12.3
Zimbabwe	14.4	60.8	52.4	$1790	12.7
Total/averages	1.1 Billion	60.9	43.4	$1517	4

[a]Data from the World Bank: https://databank.worldbank.org/source/world-development-indicators (accessed 8 April 2020)

2   Epidemiology

2.1   Extent of Self-Immolation in Sub-Saharan Africa

Based on published literature, self-immolation appears to be a relatively uncommon method for suicide in Sub-Saharan Africa except in certain regions or countries. Over the past 25 years, only six studies exist that include some reporting on cases of self-immolation, of which three reported further on the epidemiology of these cases. Four of the studies analyzed data from Durban [9, 10] and Pretoria [11, 12] in *South Africa*, while the remaining two gathered data from the cities of Harare in *Zimbabwe* [13] and Sokoto in *Nigeria* [14]. The studies in Harare and Sokoto reported on data from burn units, while the remaining studies focused on data from post-mortem investigations. For the studies based on post-mortem investigations, data were included from all mortuaries in the respective cities – three in Durban and one in Pretoria. Based on relatively more representative mortuary-based data (versus burn-unit data that is limited to non-fatal cases at admission), the largest proportion of suicide cases due to self-immolation was found in the city of Durban, accounting for 69 (9.9%) of all 696 suicides over a 5-year period from 1996–2000 [10]. While the proportion was similar across the 5 years, a further study for the city showed much lower proportions in later years of 2% (of 465 total suicides in 2006) and 1% (of 497 total suicides in 2007 [9]. For the city of Pretoria, similar proportions of 2.9% (of 1018 suicide cases over a 4-year period from 1997–2000) [12] and 2.4% (of 957 suicides over a 4-year period from 2007–2010) [11] were a result of self-immolation.

Based on reviews across various parts of the world, self-immolation is a relatively uncommon method of suicide in high-income countries of Europe and the United States, accounting for approximately 1% of all suicides, including many from immigrant populations [1, 4]. Based on burn unit data and like for earlier years in Durban, self-immolation accounted for roughly one-tenth (11%) of all attempted suicide admissions at the Harare burn unit in 1998. Additionally, of 47 patients admitted for self-inflicted burns over a 4-year period from 1995–1998, 32 (68%) were fatal [13].

2.2 Demographics of Self-Immolators in Sub-Saharan Africa

A salient feature of the epidemiology of self-immolation is the preponderance of women and persons with socio-economic disadvantage. Women account for approximately three-quarter (76.8%) and nearly two-thirds (63.3%) of self-immolation cases in the cities of Durban and Pretoria, respectively [13]. In addition, women are significantly more likely than men to use self-immolation as a method of suicide. In Pretoria, self-immolation accounted for nearly one tenth (8.4%) of all suicides in women compared to 1.4% of suicides in men [12]. Similarly, in Harare, self-immolation accounted for 14.3% of suicides in women versus 5.5% of suicides in men [13].

In Sokoto, the women to men ratio of self-immolators over a 5-year period was 6:1 [14]. Individuals from historically disadvantaged Black and Indian population groups account for the vast majority of self-immolation cases in Durban (81.2% and 17.4%, respectively). In Pretoria, roughly one-third of all suicides among Black women (16 of 47 cases) were a result of self-immolation.

The predominance of women who self-immolate in these sub-Saharan settings is consistent with that reported in many other less developed countries [1, 3, 4, 15]. The association between socio-economic disadvantage and self-immolation has also been reported in several other international settings [1, 15, 16].

3 Risk Factors for Self-Immolation in Sub-Saharan Africa

The literature on self-immolation points to a range of risk factors for self-immolation that may be considered under the following three broad categories:

1. Enabling situational factors such as social vulnerability, cultural context and availability of the means to undertake the act of self-immolation.
2. Precipitating factors such as marital conflict or political protests.
3. Individual-level predisposing factors such as psychiatric illnesses, harmful use of substances, and possibly HIV infection.

Given the extreme nature of the act of self-immolation and distinctiveness from other modes of suicide, however, it is also likely that these acts arise from a combination and interacting effect of the above factors.

3.1   Enabling Factors

In the study in Durban, all suicides occurred inside a house [10], which is distinctively different to cases in other countries where self-immolations tend to occur in public areas as an expression of public protest or political dissent. The choice of a private home setting may relate to social isolation and affective states of shame and perceived burdensomeness, as well as the person's clear intention to end life and be unlikely to be helped by others [4, 16].

The predominance of private homes as the setting for self-immolation events, along with suicidal persons generally being young women from historically disadvantaged population groups, may be indicative of living situations underpinned by *social vulnerability*. For example, low levels of education and literacy and economic disempowerment have been shown to be strongly linked to self-immolation [1, 14–16].

Social vulnerability is especially an important consideration among young married women in some cultural contexts where economic disempowerment, with women being highly dependent on their spouses or in-laws [16], is more of the driving force for suicide than experiences of absolute poverty. This experience of dependency may also be coupled with familial pressures of having a successful marriage [16], which may also relate to cultural beliefs and expectations associated with the black and Indian suicides of women in the study from Durban [10].

Easy *access to flammable liquids* is a strong correlate to acts of self-immolation [1, 3, 17]. Of note is that 83% and 98% of victims used paraffin to set themselves on fire in Durban [10] and Harare [13], respectively. Paraffin is generally used in low-income settings as a fuel for cooking and heating and is also cheaper than petrol and other variants.

3.2   Predisposing Factors

In the Harare study [13] that included findings on psychiatric history, only three cases (6.4%) had a documented psychiatric illness and all of these were diagnosed to have schizophrenia. Psychiatric conditions among persons who self-immolate that are prevalent in high-income countries include affective and psychotic disorders, major depressive disorders, psychoses, and substance use disorders [4, 15]. Adjustment disorders and posttraumatic stress disorders are frequently underdiagnosed and may be of relevance in persons who self-immolate worldwide [18, 19].

A potential predisposing factor that merits further study is the relationship between HIV infection and suicide [20], a known independent risk factor for suicide worldwide, and how this could interphase with self-immolation in Sub-Saharan African countries with high prevalence of HIV multimorbidities. There is no literature on self-immolation in HIV, but there is some literature establishing an association with fire setting, either accidental fire setting or triggered by behavioural disinhibition, in persons with HIV dementia [21–23].

3.3 Precipitating Factors

The experience of social vulnerability may also be underpinned by marital and family conflict [1, 3, 15, 16] along with associated domestic violence that would serve as a powerful precipitant to the act of self-immolation, especially among those who face other predisposing and enabling factors as discussed above. For example, from the study in Harare [13], conflict in marital, family and love relationships including problems with in-laws accounted for the majority (60%) of all circumstances leading to the self-immolation event.

The association between negative affective states and suicide (see Chap. 11) may be transdiagnostic and merits close attention. Affective states that correlate with suicide include hopelessness, anxiety, anger, perceived burdensomeness, thwarted belongingness, guilt, shame, and loneliness.

4 Transcultural Aspects of Self-Immolation in Sub-Saharan Africa

Study results of predisposing and protective factors of suicide are variable across different cultures [24]. These differences in diverse populations may also determine the various methods of suicide chosen by suicidal persons across cultures [25]. While psychosocial, economic and health related factors generally determine suicide risk, the method of suicide is usually related to access to means [26] but could also be triggered by contagion and culturally endorsed attitudes.

Self-immolation as a means of suicide has cultural and social undercurrents [1]. For instance, African-Americans and Asian-Americans living in the United States of America are more likely to choose self-immolation as a method of suicide [27]. Some studies show that suicide risk among immigrants matches that of the host country after acculturation and assimilation takes place [28–30]. Immigrants may also be at higher risk soon after arrival in their host country if faced with disappointment, loneliness, nostalgia and traumatic experiences during relocation. In addition, suicide rates of disenfranchised ethnic minorities or social groups could be elevated as a result of xenophobia and socioeconomic deprivation. Clarke and

Lester [31] propose a psychodynamic formulation of self-immolation that heavily weighs in the symbolic aspects of suicide by burning. The intensely dramatic nature of self-immolation is an impressionable means of registering protest or expressing individual personal distress or displeasure with prevailing authority [32]. Persons who experienced some form of governmental or social injustice and unsuccessfully attempted to seek rectification may choose self-immolation in an effort to release psychic tension and distress [33]. Many of the self-immolations that triggered the *Arab Spring* were not politically motivated *per se*. Dissatisfied individuals, repeatedly bullied and tormented by authorities or corrupt bureaucracies, reached their threshold of distress opting to publicly self-immolate as a fiery and rageful act of revenge and protest. The spectacle of these self-immolations ignited the collective psyche fueling revolt and manifestations that led to social and political transitions (see Chap. 9 for a description of the index self-immolations in Tunisia that spread throughout North Africa and beyond during the *Arab Spring*) [34]. Another social dynamic of self-immolation relates to self-sacrifice and altruism, although perhaps this is not a relevant psychosocial factor in suicides in Sub-Saharan Africa.

Losing touch with reality and collective states of dissociation [35] characterize isolated instances of mass immolations. In the year 2000 a mass self-immolation took place in Uganda, in a border town near Congo and Rwanda, when a cult-like sect that emphasized apocalypticism, called the Movement for the Restoration of the Ten Commandments of God and led by Joseph Kibweteere, predicted the end of times and set themselves on fire inside a church, killing up to 800 people in the largest mass suicide of this century [36, 37]. Sociocultural forces that preceded this deadly event include the political instability of the region, overthrow of Idi Amin, civil war, genocide against the Tutsi, and the AIDS pandemic, together with the rise of post-Catholic fundamentalist groups that broke away with the Roman Catholic Church.

Necklacing is of historical importance in South Africa and may persist in the collective psyche of its population, perhaps as a unique cultural factor that may encourage suicide by burning. A fate reserved for traitors by anti-apartheid activists, *necklacing* consisted of placing a rubber motor vehicle tire around a person's neck and arms, filled or doused with gasoline, and set on fire in a public execution for others to watch the person burn in agony as the tire melted and helped incinerate the body. Death by fire via *necklacing* was a powerful weapon against collaborators of the apartheid regime in the 1980s. Recent reports document that it is still practiced against common criminals as a form of punishment, mob justice and vigilantism [38].

The prevalence of self-immolation in some developing countries still surpasses that of the developed countries [3, 4, 10]. It is quite apt to assume that the prevalence of self-immolation in Sub-Saharan Africa might be underestimated due to under-reporting [39]. A major proportion of documented cases are from either postmortem or hospital based reviews [40]. Many cases of self-immolation that resulted in deaths may not have presented at the hospitals or recorded as such. Another reason for under reporting in sub-Saharan Africa is the criminalization of suicidal behavior.

Proponents of decriminalization of suicide argue that majority of persons who attempt suicide have an underlining mental illness [41]. Negative attitudes towards suicide add to the stigma of mental disorders, alienation and criminalization of the mentally ill [42].

5 Suicide Prevention in Sub-Saharan Africa

To prevent self-immolation requires a multifaceted approach including education, clinical services, legal enforcement and advocacy. Cultural standardized assessment tools are needed to screen for risk of suicide and psychiatric disorders [15]. A clinical approach to suicide prevention should consider the role of cultural differences, age and gender, imitation and intent, religion and spirituality [3].

Researchers have proposed several strategies for suicide prevention, including the training of general practitioners and community leaders in the recognition, identification and treatment of at-risk individuals such as those with mental disorders, and awareness campaigns to enhance public education help-seeking behavior. The training of gatekeepers and community facilitators in recognizing suicidality and helping at-risk people to access appropriate services is essential. Improvement of healthcare services is needed targeting people at risk, including organizational measures such as making adequate inpatient and outpatient aftercare available to people discharged from burn units or with family history of self-immolation. The training of journalists in responsible reporting of self-immolation or the imposing of media blackouts with internet and hotline support could help mitigate suicide by contagion [43–45].

Suicide prevention requires learning to elicit a thorough suicide history. The only treatment for suicide is prevention. Prevention involves reduction of psychological distress and that we establish important trusting relationships, restore hope and help individuals find meaning in life. Timely application of psychotherapeutic, psychosocial and pharmacological interventions can prevent death by suicide [20]. In the absence of trained mental health professionals, general practitioners and all healthcare workers, as well as community role models, need to take the lead to help identify persons at risk for suicide and create a safety network to protect them during a time of crisis.

6 Conclusion

Suicide by self-immolation in Sub-Saharan Africa is of concern in certain areas, as documented by studies in Zimbabwe, South Africa and Nigeria, and anecdotally or from clinical experience in other countries. Biopsychosocial correlates of self-immolation include poverty, low education, intimate partner violence, family and romantic turmoil, marital discord, HIV infection, mood disorders, psychosis, posttraumatic and stressor related disorders, and harmful use of substances. All of these are considered risk factors for suicide in other parts of the world as well. Self-immolation suicides in Sub-Saharan Africa, unlike in North Africa and some regions in Asia, are generally apolitical and not associated with self-sacrifice to protest societal injustices. A transcultural understanding of the enabling, predisposing and precipitating determinants of self-immolation may help inform suicide prevention strategies in developing countries in the continent of Africa.

References

1. Ahmadi A. Suicide by self-immolation: comprehensive overview, experiences and suggestions. J Burn Care Res. 2007;28(1):30–41.
2. Rastegar AL, Alaghehbandan R. Epidemiological study of self-inflicted burns in Tehran, Iran. J Burn Care Rehabilit. 2003;24(1):15–20.
3. Laloë V. Patterns of deliberate self-burning in various parts of the world: a review. Burns. 2004;30(3):207–15.
4. Poeschla B, et al. Self-immolation: socioeconomic, cultural and psychiatric patterns. Burns. 2011;37(6):1049–57.
5. Zarghami M, Khalilian A. Deliberate self-burning in Mazandaran, Iran. Burns. 2002;28(2):115–9.
6. Grossoehme D, Springer L. Images of God used by self-injurious burn patients. Burns. 1999;25(5):443–8.
7. Headley LA. Suicide in Asia and the near East. Oakland: Univ of California Press; 1983.
8. Rezaie L, et al. Is self-immolation a distinct method for suicide? A comparison of Iranian patients attempting suicide by self-immolation and by poisoning. Burns. 2011;37(1):159–63.
9. Naidoo SS, Schlebusch L. Sociodemographic characteristics of persons committing suicide in Durban, South Africa: 2006–2007. Afr J Prim Health Care Family Med. 2014;6(1):1–7.
10. Sukhai A, et al. Suicide by self-immolation in Durban, South Africa: a five-year retrospective review. Am J Forensic Med Pathol. 2002;23(3):295–8.
11. Engelbrecht C, et al. Suicide in Pretoria: a retrospective review, 2007–2010. South Afr Med J. 2017;107(8):715–8.
12. Scribante L, et al. A retrospective review of 1018 suicide cases from the capital city of South Africa for the period 1997–2000. Am J Forensic Med Pathol. 2004;25(1):52–5.
13. Mzezewa S, et al. A prospective study of suicidal burns admitted to the Harare burns unit. Burns. 2000;26(5):460–4.
14. Legbo JN, Ntia IO, Opara WE, Obembe A. Severe burn trauma from deliberate self-harm: the Sokoto experience. Nigerian Postgrad Med J. 2008;15(3):164–7.
15. Peck MD. Epidemiology of burns throughout the World. Part II: intentional burns in adults. Burns. 2012;38(5):630–7.
16. van de Put W. Addressing mental health in Afghanistan. Lancet. 2002;360(Suppl):s41–2.
17. Woeser T. Tibet on fire: self-immolations against chinese rule. London: Verso; 2016.
18. Sarah L, Prat S. Variation in the incidence of self-immolation according to culture and income level: a literature review. J Forensic Sci Criminol. 2017;5(2):203.
19. Rezaie L, et al. Why self-immolation? A qualitative exploration of the motives for attempting suicide by self-immolation. Burns. 2014;40(2):319–27.
20. Alfonso CA, Stern-Rodríguez E, Cohen MA. Suicide and HIV. In: Cohen MA, Gorman JM, Jacobson JM, Volberding P, Letendre SL, editors. Comprehensive textbook of AIDS psychiatry. New York: Oxford University Press; 2017.

21. Castellani G, Beghini D, Barisoni D, Margio M. Suicide attempted by burning: 1 10-year study of self-immolation deaths. Burns. 1995;21(8):607–9.
22. Cohen MA, Aladjem AD, Brenin D, Ghazi M. Firesetting by patinets with the acquired immunodeficiency syndrome. Ann Intern Med. 1990;112:386–7.
23. Alfonso CA, Cohen MA. HIV dementia and suicide. Gen Hosp Psychiatry. 1994;16:45–6.
24. Colucci E. The cultural facet of suicidal behaviour: its importance and neglect. Australian e-J Adv Mental Health. 2006;5(3):234–46.
25. Akinade EA. Cross-cultural differences in suicidal ideation between children in Nigeria and Botswana. Int Perspect Child Adolesc Mental Health. 2002;2:481–99.
26. Bilsen J. Suicide and youth: risk factors. Front Psychiatry. 2018;9:540.
27. Lester D. Suicide as a staged performance. Comprehens Psychol. 2015;4:12–8.
28. Malenfant EC. Suicide in Canada's immigrant population. Health Rep. 2004;5:9117.
29. Pavlovic E, Marusic A. Suicide in Croatia and in Croatian immigrant groups in Australia and Slovenia. Croat Med J. 2001;42(6):669–72.
30. Pérez-Rodríguez MM, Baca-García E, Oquendo MA, Wang S, Wall MM, Liu SM, Blanco C. Relationship between acculturation, discrimination and suicidal ideation and attempts against US Hispanics in the National Epidemiological Survey of Alcohol and Related Conditions. J Cin Psychiatry. 2014;75(4):399–407.
31. Clarke RV, Lester D. Suicide: closing the exits. Piscataway: Transaction Publishers; 2013.
32. Romm S, Combs H, Klein MB. Self-immolation: cause and culture. J Burn Care Res. 2008;29(6):988–93.
33. Lévy BT, et al. From querulous to suicidal: self-immolation in public places as a symbolic response to the feeling of injustice. Front Psychol. 2017;8:1901.
34. Morovatdar N, Moradi-Lakeh M, Malakouti SK, Nojomi M. Most common methods of suicide in Eastern Mediterranean Region of WHO: a systematic review and meta-analysis. Arch Suicid Res. 2013;17:335–44.
35. Beck AT, et al. Classification of suicidal behaviors: II. Dimensions of suicidal intent. Arch Gen Psychiatry. 1976;33(7):835–7.
36. BBC News. *Quiet cult's doomsday deaths*. 29 March 2000. http://news.bbc.co.uk/2/hi/africa/683813.stm. Accessed 12 Apr 2020.
37. The New York Times. *Uganda's cult mystique finally turned deadly*. https://www.nytimes.com/2000/04/02/world/uganda-cult-s-mystique-finally-turned-deadly.html. Accessed 12 Apr 2020.
38. BBC News. *Is necklacing returning to South Africa?* https://www.bbc.com/news/world-africa-14914526. Accessed 12 Apr 2020.
39. Mars B, et al. Suicidal behaviour across the African continent: a review of the literature. BMC Public Health. 2014;14:606.
40. Oladele AO, Olabanji JK. Burns in Nigeria: a review. Ann Burns Fire Disast. 2010;23(3):120–7.
41. Adinkrah MJA. Anti-suicide laws in nine African countries: criminalization, prosecution and penalization. Afr J Criminol Just Stud. 2016;9:1.
42. Lester D, Akande A. Attitudes about suicide among the Yoruba of Nigeria. J Soc Psychol. 1994;134(6):851–3.
43. Mann JJ, et al. Suicide prevention strategies: a systematic review. JAMA. 2005;294(16):2064–74.
44. Van der Feltz-Cornelis CM, et al. Best practice elements of multilevel suicide prevention strategies: a review of systematic reviews. Crisis. 2011;32(6):319–33.
45. Zalsman G, et al. Suicide prevention strategies revisited: 10-year systematic review. Lancet Psychiatry. 2016;3(7):646–59.

Self-Immolation in the Tibet Autonomous Region and Tibetan Diaspora

Warut Aunjitsakul ⑩, Poom Chompoosri, and Asher D. Aladjem

"I am giving away my body as an offering of light to chase away the darkness, to free all beings form suffering and to lead them to the paradise of the Buddha of Infinite Light. My offering of light is for all living beings ... to dispel their pain and guide them to the state of enlightenment"

Sonam Langyal (a.k.a. Lama Sobha), who self-immolated on January 8, 2012 [1]

1 Introduction

The *tulku* (reincarnate custodian) Lama Sobha recorded a message on tape, part of which is quoted above, before his self-immolation in 2012 in Darlag county, Golog Autonomous Tibetan Prefecture, Qinghai province, prior to drinking and pouring kerosene to set himself on fire, calling for the autonomy of Tibet and the reunification of the Tibetan people [1]. This particular self-immolation is of significance given the high religious profile of the now deceased Tibetan activist. Lama Sobha, a known Buddhist scholar, venerated teacher and community leader, established a

W. Aunjitsakul (✉)
Department of Psychiatry, Faculty of Medicine, Prince of Songkla University, Songkhla, Thailand
e-mail: awarut@medicine.psu.ac.th, aunjitsakul.w@gmail.com

P. Chompoosri
Department of Psychiatry, School of Medicine, Mae Fah Luang University, Chiang Rai, Thailand
e-mail: poom.cps@gmail.com

A. D. Aladjem
NYU Program for Survivors of Torture, New York, NY, USA

NYU School of Medicine, New York, NY, USA
e-mail: asher.aladjem@nyumc.org

C. A. Alfonso et al. (eds.), *Suicide by Self-Immolation*,
https://doi.org/10.1007/978-3-030-62613-6_8

Table 1 Characteristics of Tibetan self-immolations (references: [3–10])

Characteristics		Number	Percent
Sex	Male	139	83.73
	Female	27	16.27
Age	<20	45	27.11
	21–30	71	42.77
	31–40	22	13.25
	41–50	17	10.24
	>50	8	4.82
	Unknown	3	1.81
Monkhood	Former	11	6.63
	At immolation	49	29.52
	Never ordained	106	63.86
Location	Tibet Autonomous Region	8	4.82
	Sichuan	80	48.19
	Qinghai	34	20.48
	Gansu	33	19.88
	Beijing	1	0.60
	India	7	4.22
	Nepal	3	1.81

well-attended home for the elderly and a vibrant local primary school in Darlag. We know of two triggering and disappointing events prior to his self-immolation. Chinese authorities denied him a request to increase the number of students to be registered at his school and also refused him permission to travel out of Tibet to attend a Kalachakra (tantric initiation ceremony that attracts thousands) in the Bodhi Gaya pilgrimage holy site in India. The 14th and current Dalai Lama of Tibet, Tenzin Gyatso, presided over this particular historical Kalachakra in India in 2012 [2]. Lama Sobha's missed pilgrimage was the best attended Kalachakra ever, with participation of close to 200,000 monks [2].

From 1998 to January 2020, there have been 166 incidents of Tibetan self-immolations (see Table 1 and Fig. 1) [3]. One hundred twenty-four Tibetan self-immolators died in the act and many of those who survived were detained by Chinese security forces and disappeared. The high number of Tibetan self-immolations causes commotion around the world and draws intense international media attention. This chapter will attempt to place Tibetan self-immolations in a comprehensive historical, political, social and religious cultural context, understand individual and altruistic motivations, choice of suicide method, explore how Tibetans-at-large view these actions, and propose prevention strategies.

2   Tibetan People and Their History

Tibet occupies a vast surface area, equivalent to what would be the tenth largest country in the world, and the highest altitude region on Earth. It is currently incorporated into the People's Republic of China (PRC) as the Tibet Autonomous Region,

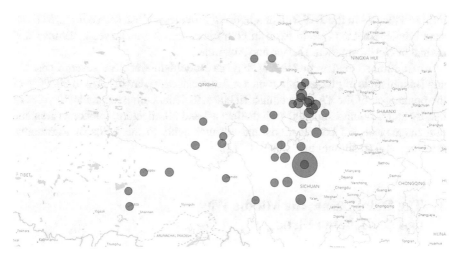

Fig. 1 Self-immolations in Tibet and adjoining provinces

or TAR. The PRC is politically subdivided into 23 provinces, five autonomous regions and four municipalities [11]. A vociferous albeit comparatively small group of Tibetan exiles and locals consider Tibet to be a separate country [12]. Prior to the Yuan dynasty (1271–1368) China and Tibet were indeed separate neighboring countries. Although the uniqueness and separateness of Tibetan culture and identity is universally recognized, the United Nations, the European Union and no individual nation officially accept the sovereignty of Tibet at present.

In 1949, the PRC claimed and annexed Tibet. Violent political and religious reforms led to revolts and bloodshed. His Holiness the 14th Dalai Lama, who ruled Tibet since 1940, was forced into exile in 1959, along with approximately 80,000 Tibetans, to Dharamshala in the North of India, where they established a shadow government [13]. Chinese officials ordered the destruction of thousands of religious temples and scriptures and undermined the Dalai Lama's role in Tibet [14]. Since the Cultural Revolution Tibetans live with restrictions of freedom of speech, press, association and religion, and those who deviate from the law could be imprisoned and tortured. The PRC lifted some restrictions in the TAR in 1976, including the ban on practicing Buddhism, but other repressive measures persisted instigating protests to date. In 1989 the Dalai Lama was awarded the Nobel Peace Prize in recognition of his endorsement of peaceful protests of Tibetans against the PRC [14, 15]. In 1999, the PRC campaigned to transform Tibet by launching an economic development plan in Western China expanding infrastructure and access from other provinces. Although a large number of ethnic Han Chinese recently migrated to Tibet, the vast majority of the population in the region remains ethnic Tibetan.

Although Chinese authorities and the Tibetan administration of the Dalai Lama and exiled groups dispute the numbers, we estimate that half of the six million ethnic Tibetans live in the TAR and half outside of TAR geographical boundaries, mostly in contiguous PRC provinces. The majority of ethnic Tibetans outside of the TAR populate Chinese provinces of Qinghai, Gansu, and Sichuan. In addition to six million Tibetans in the TAR and neighboring provinces, close to two hundred thousand ethnic Tibetans live in exile in countries such as India, Nepal, Bhutan and abroad in North America, Europe and Australia.

Most ethnic Tibetans practice Mahayana Buddhism since the seventh century, and Buddhism is of pivotal importance in Tibetans' everyday life. Up to 80–90% of the population of the TAR are ethnic Tibetans. Tibetan culture spans 5000 years of history and accomplishments, with distinct art and architecture, music, written and oral languages, and contributions and advancements to the fields of astronomy, astrology and traditional medicine [16, 17].

3   The Dalai Lama, the Middle Way, and the Tibetan Struggle

Despite the fact that the 14th Dalai Lama serves as spiritual leader and is regarded with the utmost respect by Tibetans, anger and frustration remain as a result of his response to the oppressive acts of the PRC throughout 1960s and 1970s. The Dalai Lama advocated a nonviolent approach emulating Gandhi's peaceful approach that led to India's independence, whereas many Tibetans repeatedly demonstrated a willingness to risk their lives in the pursuit of liberation and freedom [13]. As violence peaked in the region in the 1970s, the Dalai Lama unveiled and invoked the Middle Way or Middle Path approach, based on Buddhist's principles, in order to negotiate peace and the repatriation of Tibet.

The *Middle Way* (དབུ་མའི་ལམ།) is a doctrine that spans all forms of Buddhism, referring to the path of liberation and successful exit from the circuitous samsara or the cycle of rebirth. Practices that focus on alignment of *speech, views, resolve, conduct, livelihood, effort, mindfulness and meditative union* lead to body-mind balance and compassion. These eight component practices are the iconographical symbolic elements of the eight spokes of the Dharma Wheel or Dharma Chakra. Following the *Noble Eightfold Path*, or Middle Way, leads to enlightenment, emancipation, liberation and release [18]. The Middle Way for Mahayana Tibetan Buddhists results in social and political attitudes characterized by moderation and patience, invoking non-violence and renouncing extremist or anarchic positions.

Many Tibetans feel abandoned with a sense that the Dalai Lama, who has an approval rating of 65% among Tibetan refugees in exile, dismisses their struggle [13]. Popular Tibetan protest methods continue mostly in the form of peaceful marches and candlelight vigils [19]. Other peaceful methods advocated by the Middle Way approach include poster campaigns, distribution of educational materials about Tibetan history, or dissemination of popular music with a political message of commitment to the Tibetan struggle and support of the Dalai Lama [13].

An organized group of young Tibetans questioned the effectiveness of the Middle Way nonviolent strategy advocated by the Dalai Lama. This activist organization, the Tibetan Youth Congress (TYC), deviated from the nonviolent path since the

1970s across India and Nepal [19]. Dharamshala's leadership publicly condemned the TYC but the protests remained intense for decades. In 1998 the TYC escalated their protest methods from hunger strikes with the first public act of Tibetan self-immolation taking place in Delhi. Thubten Ngodrup set himself on fire on April 27, 1998 after the Indian police force broke up the hunger strike demonstrators, and died from severe burns 2 days later [20]. Since this unfortunate event, his sacrifice served as a role model encouraging other Tibetan self-immolators. Thubten Ngodrup is considered by many a Tibetan hero and martyr. It is perhaps no accident of history that Tibetan self-immolation began as a reactionary feat when a more peaceful method of protest yearning for social change was disbanded and suppressed.

The next Tibetan self-immolation in exile occurred in 2008, in Bangalore, when Lhakpa Tsering, the president of the TYC, set himself on fire to protest Hu Jintao's visit to India. A year later, in February 27, 2009, a peaceful demonstration was interrupted in a Tibetan enclave in Sichuan when authorities shot dead close to two dozen people including school age children. When the authorities demanded cancelling funeral ceremonies soon after, a young monk named Tapey doused himself with gasoline, walked to the crossroads and lit himself on fire while holding the Tibetan flag and a photo of the Dalai Lama [3]. Two years later, another Tibetan monk, Phuntsog, self-immolated also in a Tibetan region of Sichuan, on the anniversary date of the assassination of Tibetan peaceful protesters. After Phuntsog's death, self-immolation became epidemic with 166 incidents recorded to date throughout the TAR and the Tibetan diaspora (see Table 1). Self-immolators comprise all walks of Tibetan life: from religious people (monks or former monks, nuns) to lay persons, men and women, and persons of all ages [3]. Self-immolations now carry the stigma of being an antidote to silencing, oppression and subjugation, and are glorified as acts of self-sacrifice that use the body in flames as a 'political weapon' [21].

4 Tibetan Self-Immolations: Politically or Religiously Driven?

Self-immolations are internationally recognized as political or protest suicides [22]. A critical political self-immolation with global repercussions occurred in 1963 when a Vietnamese Buddhist monk named Thich Quang Duc protested South Vietnam's persecution of Buddhists by setting himself on fire on a busy street in Saigon. Vietnam at the time was almost 90% Buddhist but governed by a Catholic minority that violently forced religious conversions. To protest the persecution and oppression of Buddhists, Quang Duc sat in the lotus position in an intersection surrounded by over a hundred monks, nuns and international journalists who had been called to observe. Several other monks poured gasoline over him and retreated to a safe distance before he finally lit himself on fire. His sacrifice became an archetypal self-immolation because of the dramatic staging and wide dissemination via Malcolm Browne's Pulitzer-prize winning photograph and historic media coverage

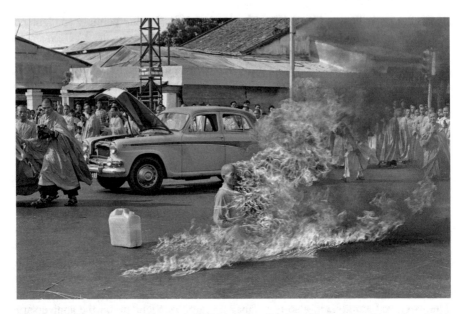

Fig. 2 Malcolm Browne's photograph of Thích Quảng Đức's self-immolation (Reproduced with permission from the Associated Press)

(see Fig. 2). Quan Duc is revered ever since as a Bodhisattva (one who attains Buddhahood for the benefit of others).

After Quan Duc's auto-cremation, self-immolation became widespread as a political symbol in many countries. Worldwide self-immolations include Norman Morrison's protesting United States' involvement in Vietnam (1965), Jan Palach's protesting the Soviet invasion of Czechoslovakia (1968), and Tarek al-Tayeb Mohamed Bouazizi's protesting his government in Tunisia (2010) and inciting the 'Arab Spring' [23, 24]. Tibetans continue to self-immolate to protest Chinese government policies. Although it is easy to link self-immolations worldwide to a symbolic attempt to escape chaotic political conflicts and oppression, occurrences in Tibet also have religious determinants, which leads us to consider that politics and religion are intertwined as driving forces of Tibetan self-immolations.

Tibetans follow traditional Buddhist values as core to their existence, including compassion, karma, and the bond between Tibetans and Avalokiteshvara [25]. Mahayana Buddhists believe that Avalokiteshvara, (Sanskrit: avalokita, "looking on"; ishivara, "lord") supremely exemplifies the Bodhisattva ("buddha-to-be") of compassion and mercy. Avalokiteshvara postpones his own Buddhahood until he has helped every sentient being on Earth achieve liberation (moksha; literally, "release") from suffering (dukkha) and escape the process of death and rebirth (samsara). In Tibetan Buddhism the Dalai Lamas are believed to be personifications of Avalokiteshvara and monks who self-immolate are revered as Bodhisattvas.

Tibetan politics and religion are inherently fused. The identity of the state is legitimized based on religious influences, and Tibetan leadership is passed down, not through heredity, but through the reincarnation of its religious teacher. Additionally, the Tibetan government has a religious system of government [26] that stipulates the superiority of the path to enlightenment warranting and legitimizing political power [27]. The Dalai Lama is the legitimate leader and the monasteries are centers of social, political, religious, and economic life in Tibetan society. As religion overlaps with politics, protest methods, either nonviolent or violent, seem to have inseparable links to both politics and religion.

The complexity of interactive politics and religion is expressed in different ways of protesting. In nonviolent protests, endorsed by the 14th Dalai Lama, Tibetan protesters, including monks and nuns, engage in frequent peace vigils and marches in Dharamshala against the Chinese government. Furthermore, the religious rituals have been cleverly transformed into forms of political protest. For example, monks conduct a traditional circumambulation as a political statement; groups execute the religious act of humility by bowing the body to the floor over long distances in an act of political protest; and the monastic debate of Buddhist dialectics, which Tibetan monks normally perform to seek truth and profound understanding, is sophistically applied to political debate [13]. Many, if not most Tibetan protesters, follow the Middle Way approach in consonance with Mahayana Buddhist principles and practices.

Violent resistance dramatically increased since 2009, from hunger strikes to self-immolations. Some TYC leaders in Dharamshala pressure activists to believe that spiritual beliefs need to be kept separate from political aims and methods, with compassion and passivity not being effective political strategies [19]. However, activists struggle differentiating politics from religious acts, as the TYC continues to emphasize that the side-lining of religious principles is a necessarily pragmatic approach to effectively deal with the current political situation. The TYC substantiates self-immolation as plausible within the Tibetan religious framework, as a political self-sacrifice that is both noble and meritorious. From a mental health and suicide prevention perspectives, this is problematic.

5 States of Mind of Tibetan Self-Immolators

Ethnographic studies examined last words, writings and manifestos of self-immolators to understand their affective states and thought processes. A study of last words from hand-written notes, video and verbal communications to friends and family of 26 self-immolators concluded that there are three common features related to political demands behind acts of religious dedication [28]. First commonality is that there is a high incidence of Tibetan self-immolators living in exile or outside of TAR boundaries given their intolerance of perceived oppression and subjugation in the TAR region. Second, self-immolations are expected to draw international attention to the Tibetan cause. Third, violent self-immolations aim to attain the political goal of Tibetan independence. Last words linking political demands were, for example, "let the Dalai Lama return"; "release the 11th Panchen Lama"; "freedom for Tibet"; and "freedom of speech" [29].

Another study analyzed 49 last statements of self-immolators and showed that 30.4% prayed for the return of Dalai Lama. This study concluded that "self-immolation is a religious offering, as well as a protest against the state" and "self-immolation is intended to express the spiritual strength of the Tibetan people" [30]. Ngawang Norphel's recorded last words were as following:

> We do not have the ability to help Tibetan's religion and culture. We do not have the economic means to help other Tibetans. For the sake of our Tibetan race, in particular for the return of His Holiness Dalai Lama to Tibet, we choose self-immolation. We want to tell all the Tibetan youth, swear to yourself, never fight against each other, among Tibetans, we have to be united and protect our race. [31]

Last words' analyses of self-immolators show the interconnectedness of religion and politics of the Tibetan cause, in spite of Dalai Lama's encouragement of nonviolent protests. Nonetheless, we and others suggest that self-immolations should not be strictly assessed only on the basis of religion, as these acts convey a sense of despair, helplessness, and a misguided and perhaps extreme altruistic wish to self-sacrifice for a greater cause. Psychological distress may be veiled as actions that press for social change [30]. To date, there are no studies examining psychiatric disorders in Tibetan self-immolators.

6 Tibetan Self-Immolations, Predicament Suicides, Self-Sacrifice and Mental Health

We discussed in previous sections self-immolation as protest suicides to advance political causes, either linked or unlinked to religious motivations [22]. An unanswered question remains if Tibetan self-immolators have treatable psychiatric disorders. *Predicament suicides* affect people without psychiatric diagnoses that face unacceptable social and/or environmental stressors [32]. *However, persons engaging in predicament suicides may have subsyndromal or undiagnosed trauma and stressor related disorders*, such as adjustment disorders and posttraumatic stress disorders. Tension among PRC and TAR leaders, fueled by groups such as the TYC, trickles down to ordinary Tibetans, monks, nuns and community leaders, who may opt to escape distress and social discontent by becoming politically active and self-immolating. A dimension of meaningfulness of Tibetan public suicides may extend beyond sociopolitical and religious formulations and have personal valence. Self-immolations, therefore, could be prevented with mental health interventions.

Tibetans' answers when asked if self-immolation is an act of suicide include the following: "No it's not a suicide, it's for all Tibetans. They give their life for us. It's good merit."; "Well, not really a suicide, someone brave like this, and so selfless, will have a good rebirth, so it's not like a suicide."; or "It's a suicide, but it's not like other suicides." These answers reflect the importance of the cultural context when studying suicide ethnographically but could also be interpreted as a maladaptive idealization of suicidal behavior.

Self-immolation is the act of burning of one's own body, and is also referred to as 'auto-cremation' [33]. The Latin etymology of immolation refers to killing or offering as a sacrifice, and sacrifice implies an act of giving up something of value for the sake of something that is of greater value or importance. Hence, self-immolation literally suggests self-sacrifice [34]. To understand acts of Tibetan self-sacrifice, there are two influential Buddhist narratives to consider, the *Lotus Sutra* and *Jataka Tales*, that are part of the Tibetan cultural background and could be of significance in the collective psyche of its people.

Tibetan Mahayana Buddhists believe that 'abandoning the body' through drowning, starvation, being fed to an animal or auto-cremation represent spiritual ways of sacrifice [33]. An instance of self-immolation mentioned in the Lotus Sutra is when the Buddha describes the Medicine King, the Bodhisattva Bhaisajyaraja, telling the story that in a previous life he showed his devotion by burning his body as a sacrificial offering. The Lotus Sutra is one of the most important Mahayana *sutras* (aphorisms) containing central teachings of the Buddha [35].

The Jataka Tales are a collection of popular Theravada fables in verse with annotated prose, translated into may languages worldwide and with regional variants in the oral tradition of Buddhist countries. A popular tale is that of Prince Sattva, one of the previous incarnations of Buddha, who commits altruistic suicide. The fable tells the story of the Prince strolling along with a disciple approaching the edge of a precipice. Looking down they noticed a hungry tigress trapped on a small platform of rocks about to devour her cubs in desperation. The Prince sends out his disciple to search for fare to feed the tigress but as the disciple leaves, the Prince realizes that time is critical and makes the altruistic decision of throwing himself down the precipice for his body to be devoured by the tigress and save the cubs. Upon his return his disciple realizes the magnanimous compassion of Prince Buddha in this act of self-sacrifice, gathers other disciples, and showers the spot with an offering of lotus flowers. This compassionate act in the Prince Sattva and the Tigress story may serve as motivational inspiration in Tibetan altruistic self-sacrifices [35], and Tibetans who were asked about self-immolations frequently referred to this tale [19].

In keeping with Tibetan practices, an offering of light signifies removing and dispelling ignorance in a positive and pure way, as when the Lama (teacher, guru) lights up a butter lamp. Additionally, fire and light are transcultural symbols of wisdom, which for Buddhists refers to the teachings of Buddha as a path to enlightenment [36]. Since Quan Duc's self-immolation in 1963, lighting up or igniting the body becomes a symbolic representation of spiritual dedication to affirm human rights. The Vietnamese monk Thich Nhat Hanh sent a letter to Martin Luther King and explained that self-sacrifice by immolation is a non-violent 'act of construction, that is, to suffer and to die for the sake of one's people' [37]. A last statement written before a Lama's self-immolation states:

> The immolation of one's precious body was for the return of Gyalwang Tenzin Gyatso [the Dalai Lama] to his homeland; for the release of the Panchen Nangwa Thaye [the Panchen Lama] from prison; for the welfare of the six million Tibetans. My body has been offered to the fire for these. [38]

Buddhist teachings promulgate the importance of dying well, as death is part of the normal process of life and one should seek to understand the reality of death. Furthermore, Buddhists assert that persons should spend their lifetime thinking about eventual death and preparing for it without fear or apprehension. By paradigmatically shifting death from distressing to harmonious, life is experienced as more valuable [39]. The fluidity of the Buddhist belief in the life-death-rebirth or enlightenment cycle destigmatizes suicide and may provide comfort and motivate self-immolation when other sociopolitical circumstances are aligned, as Tibetan Buddhism is an essential component of the construction, practice and rhetoric of Tibetan nationalism [40].

Differences exist among Buddhist practices in Asia and abroad. In Theravada Buddhism tradition (practiced nowadays primarily in Southeast Asia), the idea that one should not commit acts of violence to the self is important for the harmony of future rebirths, thus self-immolation is considered taboo. In Mahayana Buddhism (practiced in the Tibetan plateau) the notion of giving oneself up for others selflessly is of utmost importance [41]. The PRC publicly labeled self-immolations as acts of terrorism [13], and reiterates that Buddhist doctrines view all suicides as sinful, quoting various scriptures and religious scholars in a document published online in 2012 as 'Sin of Suicide' [42]. Although the PRC is persuasive in its argument, self-immolations are idealized by Mahayana and other religious traditions, so that even if not ego-syntonic they are socially sanctioned in the TAR as purposeful and altruistic. Self-immolation suicide prevention strategies may need to consider bridging these extreme views in creative ways.

7 Tibetans' Views on Self-Immolation

Although the 14th Dalai Lama consistently supports peaceful solutions to conflict suggesting that self-immolations are violent methods of protest, many Tibetan insist that self-immolations are altruistic actions that could advance the welfare, freedom, and independence of the Tibetan people [43]. When a journalist interviewed a Tibetan refugee asking what motivates self-immolation he answered the following way:

> Burning oneself for the freedom of six million Tibetans cannot bring negative karma. They do it for a selfless cause … this is not against Buddhist beliefs … Gandhi also declared hunger strike unto death on many occasions. Does that make him violent? In every freedom struggle, violent or non-violent, people lose a part of themselves to attain a larger goal. [44]

A survey of the opinions of Tibetan people in Dharamshala about the nature of self-sacrificial resistance methods revealed that 77.5% view self-immolations as nonviolent, and 77.8% viewed hunger strikes as a nonviolent form of protest as well [19]. Nonetheless, 46.1% strongly disagreed with using violence in pursuit of Tibetan freedom [19]. An obvious limitation of this survey is that it was conducted only amongst Tibetans in exile while most immolations occur in PRC Tibetan enclaves bordering the TAR.

Thich Nhat Hanh, when addressing the purposefulness of self-immolation, states:

> To burn oneself by fire is to prove that what one is saying is of the utmost importance. There is nothing more painful than burning oneself. To say something while experiencing this kind of pain is to say it with the utmost courage, frankness, determination and sincerity. [37]

His Holiness the Dalai Lama, a central figure invoked in every protest, continues to encourage Tibetans to adhere with the Middle Way precepts when faced with conflict. However, it is curious that *he has never made a direct appeal to the people of Tibet to stop self-immolating*. We do not know what motivates the 14th Dalai Lama not to directly condemn self-immolators. Some speculate that he would alienate the family and community of the self-immolators and lose political traction if categorically condemning it and going against a majority opinion [45, 46]. He stated the following in an interview in 2013:

> Actually, suicide is basically a type of violence but the question of good or bad depends on the motivation and goal. I think as goal is concern, these self-immolators are not drunk, don't have family problems this is for Buddha Dharma for Tibetan National interest but then I think that the ultimate factor is the individual motivation.... If motivation consists of too much anger, hatred, then it is negative but if motivation is more compassionate, calm mind, then such acts can be positive... [45]

The refusal to directly condemn self-immolation is problematic from the perspective of suicide prevention.

8 Prevention of Self-Immolation in the Tibet Autonomous Region and Tibetan Diaspora

While most Tibetans view self-immolation as self-sacrifice and a form of protest, clinicians are ethically inclined to consider it suicide, and thus, make preventive efforts [47, 48]. Clinical efforts must be culturally informed to improve suicide prevention outcomes and foster a therapeutic alliance. The World Health Organization (WHO) published comprehensive suicide prevention strategies and guidelines (see Chap. 1, Sect. 7, and Table 1) highlighting that interventions need to be designed to protect vulnerable groups, individuals at risk, and bereaved families and significant others [48].

To our knowledge, there are no specific strategies proposed to prevent self-immolations of Tibetans, regionally in the TAR or in the diaspora. Self-immolation is prevalent and almost always a lethal method of suicide in low-and-middle-income countries and specific regions of the world, including populous countries in Central and South Asia [49]. Prevention efforts in neighboring countries with relative success include responsible reporting of suicides, increased access to mental health care, community support for those at risk and the bereaved, and sensible legislation addressing psychosocial political factors that may increase suicide risk. Some prevention strategies that may have a positive impact on decreasing deaths by suicide, such as restricting access to means, may be difficult to implement given the wide availability of solvents and flammable liquids. Other efforts may be more intuitively effective, such as liaising with political and community leaders who could engage individuals in other forms of protest, allowing the disenfranchised to be heard while not placing lives at imminent risk.

One of the chapter authors (AA) is a liaison psychiatrist delivering services to persons seeking asylum in the United States after escaping political persecution and torture in their countries of origin. The following clinical vignette describes a carefully crafted and effective suicide prevention intervention of Tibetans in exile.

Clinical vignette: In the spring of 2012 three Tibetan activists sat in front of the United Nations headquarters in New York City for 30 consecutive days in a hunger strike. Their demands seemed unattainable at first, and in a letter to the United Nations requested that the organization send an official delegation accompanied by international media to independently investigate human rights violations in Tibet that was inciting an epidemic of self-immolations, to have the PRC free political prisoners, and put an end to patriotic reeducation of Tibetans [4, 50]. The New York City Police Department requested a psychiatric consultation from the New York University/Bellevue Program for Survivors of Torture (PSOT) to assess the competency of the Tibetan strikers, asking if they were striking on their own free will and if they remained competent after a month of food deprivation. After a careful and therapeutic evaluation, the psychiatrist determined that the Tibetans had decisional capcity and were striking independently of undue influence by the TYC organizers. Furthermore, the psychiatrist concluded that they were not acutely suicidal, understood that the hunger strike could result in death, but that self-inflicted death was not their intention. The results of the evaluation leaked to social media and validated the strikers' plight for justice. Validation of suffering and compassion, key elements of empathic attunement essential to cement a therapeutic alliance, served to catalyze a series the ensuing events that ended the strike. After a dialogue with the psychiatrist the strikers accepted medical assistance, the United Nations furnished a letter in support of their cause, and the strikers broke their fast. This peaceful negotiation among clinicians, law enforcement agents and political groups demonstrates how acts of self-sacrifice can be rechanneled to prevent premature deaths and promote social change in non-violent ways.

A program similar to the NYU/Bellevue PSOT is the Tibetan Torture Survivors' Program (TTSP), established by the Central Tibetan Administration (Tibetan government in exile), providing comprehensive psychosocial care to survivors of trauma in India and Nepal. This program delivers cost-free medical and psychological treatments and refers those with severe complications to hospitals in India that offer a higher level of care. The TTSP distributes financial support and serves all traumatized refugees, regardless of political affiliation, offering group therapy led by senior Buddhist monks [50].

Programmatic efforts to improve quality of life and region-specific interventions are needed across the Tibetan diaspora. These could be effective in preventing or extinguishing self- immolations, in our opinion, only if carefully crafted and coordinated with political groups in conflict. Responsible reporting of suicides is essential, using the media as a vehicle to educate about suicide and how to seek help. Reporting of suicides should avoid language that sensationalizes, prominent placement of stories, and undue repetition [48]. A Tibetan national and regional strategy must involve the following components: *surveillance, responsible media reporting, access to treatment and education, crisis intervention, postvention, stigma reduction, oversight coordination* of efforts by NGOs and governmental organizations, and *measuring outcomes* [48].

9 Conclusion

Unique sociopolitical and transcultural circumstances serve as precursors and create a meaningful context for Tibetan self-immolations, which are highly prevalent with deaths by suicide rapidly increasing since 2011. Up to date, there are 166 accounts of Tibetan self-immolations, almost all in this geographically sequestered region of the world. International communities show grave concern and are intrigued as to what motivates self-immolation protests in Tibet. The Tibetan plateau is an isolated region where the practice of Mahayana Buddhism flourished over thousands of years. In this chapter, we comprehensively summarized plausible determinants of self-immolations in Tibet, including the ongoing conflict between PRC and TAR politicians, and between the Tibetan surrogate government in exile and TYC leadership. Religious Mahayana Buddhist traditions and political realities in Tibet seem inseparable and also may influence acts of self-immolation.

The 14th Dalai Lama is respected as a representative of God, reincarnation of Buddha, and a spiritual leader, and developed over decades of political experience a peaceful protest style based on the doctrines of the Middle Way, emulating Gandhi's non-violent methods, while staying on course demanding political autonomy of Tibet and protection of human rights. However, he has failed to publicly condemn self-immolations, perhaps erring on political correctness not realizing that this compromises Tibetans' mental health.

This chapter described Tibetan self-immolations as a form of political protest and resistance, as altruistic suicides to promote a cause, as predicament suicides, and as a result of subsyndromal psychiatric disorders and trauma and stressor related disorders. The vast majority of Tibetans do not view self-immolation as suicide and people who self-immolate are glorified as heroic. Viewing self-immolations as predicament suicides may have roots in Mahayana traditions where death is considered an integral part of the life cycle, the belief that enlightenment and freedom can be attained from self-sacrifice and compassion, and encouragement of altruistic actions.

Prevention strategies of self-immolations of Tibetans need to take into account interrelated clinical, sociocultural and political factors. We propose that mental health clinicians, suicidologists, community activists, law enforcement agents, and politicians work in consonance with aligned and clearly stated efforts, offering altruistic alternatives to suicide and politically compromising to combat the unexpressed and latent hopelessness and helplessness of Tibetan self-immolators.

References

1. Cabezón J. On the ethics of the Tibetan self-immolations. 2013 [updated June 18, 2013]. https://religiondispatches.org/on-the-ethics-of-the-tibetan-self-immolations/.
2. Lama TD. Introduction to the Kalachakra. https://www.dalailama.com/teachings/kalachakra-initiations.
3. Self-Immolation Fact Cheet. 2019 [updated December 2, 2019]. https://savetibet.org/tibetan-self-immolations/.
4. Data T. Self-immolations in Tibet. 2015. https://tibetdata.org/projects/selfimmolationData/index.html.
5. Burning T. Self-immolations for Tibet. 2018. https://tibetburning.in/2006/11/23/lhakpa-tsering/.
6. Gill HK. Tibetan self-immolations: sacrifice and the Tibetan freedom struggle in exile, India. Oslo: University of Oslo; 2015.
7. Congress TY. 16. Sonam Wangyal. 2014. https://www.tibetanyouthcongress.org/2014/10/16-sonam-wangyal/.
8. Tibet UF. Projects filed under: Protesters. 2014. https://unitefortibet.org/protesters/sonam-rabyang/.
9. Asia RF. Tibet: clampdown imposed as nun secretly cremated after burning protest. 2013. https://www.refworld.org/docid/51cbfbfa18.html.
10. Free Tibet. Court sentences Tibetan monk to three years in prison. 2019. https://www.freetibet.org/news-media/na/china-sentences-tibetan-monk-three-years-prison.
11. Agency CI. East Asia/Southeast Asia: China 2020. https://www.cia.gov/library/publications/resources/the-world-factbook/geos/ch.html.
12. Tibet F. Introduction to Tibet. https://freetibet.org/about.
13. Kohn S. Tibetan nonviolence. Peace Rev. 2014;26(1):62–8.
14. Hartnett SJ. "Tibet is burning": competing rhetorics of liberation, occupation, resistance, and paralysis on the roof of the world. Q J Speech. 2013;99(3):283–316.
15. History.com. Dalai Lama begins exile. 1959. https://www.history.com/this-day-in-history/dalai-lama-begins-exile.
16. Center CII. Tibet facts and figures 2007. 2007. http://www.china.org.cn/china/tibetfactsandfigures/node_7043566.htm.
17. Megazine NYT. Exploring the mysteries of Tibetan medicine. 1981. https://www.nytimes.com/1981/01/11/magazine/exploring-the-mysteries-of-tibetan-medicine.html.
18. Brekke T. The religious motivation of the early buddhists. J Am Acad Relig. 1999;67(4):849–66.
19. Ramsay Z. Religion, politics and the meaning of self-sacrifice for Tibet. Contemp South Asia. 2016;24(1):75–93.

20. Norbu J. Rite of freedom: the life and sacrifice of Thupten Ngodup. 1998 [updated May 12, 2008]. https://www.jamyangnorbu.com/blog/2008/05/12/remembering-thupten-ngodup/.
21. Fierke KM. Political self-sacrifice: agency, body and emotion in international relations. Kindle Edition. Cambridge: Cambridge University Press; 2013.
22. Biggs M. Making sense of suicide missions. 2005.
23. Lester D. Suicidal protests: self-immolation, hunger strikes, or suicide bombing. Behav Brain Sci. 2014;37(4):372.
24. Walter SPG. Protest suicide. Australasian Psychiatr. 2012;20(6):533–4.
25. Dreyfus G. Tibetan Studies: Proceedings of the 6th Seminar of the International Association for Tibetan Studies. Fagernes, editor 1992.
26. Cuppers C. The relationship between religion and state (chos srid zun brei). In: Ruegg DS, editor. Traditional tibet proceedings of a seminar held in Lumbini Nepal March 2000. Lumbini: Nepal Lithographing Co (P) Ltd; 2004.
27. Paldron TM. Distinguishing between lamas and leaders. Tibetan Political Review. 2011.
28. Lixiong W. Last-words analysis—why Tibetans self-immolate? By Wang Lixiong. 2012 [updated December 27, 2012]. http://www.phayul.com/news/article.aspx?id=32726.
29. Sun Y. Ethnic, sectarian, or localized grievances? On Wang Lixiong's analysis of Tibetan self-immolation. Asian Ethnicity. 2013;14(3):376–80.
30. Woeser T. Tibet on fire: self-immolations against chinese rule. London: Verso; 2016.
31. Tsering T. Ngawang Norphel passes away in a Chinese hospital. 2012 [updated July 30, 2012]. http://www.phayul.com/news/article.aspx?id=31810&t=1.
32. Pridmore S. Predicament suicide: concept and evidence. Australas Psychiatry. 2009;17(2):112–6.
33. Benn JA. Burning for the Buddha: self-immolation in Chinese Buddhism. Hawaii: Hawaii University Press; 2007.
34. Scott Kouri JW. Thinking the other side of youth suicide: engagements with life. Int J Child Youth Family Stud. 2014;5(1):180–203.
35. Davis LS. Enacting the violent imaginary: reflections on the dynamics of nonviolence and violence in buddhism. Sophia. 2016;55(1):15–30.
36. Harvey P. An introduction to buddhism: teachings, history and practices. 2 edn. Cambridge: Cambridge University Press Textbooks; 2012.
37. Nanh TN. African-American involement in the Vietnam war letter. Saigon: La Boi; 1965. http://www.aavw.org/special_features/letters_thich_abstract02.html
38. Monks gather to pray after self-immolation of respected Tibetan monk in Amchok. 2013 [updated December 20, 2013]. https://www.savetibet.org/monks-gather-to-pray-after-self-immolation-of-respected-tibetan-monk-in-amchok/.
39. Vehaba A. Buddhism, death, and resistance: what self-immolation in Tibet has borne. Polit Relig Ideol. 2019;20(2):215–43.
40. John W-B. Tibet on fire: buddhism, protest, and the rhetoric of self-immolation. 1st ed. New York: Palgrave Macmillan; 2015.
41. Gouin M. Self-immolation and martyrdom in Tibet. Mortality. 2014;19(2):176–83.
42. Online CT. Sin of suicide. 2012 [updated March 16, 2012]. http://chinatibet.people.com.cn/96069/7759971.html.
43. Network IT. Self-immolations increase as Chinese leadership changes 2012. http://tibetnetwork.org/self-immolations-increase-as-chinese-leadership-changes/.
44. Jazeera A. Tibet's burning protest. 2012 [updated Jun 1, 2012].
45. Phayul. Dalai Lama talks about self-immolation. 2013 [updated March 26, 2013]. http://www.phayul.com/news/article.aspx?id=33263.
46. BBC. 'The Human Torches of Tibet': BBC's Our World Documentary Series. 2012 [updated May 27, 2012]. https://www.youtube.com/watch?v=FMwhl-Cfyyc.
47. Zarghami M. Selection of person of the year from public health perspective: promotion of mass clusters of copycat self-immolation. Iran J Psychiatr Behav Sci. 2012;6(1):1–11.

48. WHO. Preventing suicide: A global imperative. 2014. https://apps.who.int/iris/bitstream/handle/10665/131056/9789241564779_eng.pdf;jsessionid=9478E002BDC3F065E43053273FB EFC9D?sequence=1.
49. Rezaeian M. Epidemiology of self-immolation. Burns. 2013;39(1):184–6.
50. Administration CT. Department of Health: Tibetan Torture Survivors Program. 2020. https://tibet.net/department/health/#code0slide1.

Self-Immolation in the Arab World After the *Arab Spring*

Reham Aly and César A. Alfonso

> *"(My sons) are both victims of the state…"*
>
> *Zeina, Husseini and Saber Kalai's mother, commenting on her two sons who self-immolated in Tunisia, as reported in a Time magazine interview published 6 October 2016.*

1 Introduction

Suicide is globally recognized as a public health priority. The World Health Organization (WHO) estimates that almost 1.53 million people will die from suicide in 2020. This means that there is an average of three suicides occurring per minute at any point in time. Suicide is the second leading cause of death among young people worldwide and up to 80% of all suicides occur in low-and middle income-countries [1].

The Arab world, with a relative cultural and geographical similarity, covers a population of over 500 million and extends from Morocco to Afghanistan. It

R. Aly
Ministry of Health, Cairo, Egypt

World Psychiatric Association Special Interest Group on Cultural Adaptations of Cognitive Behavioral Therapy, Geneva, Switzerland
e-mail: rehamaaly@hotmail.com

C. A. Alfonso (✉)
Columbia University Medical Center, New York, NY, USA

Universitas Indonesia, Jakarta, Indonesia

National University of Malaysia, Kuala Lumpur, Malaysia

World Psychiatric Association Psychotherapy Section, Geneva, Switzerland
e-mail: cesaralfonso@mac.com, caa2105@cumc.columbia.edu

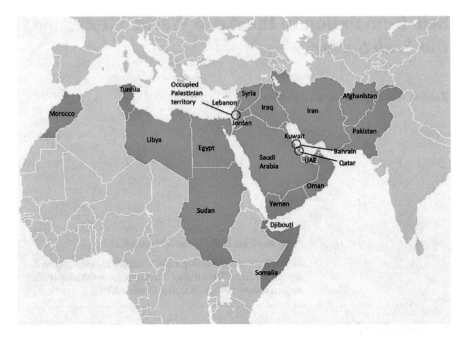

Fig. 1 The Eastern Mediterranean Region (EMR) countries

includes 22 countries (see Fig. 1). The majority of the population in these countries is Muslim [2]. Most Arab countries are in the low-and-middle income category as defined by the World Bank [3]. Countries of low-and-middle income are home to the majority of the world's young people and account for the majority of suicides [4]. The WHO classifies the Arab world as the Eastern Mediterranean Region (EMR) [5]. Although some EMR countries do not officially belong to the Arab League (The League of Arab States), the country distribution is predominantly aligned in both.

Based on burden-of-disease data from 2000, an analysis of patterns of suicide among people aged 15 or above in the countries of the WHO-EMR reports that the peak age for suicide among women is 15–29 years and that suicide accounts for 20% of all deaths among women in this age-group [6]. Within the Arab world, suicide rates among women and men were lowest in high-income countries (Bahrain, Kuwait, Oman, Qatar, Saudi Arabia and United Arab Emirates). Official statistics are likely to underreport actual rates, given sociocultural and religious taboos; likewise, mental conditions result in underreporting because of the attached stigma [7].

This chapter will offer an overview of suicide in the Arab world, with special emphasis on understanding the determinants of suicide by self-immolation in this region. Although frequently associated with the *Arab Spring* and viewed as protest, altruistic or predicament suicides, we will describe additional predisposing psychosocial factors and commonalities of self-immolations in order to formulate effective clinical approaches and prevention strategies.

2   Suicide in the Arab World

The most common suicide methods in the EMR are hanging (39.7%), poisoning (20.3%), self–immolation (17.4%), firearms (7%), drowning (3.1%), drug overdose (2.5%), and jumping from heights (0.8%). These methods account for 77.4% of all suicides in this region. The most common methods for men and women were hanging and poisoning, respectively. Self-immolation is the second most common suicide method for women in the EMR [6].

In the EMR, according to a WHO report from 2008, the difference in suicide methods is much larger between countries than between genders. Exceptions include very high incidence of self-immolations occurring almost exclusively by women in Afghanistan (see Chap. 4) and men in Tunisia. Choice of suicide methods varies across different cultures, depending on factors such as knowledge about effective lethal ways, which are sometimes culture-specific, and access to means [8]. Determining the prevalence of common methods of suicide is important from the perspective of prevention in order to and decrease suicide rates.

Worldwide and also regionally in the EMC, there is variability in frequency of self-immolation between genders. A study from Iran found that suicide by self-immolation is more prevalent in females (29.4%) than males (11.3%) [9]. In Afghanistan almost all self-immolators are young women (see Chap. 4). A reasonable generalization is that within the EMR, there is a high incidence of self-immolation in Muslim young women [6]. The fuel commonly used for burning is cooking and heating oil, which women have easy access to [6]. Self-immolation is considered a violent expression of distress and women who choose this method communicate rage and vengeance at their abusive spouses and families. Men who self-immolate in the Arab world do so in the context of political and national turmoil, and specifically as a reaction to shaming, brutality perpetrated by government officials and law enforcement agents, unemployment and financial distress. Self-immolation becomes an expression of impulsive protest against injustices, especially when rage, discontent, hopelessness and helplessness reach a threshold and no other solution seems effective to escape distress.

Like other religions, suicide is viewed as sinful by Islam, and killing oneself and others are considered transgressions. There are cultural precedents, however, that could encourage self-immolation in times of despair. The allegory of Ibrahim recounts how he survived execution by immolation with divine intervention. Ibrahim was sentenced to death and while being burned, having accepted his fate, was miraculously saved by Allah. The fire burned his chains freeing him and he was able to walk out of the flames unharmed. Many could rationalize that Allah's capacity to forgive all sins could justify acts of suicide, especially self-immolations, when suicide occurs in an environment of oppression, despair and helplessness. There are other cultural factors, nevertheless, that exalt martyrdom and self-sacrifice, not rooted in religion, that serve to endorse acts of self-immolation as heroic.

3   Self-Immolation: A Global Perspective

Self-immolation occurs more frequently in low-and-middle income countries. Countries with a high prevalence of self-immolation include Iran, Iraq, Afghanistan Tunisia and India. Common are also self-immolations in the Tibetan diaspora (see Chap. 8) and protest suicides during and after the *Arab Spring*, which attract international media attention. Self-immolators in countries with lower socioeconomic and education status tend to be young women experiencing human rights violations and extreme forms of abuse and oppression [10, 11].

Psychiatric diagnoses among self-immolators in high-income countries include psychotic disorders, substance use disorders, major depression, posttraumatic stress disorder and adjustment disorders [11–13]. Recent unemployment is a predisposing factor for self-immolation in high-income countries, especially in those with adjustment disorders [11, 13]. In low-and-middle-income countries self-immolation is highly prevalent, primarily affects women, and may be one of the most common suicide methods in regions of Central and South Asia and parts of Africa [11–14]. While in high-income countries self-immolation constitutes 0.6–1% of all suicides, in some low-income countries it comprises 40–70% of suicides [10, 12, 13]. In low-and-middle income countries, trauma and stressor-related disorders are the most common psychiatric diagnoses associated with self-immolation suicides [12, 13].

Self-immolation is widespread. Since 1940s, reports of self-immolations in the scientific literature include frequent incidents in China, India, Vietnam, United States of America, Czech Republic, Israel, Bulgaria, Germany and the United Kingdom [15–19]. In other countries it is a rare occurrence, with isolated reports in Japan, Spain, France, Sweden, Turkey, Italy, and Mexico [19].

The 17th of December 2010 marks a pivotal time in the Arab World when a Tunisian street vendor, Mohamed Bouazizi, set himself on fire being plagued by anger, humiliation and disgust, in protest against government officials. This event revolutionizied the Arab world and catalyzed the *Arab Spring*. His self-immolation was enacted by others soon thereafter in Algeria, Saudi Arabia, Mauritania, and Egypt [20–22]. Despite their relative infrequency at the time, these cases of self-immolation in the Arab world were of great significance given the fact that political uprising leading to major socio-political changes in the region followed in most of the corresponding countries.

4 Self-Immolation and the *Arab Spring*

Many historical accounts exist of self-immolation as politically driven or protest suicides acts [23, 24]. Politics and religion seem to be intertwined in Tibetan self-immolations more so than in most other politically driven suicides in other regions of the world. In the self-immolations that triggered the *Arab Spring* there seems to be a relative absence of religious motivations, and impulsivity, anger, poverty, despair, a sense of foreshortened future, and dissatisfaction with class differences and corrupt politicians served as triggering factors. The *Arab Spring* included a series of uprisings beginning with the index self-immolation of Bouazizi in Tunisia and spreading throughout Arab world countries, including Libya, Yemen, Syria, Bahrain, Morocco, Iraq, Algeria, parts of Iran, Lebanon, Jordan, Kuwait, Oman, Sudan, Western Sahara, and to a lesser extent Djibouti, Mauritania and Saudi Arabia.

On the 17th of December 2010, Tarek el-Tayeb Mohamed Bouazizi, a Tunisian street vendor, self-immolated in response to the confiscation of his wares and the harassment and humiliation inflicted upon him by a municipal official and her aides. Bouazizi was the victim of bullying and police brutality for years. He survived self-immolation but agonized for almost 3 weeks in a burn unit until his death on the fourth of January 2011 at the age of 26. Following Bouazizi's death, public anger and outcry intensified. Protests began within hours of his self-immolation and did not stop for weeks until the president of Tunisia, Zine El Abidine Ben Ali, stepped down after 23 years in power on 14 January 2011. He now lives in exile in Saudi Arabia [25]. In the 6 months following Bouazizi's death, there were 107 Tunisian self-immolations. Most were young unmarried men from poor, rural areas, with only basic education [26]. Since the *Arab Spring*, an average of 80 people per year self-immolate in Tunisia, *with close to one thousand deaths by self-immolation recorded in this small Arab country in the last decade* [27].

The success of the Tunisian protests, known as the *Jasmine Revolution*, inspired demonstrations in other Arab and non-Arab countries. The protests included copy-cat suicides (*Werther effect*) of several men who emulated Bouazizi's action in an attempt to bring an end to their own autocratic governments [28].

The first reported self-immolation following Bouazizi's death was that of Mohsen Bouterfif on 13 January 2011, a 37-year-old Algerian, who set himself on fire when his town's mayor refused to meet with him and others regarding employment and housing requests. According to the press, the mayor challenged him saying that if he had courage he would self-immolate as Bouazizi had done. He self-immolated and died on 24 January 2011 [29]. In a nearby Algerian Province, Maamir Lotfi, a 36-year-old unemployed father of six, was denied a meeting with the governor and self-immolated in front of the of El Oued's Town Hall on 17 January, dying on 12 February 2011 [30].

In Egypt, Abdou Abdel-Moneim Jaafar, a 49-year-old restaurant owner, self-immolated in front of the Egyptian Parliament. His act of protest helped instigate weeks of demonstrations leading to the resignation of Egyptian President Hosni Mubarak on 11 February 2011 and a change of government [31].

The wave of suicide by contagion reached Europe on 11 February 2011, in a case very similar to Bouazizi's. Noureddine Adnane, a 27-year-old Moroccan street vendor, set himself on fire in Palermo, in protest of the confiscation of his wares and the harassment that inflicted on him by municipal officials. He died 5 days later [32]. In Amsterdam, Kambiz Roustay, a 36-year-old asylum seeker from Iran, set himself on fire on Dam Square in protest of being rejected asylum. Roustay fled Iran after publishing works undermining the regime and feared being tortured [33]. Subsequently, self-immolations occurred in several other Arab countries including Saudi Arabia, Yemen, Lebanon, and Jordan. However, these suicides did not provoke the same kind of popular reaction and solidarity that Bouazizi's did in Tunisia or Jaafar's in Egypt [34–36].

The *Arab Spring* took place in the year 2011 with a wave of protests, uprisings and unrest powered by social media, that spread across Arabic-speaking countries in North Africa and the Middle East. It toppled governments in Tunisia, Egypt, Libya and Yemen, led to armed conflict and civil war in Syria, Libya, Iraq and Yemen, and created international awareness of the inequalities that fuelled the civil unrest throughout this region of the world [37].

5 Psychosocial and Psychiatric Aspects of Self-Immolation in Arab countries

Predisposing psychiatric, psychological and social determinants associated with self-immolation suicides in low-and-middle income countries are multifactorial and multidimensional. Some that are relevant in the Arab world include forced marriage at a young age, living in war-torn regions and countries, violence in the household, poverty, hunger, overcrowding, human rights violations, impulsivity, low education, unemployment, affective states of hopelessness and helplessness, and adjustment, depressive and syndromal or subsyndromal posttraumatic stress disorders (see Chap. 1, Table 1 and Sect. 3).

Although there is an anachronistic idealization of the *Jasmine Revolution* and *Arab Spring* self-immolators viewing them as martyrs or heroes, our clinical opinion is that most of these individuals were overwhelmed in states of despair, hopelessness and helplessness. There is no doubt that these law-abiding and secular struggling citizens triggered an extraordinary international movement. But their intentions may have been far from religious or political. A family member, Naafil Harshani, commented of the now iconic Mohamed Bouazizi: "what was important to Mohamed was putting food on the table, and football. He had nothing to do with politics and wanted nothing to do with politics" [38].

In the psychiatric literature there are three broad categories of motivational factors for suicide by self-immolation: political, cultural/religious, and mental health/substance abuse/relationship conflicts [39]. Although the perception is that most self-immolations are politically motivated, the majority are easily explained within the psychosocial and psychiatric framework [40]. Overall, adjustment disorder is a major risk factor for suicide by self-immolation. More broadly, psychopathology presents an increased risk of self-immolation. In male patients, adjustment disorders, harmful use of drugs, and depressive disorders increase the risk of self-immolation. Among females, posttraumatic stress disorder, adjustment disorders and depressive disorders increase the risk. As a result, access to mental health services, violence prevention programs designed for men, mental health awareness programs, support services for disenfranchised women, and alcohol and drug treatment programs for men are appropriate and imperative for suicide prevention [41].

6 Medico-Legal Aspects of Suicide

It is in the interest of public safety and proper functioning of the legal system that every case of suicide be confirmed and unambiguously differentiated from natural death, homicide, or accident [13]. This awareness is not yet integral to usual judicial practice and is one of the aims of collaboration between physicians and those involved in justice. On the other hand, workers in intensive burn care units face many challenges in assessing such medico-legal situations, especially in cases of self-immolation [42].

Many law articles across the Arab world address suicide. Egyptian Law does not punish suicide, yet it criminalizes and punishes anyone who assists suicide, according to Article 47, by imprisonment of no more than 3 years and/or financial penalty of no more than 3000 L.E [43]. Paragraph 3 of Article 408 of the Iraqi Penal Code expressly states that the attempt to commit suicide should not be criminalized as a punishment. The Iraqi legislation, Article 408, paragraph 1, imposes a prison sentence of no more than 7 years to anyone who incites or assists in suicide [44]. The law requires, in some cases, that suicide and killing of the soul be punished, as in Kuwaiti, Syrian and Iraqi law. In Jordanian law attempting suicide is not punishable unless the person is a soldier and attempts suicide to escape from military service [45].

Other Arab legislations take a different stance in this regard. Omani Law punishes attempt to commit suicide, stipulating that "he shall be punished by imprisonment for a period not exceeding 6 months and by a fine not exceeding three thousand Omani riyals, or by either of these two penalties. The same is true for Qatari law, as Article 157 of the Qatari Penal Code states that "anyone who commits suicide by taking any of the actions that may lead to his death shall be punished with imprisonment for a period not exceeding 1 year or a fine not exceeding one thousand riyals, or with two penalties. Sudanese law similarly stipulates in Article 133 that" whoever commits suicide by trying to kill himself by any means shall be punished with imprisonment for a period not exceeding 1 year or by a fine or by both."

The WHO's position [46] and the opinion of these authors is that decriminalization of suicide helps combat stigma and makes it easier for suicidal persons to seek help. Additionally, countries should develop and enact into law *comprehensive national suicide prevention strategies.* These usually include a clear set of best practices and evidence-based treatment guidelines. National strategies comprise surveillance, means restrictions, stigma reduction, raising awareness, media reporting guidelines, and training of healthcare workers and community volunteers. As of 2018, only 28 countries in the world had a national suicide prevention strategy. None of these are EMR countries [46].

7   Social Media and Suicide

The relationship between social media and suicide is a relatively new phenomenon that influences suicidal behavior. There is increasing evidence that social media affects and changes people's lives, especially teenagers, and sometimes adversely. Excessive use can become addictive causing dissociation, inattention, fatigue, dysphoria and, paradoxically, social isolation [47]. Of relevance is the cause and effect relationship between social media advertised suicides and younger generations being influenced by them. The first person who committed suicide live on a social media platform, Océane Ebem, an 18-year-old woman from Égly in the suburbs of Paris, explicitly said "I want to communicate a message, and I want it to be passed around, even if it is very shocking" [48]. In 2019, Nader Mohamed, 20, an engineering student at Helwan University in Cairo, reportedly was going through a psychological crisis. Nader informed a friend and posted on Twitter that he intended to commit suicide. A video from surveillance cameras showing him jump from Cairo Tower was leaked and became viral [49]. Those who post suicide notes online tend not to receive help [50]. Lately, Facebook and other social network platforms enforced policies to prevent glorification of such misfortunate events. Yet, research indicates that providing more online support for suicidal people would be more effective than shutting down pro-suicide websites [51].

The WHO emphasizes the role of Ministers of Health in providing leadership and bringing together stakeholders from other sectors to achieve effective suicide prevention. It is also important to improve surveillance at this stage [46]. In Egypt, hotlines such as the General Secretariat of Mental Health's hotline, receive psychological inquiries and offer psychological support, particularly to preventively engage those who wish to commit suicide. The National Council for Mental Health also runs a hotline to respond to psychological inquiries and crises [52].

8   Region-Specific Suicide Prevention

Self-immolation remains a significant contemporary problem in Arab countries. Its epidemiology, causes, and prevention intervention strategies require adjustment between higher- and lower-income countries. This classification by income is not arbitrary, as it correlates with other measures of development. The epidemiologic patterns revealed demonstrate distinct differences, suggesting differing causes and intervention strategies. We need more studies to distinguish associations from underlying causes and identify efficient points of intervention [40].

Prevention strategies are manifold. First and foremost, it is important not to idealize self-immolation suicides as heroic, altruistic or purely as predicament suicides. Other peaceful and less violent ways of protest can be effective in achieving social changes.

We are not trying to be dismissive of the cultural and religious context of populations with high prevalence of self-immolation, as a transcultural framework is essential to engage persons in suicide prevention efforts. Severe psychosocial stressors need to be recognized and creative clinical efforts that are culturally informed implemented to alleviate distress, increase interconnectedness, reduce alienation and help suicidal persons find hope and accept help.

The first and last chapter of this book summarize WHO suicide prevention strategic guidelines (see Table 2 in Chap. 1 for a detailed description) [46]. Universal, selective and indicated interventions should be realized in Arab countries. These could include increasing access to mental health care, decreasing harmful use of substances, promoting responsible media reporting and implementing mental health policies that protect individuals prone to victimization by shaming, humiliation and violence. Training religious and community leaders is as important as training clinicians to identify persons at risk. Most importantly, legislation needs to be decreed to safeguard vulnerable groups, preserve social ties and protect individuals from feeling alienated and expendable. Lastly, countries in the EMR/Arab world need to design and implement national suicide prevention strategies.

9 Conclusion

Historically associated with protest and political uprising, self-immolations in the Arab world are perhaps more commonly the result of trauma and stressor related disorders, intolerable affective states, social oppression, human rights violations, and experiencing severe and enduring psychosocial stressors. Within the EMR, there is a high incidence of self-immolation in Muslim young women. Self-immolation is considered a violent expression of distress and women who choose this method communicate rage and vengeance to abusive spouses and families. Men who self-immolate in the Arab world seem to do it as an expression of impulsive protest against injustices, especially when rage, discontent, hopelessness and helplessness reach a threshold and no other solution seems effective to escape distress.

Nowadays, there is an urgent need to work in suicide research and prevention. Despite the fact that countries throughout the world achieved important developments in understanding and preventing suicide, the Arab world still faces extraordinary challenges. Several indicators urge to move the field forward in the region. These include the emergence of social media as a new voice for suicide, the observed social effect of suicide in the community, novel techniques improving the prediction of suicidal behavior, harnessing new technologies to monitor and intervene when there is suicide risk, moving toward a more refined understanding of people at risk and developing tailored prevention interventions that are culturally informed. However, many challenges remain, as the ability to predict suicide is still not much better than chance. The work presented in this chapter only hopes to encourage new synergies and opportunities for interdisciplinary research in the field of suicide prevention in the Arab world.

References

1. World Health Organization. Global Health Estimates 2016: deaths by cause, age, sex, by country and by region, 2000–2016. Geneva: World Health Organization; 2018. https://www.who.int/news-room/detail/09-09-2019-suicide-one-person-dies-every-40-seconds.
2. Arab human development report 2016. https://www.undp.org/content/dam/rbas/report/AHDR%20Reports/AHDR%202016/AHDR%20Final%202016/AHDR2016En.pdf. Accessed 10 Mar 2020
3. World Bank. https://data.worldbank.org/indicator/SH.STA.SUIC.P5. Accessed 25 Mar 2020
4. McKinnon B, Gariépy G, Sentenac M, Elgar FJ. Adolescent suicidal behaviours in 32 low-and middle-income countries. Bull World Health Organ. 2016;94:340–50.
5. World Health Organization. www.emro.who.int/ar/emhj-vol-20-2014/volume-20-issue-10/invited-review-injuries-and-violence-in-the-eastern-mediterranean-region-a-review-of-the-health-economic-and-social-burden.html. Accessed 25 March 2020.
6. Morovatdar N, Moradi-Lakeh M, Malakouti SK, Nojomi M. Most common methods of suicide in Eastern Mediterranean Region of WHO: a systematic review and meta-analysis. Arch Suicide Res. 2013;17:335–44.
7. Malakouti SK, Davoudi F, Khalid S, Ahmadzad-Asl M, Khan M, Alirezaie N, Mirabzadeh A, De Leo D. The epidemiology of suicide behaviors among the countries of the Eastern Mediterranean Region of WHO: a systematic review. Acta Med Iran. 2015;53:257–65.
8. Bachmann S. Epidemiology of suicide and the psychiatric perspective. Int J Environ Res Public Health. 2018;15(7):1425.
9. Ahmadi M, Ranjbaran H, Azadbakht M, Heidari Gorji M, Heidari Gorji A. A survey of characteristics of self-immolation in the northern iran. Ann Med Health Sci Res Sep. 2014;4(Suppl 3):S228–32.
10. Laloë V. Patterns of deliberate self-burning in various parts of the world: a review. Burns. 2004;30(3):207–15.
11. Zamani SN, Bagheri M, Nejad MA. Investigation of the demographic characteristics and mental health in self-immolation attempters. Int J High-Risk Behav Addict. 2013;2(2):77–81.
12. Suhrabi Z, Delpisheh A, Taghinejad H. Tragedy of women's self-immolation in Iran and developing communities: a review. Int J Burn Trauma. 2012;2(2):93–104.
13. Poeschla B. Self-immolation: socioeconomic, cultural and psychiatric patterns. Burns. 2011;37(6):1049–57.
14. Sheth H, Dziewulski P, Settle JAD. Self-inflicted burns: a common way of suicide in the Asian population. A 10-year retrospective study. J Burns. 1994;20(4):334–5.
15. Hanna VN, Ahmed A. Suicide in the Kurdistan region of Iraq, state of the art. Nordic J Psychiatr. 2009;63:280–4.
16. Shadow Tibet: Jamyang Norbu » Blog Archive » Self-immolation and buddhism. https://www.nytimes.com/2013/02/15/world/asia/100th-self-immolation-inside-tibet-is-reported.html. https://www.jamyangnorbu.com. Accessed 25 Mar 2020.

17. Lensman attempts suicide. https://timesofindia.indiatimes.com/ show/7536272.cms. The Times of India. February 20, 2011. Accessed 25 Mar 2020.
18. Zarghami M. Selection of person of the year from public health perspective: promotion of mass clusters of copycat self-immolation. Iran J Psychiatry Behav Sci Spring. 2012;6(1):1–11.
19. List of political self-immolations. http://en.wikipedia.org/wiki/List_of_political_self-immolations. Accessed 12 Mar 2020.
20. Algerian dies from self-immolation. https://www.aljazeera.com/news/africa/2011/01/20111162363063915.html. Al Jazeera English. Accessed 25 Mar2020.
21. Man dies in Saudi self-immolation. https://www.news.com.au/world/breaking-news/saudi-man-dies-from-self-immolation/newsstory/d4c0b7f94fe1b5a37bfa022ee4fe732012260465. BBC News. 2011. Accessed 25 Mar 2020.
22. Mauritanian man sets himself ablaze in capital. https://www.foxnews.com/world/second-egyptian-sets-himself-on-fire. Accessed 25 Mar 2020.
23. LaFraniere S (January 9, 2012). More Monks Die by Fire in Protest of Beijing. https://www.nytimes.com/2012/01/10/world/asia/3-monks-deaths-show-rise-of-self-immolation-among-tibetans.html. The New York Times. Accessed 1 Mar 2020.
24. Shadow Tibet: Jamyang Norbu » Blog Archive » Self-immolation and Buddhism. http://www.jamyangnorbu.com/blog/2012/01/03/self-immolation-and-buddhism/. https://www.jamyang-norbu.com. Accessed 1 Mar 2020.
25. Fahim K (21 January 2011). Slap to a Man's Pride Set Off Tumult in Tunisia. https://www.nytimes.com/2011/01/22/world/africa/22sidi.html?_r=1&pagewanted=2&src=twrhp. New York Times. p. 2. Accessed 23 Jan 2011.
26. BBC News—Tunisia one year on: New trend of self-immolations. https://www.bbc.co.uk/news/world-africa-16526462. Bbc.co.uk. 12 January 2012. Accessed 12 Mar 2020.
27. Blaise L. Self-immolation, catalyst of the Arab Spring, is now a grim trend. https://www.nytimes.com/2017/07/09/world/africa/self-immolation-catalyst-of-the-arab-spring-is-now-a-grim-trend.html. Accessed 23 Mar 2020.
28. Worth RF. (21 January 2011). How a Single Match Can Ignite a Revolution. https://www.nytimes.com/2011/01/23/weekinreview/23worth.html. New York Times. Accessed 26 Mar 2020.
29. Xinhua (25 January 2011). Algeria reports 2nd death of self-immolation. https://en.wikipedia.org/wiki/2011_Algerian_self-immolations. China Daily. Accessed 25 Mar 2020.
30. Quatrième décès par immolation en Algérie, à la veille de la marche du 12 février. http://www.jeuneafrique.com/Article/ARTJAWEB20110212105526/algerie-pauvrete-tunisie-manifestationquatrieme-deces-par-immolation-en-algerie-a-la-veille-de-la-marche-du-12-fevrier.html. Jeune Afrique (in French). 12 February 2011. Accessed 25 Mar 2020.
31. In Egypt, man sets himself on fire, driven by economic woes. http://english.ahram.org.eg/NewsContent/1/2/4115/Egypt/Society/In-Egypt,-man-sets-himself-on-fire.aspx. English Al-Ahram. 17 January 2011. Accessed 25 Mar 2020.
32. Street Vendor Sets Himself on Fire in Palermo, Critical. https://listverse.com/2011/03/10/10-horrifying-acts-of-self-immolation/. Accessed 25 Mar 2020.
33. Iraniër waarschuwde al voor wanhoopsdaad. https://www.at5.nl/artikelen/60029/iranier-waarschuwde-al-voor-wanhoopsdaad. At5.nl. 7 April 2011. Accessed 4 Mar 2020.
34. Man dies after setting himself on fire in Saudi Arabia. https://www.bbc.co.uk/news/world-middle-east-12260465. BBC News. 23 January 2011. Accessed 20 Mar 2020.
35. Man dies in possible first self-immolation in Saudi https://en.wikipedia.org/wiki/Timeline_of_the_2011–12_Saudi_Arabian_protests_(January–April_2011). Accessed 25 Mar 2020.
36. Corporatist Collapse in Tunisia. 2018. Labor Politics in North Africa, 94–122.
37. Burhani AN. Fatwās on Mohamed Bouazizi's Self-Immolation: Religious Authority, Media, and Secularization. In: Daniels T, editor. Sharia dynamics. Cham: Contemporary Anthropology of Religion. Palgrave Macmillan; 2017.
38. The Arab Spring- Facts and information–National Geographic. https://www.nationalgeographic.com/culture/topics/reference/arab-spring-cause/. Accessed 25 Mar 2020.

39. Jordan Times. The (Amman, Jordan) 18 December 2011, NEWS. NewsBank. Web. 26 October 2016.
40. Ahmadi A, Mohammadi R, Schwebel DC, et al. Psychiatric disorders (Axis I & II) and self-immolation: a case–control study from Iran. Inj Prevent. 2010;16:A7.
41. Gray SJ. Thesis submitted in partial fulfilment of the degree of Doctor of Psychology. Victoria: College of Arts, Victorian University; 2014.
42. Ermenc B, Prijon T. Suicide, accident? The importance of the scene investigation. Forensic Sci Int. 2005;147:S21–4.
43. Yasti AC, Tumer AR, Atli M, Tutuncu T, Derinoz A, Kama NA. A clinical forensic scientist in the burn's unit: necessity or not? A prospective clinical study. Burns. 2006;32:77–82. (Penal Code. Article 47. Government of Egypt.
44. Iraqi Penal Code. https://wikimili.com/en/Iraqi_Penal_Code. Accessed 25 Mar 2020.
45. Criminal Code, Article 339. Government of Jordan.
46. WHO. Preventing suicide: a global imperative. Geneva: World Health Organization; 2014. https://apps.who.int/iris/bitstream/handle/10665/131056/9789241564779_eng.pdf;jsessionid=4DB114A485E61068593DDC2ACC1BEB4F?sequence=1.
47. Tingle J. Preventing suicides: developing a strategy. Br J Nurs. 2015;24(11):592–3.
48. Dasgupta R. The first social media suicide. The Guardian. (August 29, 2017).
49. Memo Middle East Monitor. https://www.middleeastmonitor.com/20191202-engineering-student-jumps-from-187-metre-cairo-tower/.
50. Severson G. Facebook trying to prevent suicide by tracking what we post. KARE. 2019-01-01.
51. Science Alert. https://www.sciencealert.com/online-suicide-support-needed. Accessed 18 Mar 2020.
52. Egyptian Ministry of Health. http://www.mohp.gov.eg/. Accessed 16 Mar 2020.

Self-Immolation in High-Income Countries

Renato Antunes dos Santos, Bipin Ravindran, Saulo Castel, and Eduardo Chachamovich

"Vous avez détruit la beauté du monde!"
Huguette Gaulin Bergeron, (1944–1972), French Canadian novelist.
"You have destroyed the beauty of the world!"
Said Huguette while committing suicide by self-immolation in a major street of Montréal, in 1972. Huguette expressed deep concerns about ecological issues. The Questions about mental health can't diminish her message. Still, her words can be heard in the song in her tribute [1, 2].

Hymne À La Beauté Du Monde
De Christian Saint-Roch
Interpreté pour Diane Dufresne

R. A. dos Santos (✉)
Department of Psychiatry, The University of Toronto, Waypoint Centre for Mental Health Care, Toronto, ON, Canada
e-mail: renato.psiquiatria@gmail.com

B. Ravindran
Hunter New England Mental Health Service, Newcastle, NSW, Australia

School of Medicine and Public Health, The University of Newcastle, Callaghan, NSW, Australia
e-mail: Bipin.Ravindran@health.nsw.gov.au

S. Castel
Sunnybrook Health Sciences Centre, Toronto, ON, Canada

Department of Psychiatry, University of Toronto, Toronto, ON, Canada
e-mail: saulo.Castel@sunnybrook.ca

E. Chachamovich
Department of Psychiatry, McGill University, Montreal, QC, Canada

Northern Mental Health Program, McGill Group for Suicide Studies (MGSS), Douglas Mental Health University Institute, Montreal, QC, Canada
e-mail: eduardo.chachamovich@mcgill.ca

© The Author(s), under exclusive license to Springer Nature Switzerland AG 2021
C. A. Alfonso et al. (eds.), *Suicide by Self-Immolation*, https://doi.org/10.1007/978-3-030-62613-6_10

Ne tuons pas la beauté du monde /
Ne tuons pas la beauté du monde /
Ne tuons pas la beauté du monde /
Chaque fleur, chaque arbre que l'on tue /
Revient nous tuer à son tour /
Ne tuons pas la beauté du monde /
Ne tuons pas le chant des oiseaux /
Ne tuons pas le bleu du jour /
Ne tuons pas la beauté du monde /
Ne tuons pas la beauté du monde /
Ne tuons pas la beauté du monde /

La dernière chance de la terre /
C'est maintenant qu'elle se joue /
Ne tuons pas la beauté du monde /
Faisons de la terre un grand jardin /
Pour ceux qui viendront après nous /
Après nous /
Ne tuons pas la beauté du monde /
La dernière chance de la terre /
C'est maintenant qu'elle se joue /
Ne tuons pas la beauté du monde /
Faisons de la terre un grand jardin /
Pour ceux qui viendront après nous /
Après nous

1   Introduction

The World Bank defines a high-income country as one where the Gross National Income (GNI) divided by the number of inhabitants is 12,376 US dollars or more *per capita* [3]. This definition does not take into consideration distribution of wealth or inequality within the country. A country with a large number of struggling persons facing considerable social and economic hardship coexisting with extremely wealthy individuals would still be classified as a high-income country. The *Gini index* measures wealth distribution within a country or region, where 0 represents perfect equality and 100 represents gross inequality. Countries with an index lower than 30 are thought to have more equitable income distribution. Countries like Panama or the United States, while both listed as high-income, have a Gini index close to 50, while countries such as Slovenia, Finland, Belgium, Norway, Iceland, Czech Republic and Netherlands are high-income countries with a Gini index of 25–28 and more equitable wealth distribution [4]. Figure 1 shows the 80 high-income countries in the world and Table 1 lists all high-income countries with their respective Gini coefficients categorized by continent.

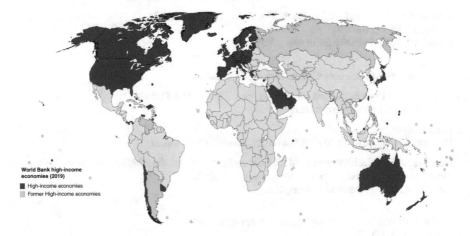

Fig. 1 World Bank high-income countries

Table 1 High-income countries and Gini indices[a], categorized by continent

Continent	Country	Population	Gini index
Africa	Seychelles	98,347	46.8
Asia	Bahrain	170,175	N/A
	Brunei	437,479	N/A
	Cyprus	120,759	31.4
	Hong Kong	749,681	54.0
	Israel	8,655,535	39.0
	Japan	126,476,610	32.9
	Kuwait	4,270,571	N/A
	Oman	510,626	N/A
	Qatar	2,881,053	41.1
	Saudi Arabia	34,813,871	45.9
	Singapore	585,042	45.8
	South Korea	51,269,850	31.6
	Taiwan	23,816,775	33.8
	U.A. E	9,890,402	32.5
Europe	Andorra	77,265	N/A
	Austria	9,006,398	29.7
	Belgium	11,589,623	27.4
	Croatia	4,105,267	30.4
	Czech Republic	10,708,981	24.9
	Denmark	5,792,202	28.7
	Estonia	1,326,535	30.4
	Finland	5,540,720	27.4
	France	65,273,511	31.6
	Germany	83,783,942	31.9
	Greece	10,423,054	34.4
	Hungary	9,660,351	30.6
	Iceland	341,343	26.8
	Ireland	4,937,786	32.8
	Italy	60,461,826	35.9
	Latvia	1,886,198	35.6
	Liechtenstein	38,128	N/A
	Lithuania	2,722,890	37.3
	Luxembourg	625,978	34.9
	Malta	441,543	29.2
	Monaco	39,542	N/A
	Netherlands	17,134,872	28.5
	Norway	5,421,241	27.0
	Poland	37,846,611	29.7
	Portugal	10,196,709	33.8
	San Marino	33,931	N/A
	Slovakia	5,459,642	25.2

(continued)

Table 1 (continued)

Continent	Country	Population	Gini index
	Slovenia	2,078,938	24.2
	Spain	46,754,778	34.7
	Sweden	10,099,265	28.8
	Switzerland	8,654,622	32.7
	United Kingdom	67,886,011	34.8
North America	Antigua and Barbuda	97,929	N/A
	Aruba	106,766	N/A
	Bahamas	393,244	57.0
	Barbados	287,375	32.0
	Bermuda	62,278	N/A
	B.V.I.	30,231	N/A
	Canada	37,742,154	33.8
	Cayman Islands	65,722	N/A
	Panama	4,314,767	49.2
	Puerto Rico	2,860,853	57.0
	Saint Kitts	53,199	N/A
	Sint Martin	38,666	N/A
	Saint Maarten	42,876	N/A
	Trinidad Tobago	1,399,488	40.3
	Turks and Caicos	38,717	N/A
	United States	331,002,651	41.4
Oceania	Australia	25,499,884	34.4
	French Polynesia	280,908	N/A
	Guam	168,775	N/A
	New Caledonia	285,498	N/A
	New Zealand	4,822,233	32.5
	Northern Mariana	57,559	N/A
	Palau	18,094	N/A
South America	Chile	19,116,201	44.4
	Uruguay	3,473,730	39.7

[a]A higher GINI index generally indicates problematic income inequality

High-income countries are a heterogeneous group with differences that may impact access to health care and quality of education, social and economic life. Moreover, high-income countries have countless cultural differences, languages, social and economic structures, population size, climate zones, and ecological distributions [5, 6]. Social and economic inequality within a country might be important in terms of life impact and perception of burden [7].

Factors that include mental health disorders, social isolation, financial problems, political protest, protests against unfair situations, and gender inequalities might act as precipitants or predispose persons to suicide by self-immolation. But how does one explain, for example, that the number of admissions for self-inflicted burns to a burns' unit is ten times higher in Israel than in the United Kingdom? [8]. The majority of persons who self-immolate in low- and-middle-income countries tend to be married women, living in poverty, with low levels of education, limited employment opportunities, facing violence at home and struggling in conflictual marital relationships [9]. While we understand disproportions in the determinants of self-immolations when comparing high-income to low-and-middle-income countries, psychosocial differences that predispose to suicide in high-income countries elude social scientists and clinicians.

Self-immolation is a particularly violent form of suicide that inflicts enormous pain on the victim and becomes tangible to witnesses of the act [10]. Unlike other forms of suicide, self-immolation organically disintegrates the physical border between self and other, creating a continuum between the person engulfed in fire and his or her audience that transcends the proxemic interpersonal space in an impactful way.

Etymologically, immolation relates to sacrifice [11]. The symbolic representations of suicide by self-immolation in Western philosophy includes accounts of Empedocles who threw himself into Mt. Etna, an act which inspired drama and poetry, and Peregrinus Proteus who self-immolated on a funeral pyre during the 165 AD Olympian Games after being ex-communicated from the Christian community. Self-immolation is also represented iconographically in the arts. In the final book of *Lord of the Rings,* Denethor orders his men to set him alight after pouring an accelerant over himself. Similarly, in the final scene of Wagner's opera, *Der Ring des Nibelungen*, Brünnhilde rides her horse into the pyre she has lit for her lover [12].

The aim of this chapter is to better understand what motivates self-immolation in high income countries. We will review data gathered from scientific sources (PubMed, Web of Science, Embase) and grey literature (documents, web news and articles) to better address the complexities of this important and often neglected topic.

2   Characteristics of Self-Immolations in High-Income Countries

Table 2 summarizes characteristics of self-immolation in high-income countries in Europe, North America, Australia and New Zealand.

2.1   Demographics

Although suicide is a common cause of death in high-income countries [22], self-immolation appears to be infrequent. Most studies show that self-immolation constitutes about 1% of all suicides. These studies tend to be retrospective forensic examinations that include details such as the extent of burn lesions, presence of smoke intoxication and burn shock [19].

Table 2 Characteristics of self-immolations in high-income countries

Country	Study period	Prevalence	Gender distribution	Average age	Other demographics	Location and accelerant
Australia and New Zealand [13, 14]	2009–2013	17.7% of admissions to Burns Unit	M > F	–	–	Indoor and petrol
	2005–2009	2.2% of admissions to Burns Unit	M > F	36	Majority are NZ and Australian nationals	–
Canada [15]	1986–1988	1% of all suicides	M > F	38	–	Familiar place or remote location
England [15, 16]	2005–2014	2% of admissions to Burns Unit	M > F	35	Majority are Caucasian; 36% are unemployed	–
	1978–1992	1–2% of all suicides	M > F	43	Majority are British; unmarried	Indoor or Outside (often alone)
Germany [17]	1990–2000	0.76% of all suicides	M > F	42	Majority are Germans	Outside and petrol
France [18]	2004–2008	14.7% of admissions to Burns Unit	F > M	38	Majority married	Indoor and petrol
Ireland [8]	12 years (unspecified)	4.2% of admissions to Burns Unit	F > M	38	Majority are Irish; 65% are unemployed, 75% are single or separated	–
Italy [19]	1993–2016	0.8% of all suicides	M > F	48	Majority are Italian nationals	–
Switzerland [20]	2000–2010	1.02% of all suicides	M > F	42	Majority are Swiss nationals, employed or on a pension	Indoor and petrol
United States [21]	1994–2002	1.5% of admissions to Burns Unit	M > F	36	Majority are Caucasian	–

Epidemiological studies in high-income countries clearly establish that suicide in general is more common in men than women. This does not apply to gender differences of self-immolations around the world, where the majority occur in low- and middle-income countries and women choose this method of suicide more often than men. In the high-income countries of Ireland and France, women self-immolate more often than men [18, 23]. Yet, in other high-income countries up to 70% of people who self-immolate are men, and the majority are unmarried (single, separated, divorced, or widowed) [20]. In contrast, in Ireland and France 75% of women who self-immolate are single or separated [8]. Male self-immolators in high-income countries tend to be older. From a socioeconomic perspective, data sets point in different directions. In Switzerland the majority of self-immolators are employed or on a fixed income, while in Ireland they are unemployed.

2.2 Place and Method

In Germany, about 65% of self-immolators choose an outside location [17]. In contrast, in England, self-immolations usually occur at home, in a car, or garden [10]. The majority of the individuals doused themselves using a liquid accelerant, usually petrol. The percentage of alcohol, medication or other psychoactive drugs found in toxicology analyses of self-immolators also varies widely [23].

2.3 Associations, Motivations and Mental Health

Research studies on self-immolation in the *United States* indicate an association with psychiatric disorders, including substance use disorders, along with poor impulse control and impairment of judgement. Up to one third of persons who self-immolate in the United States have a pre-existing documented psychiatric disorder [9, 23, 24]. In *England*, 45% have a psychiatric diagnosis, and up to one third are in a state of acute decompensation prior to the time of death [16]. Psychiatric multi-morbidities are common, including major depression, schizophrenia, personality disorders, and anxiety disorders [10]. In *Ireland*, 79% of those who self-immolate have mental disorders, mostly major depression and alcohol dependence, and 63% had prior history of suicide attempts. In the same study, 22% of self-immolation suicides were clearly planned, and 13% occurred in states of acute alcohol intoxication. The remaining cases included explicit acts of protest of human rights violations of minority groups, resisting discharge from a hospital, or avoiding a court appearance [8].

A study from *Germany* reports that very few self-immolators leave a farewell note. Psychological autopsies showed that separation from a partner and financial problems were the leading precipitants in about 60% of cases. General health problems occurred in 26%, mental health disorders in 65%, and prior suicide attempts in

36% of cases [17]. In *Australia*, 75% of self-immolators had a psychiatric disorder, including mood disorders, anxiety disorders and personality disorders. In addition, about 75% also had an identified contributing stressful life event [25]. In *France*, 42% of the patients with self-inflicted burns had a depressive disorder and two-thirds a previous suicide attempt [18]. In *Canada*, 40% of self-immolators had a previously diagnosed psychiatric illness and 1% a diagnosis of schizophrenia [15]. We believe that in high-income countries, as in low-and-middle-income countries, posttraumatic and stressor related disorders may be underdiagnosed and could be relevant in persons who suicide by self-immolation.

In a study of suicide by self-immolation in Washington State in the United States, during an 11-year period between 1996 and 2009, persons with Asian or Pacific Islander background were over-represented compared to other ethnicities [26]. In England, a retrospective study on self-immolations similarly found that people having an Asian background were at greater risk, in particular women [10]. Another study of immigrants from the Indian subcontinent, East Africa and the Caribbean who relocated to England and Wales, found that 20% of all suicides were women immigrants [27]. The authors of this study suggested that contributors to the higher suicide rate may include the traditional role that immigrants from the subcontinent place on academic and economic success, the stigmatization of failures, and the continued assignment of women to rigid social and familial hierarchical roles post migration, along with the pressures exerted on them and their families by the dowry system [27].

3   The Mind and the Environment: Psychodynamics

Some assert that self-immolation is often an impulsive act, and impulsivity is a trait found in persons who suicide [25]. Studies in high-income countries found a positive correlation between suicide by self-immolation and personality disorders [10, 28]. While mood disorders are commonly associated with death by suicide, personality disorders are present in a significant proportion of patients who self-mutilate [28, 29]. Drawing on Linehan's seminal work on borderline personality disorder [30], Wiechman and colleagues discuss how burning the body may have "important mood regulatory properties" and how both parasuicidal and suicidal burns can be seen as a "maladaptive solution to the problem of overwhelming, uncontrollable, and intensely painful negative feelings". The authors discuss how an important challenge of care provision for patients with borderline personality disorder can be the very component of effective burn care. The compassion and attention to the patient's emotional and physical distress offered in the burn unit can reinforce the dysfunctional coping strategy of self-harm, encouraging a "return to the emotional sanctuary provided by the burn unit" [28]. Other studies explored links between neuroticism and self-immolation, a trait that can be a risk factor for "postburn psychosocial complications, ineffective coping strategies, heightened scar related perceived stigmatization, and the development of psychopathology" [31].

4 Challenges to Mental and Physical Health

Rashid and Gowar examined the admission trends of patients in the Birmingham Burns Centre in the UK over a 20-year period between 1979 and 1998 [32]. They found that patients with self-inflicted burns had a significantly higher average burn size (67% Total Burn Surface Area -TBSA) and an associated mortality of 44% when compared to accidental burns, and accelerant dousing was more common in this group, leading to deeper and more extensive burns. The authors also noted a steady increase of admissions over a 20-year period for this group of patients.

A study on self-inflicted burns over a 40-year period at a Zurich Burns' Unit revealed that suicide attempts significantly increased the risks of mortality in burns patients and were statistically even better at predicting mortality than standardised tools like ABSI (The Abbreviated Burn Severity Index) [9]. The factors increasing the risk of mortality included co-morbid physical and psychiatric illness increasing likelihood of polypharmacy, drug and alcohol use, delirium from substance withdrawal, medication interactions and major side-effects of psychotropic medications, and inflammatory processes associated with depression that could compromise immune function and survival. Mortality risk seem highest in the early phase of treatment when the patient, often being sedated and intubated, is unable to participate in the treatment process.

5 Challenges of Care for Patients after Self-Immolation

People who self-immolate and are hospitalized in burn units have extensive burns requiring additional resources and attention from staff in burn centers [32]. For this reason, the team managing the care of self-inflicted burn patients should be multidisciplinary, including mental health professionals, and involving trained specialised nurses, given that patients tend to be agitated and potentially aggressive during change of dressings. Psychological challenges and psychiatric complications in patients being treated with self-immolation burns include the profound levels of stress experienced by their families who often face significant shame and guilt, challenges of psychiatric interviewing due to patients being too sick to fluently engage in the process, scarce availability of psychiatric records and collateral history, and complex interactions between psychotropics and other medications [33].

It is important to recognise the ongoing suicide risk of patients being treated following self-immolation. Psychiatric care for these patients by experienced consultation and liaison teams may be a critical component of care [34]. Factors responsible for increased suicide risk in suicidal burn patients after discharge include isolation and depression complicated by pain and disfigurement from burn injuries [35]. The early involvement of psychiatric consultation liaison services along with assertive psychiatric treatment improves outcomes [24].

An important aspect of treatment of suicidal persons in burn units is the negative countertransference of caregivers and staff, including pervasive feelings of grief and horror, irritation and anger towards the patient, and feelings that the patient may be undeserving of attention and time [13, 33].

Strategies that could be employed for effective management of self-inflicted burn injuries in patients with emotionally unstable personality disorders include validating the patient's suffering without reinforcing behaviours that are negative, consistency of care, avoiding excessive limit setting and providing a psychiatric care plan after discharge from the burn unit [28]. If possible, joint medical-surgical–psychiatric rounds should take place and dedicated specialised mental health providers should be involved in treatment, as well as chaplains offering spiritual counselling [33].

Caring for patients who self-immolate involves bioethical principles of beneficence, nonmaleficence, autonomy, collaboration and self-determination. At times, the ongoing suffering of the patient associated with an increasingly poor prognosis poses clinical challenges. Palliative interventions and comfort care are essential to optimize quality of life. Decisions to forgo life-sustaining treatments in consultation with ethics committees need to involve patients or their surrogates, after medical futility is thoroughly explained and clearly, respectfully and collaboratively processed [33].

6   Refugees and Asylum Seekers in High-Income Countries

Cases among asylum seekers who self-immolate in high-income countries attract media attention. Some high-income countries maintain people seeking asylum in detention centres, others pay less developed countries to manage their refugees and asylum seekers. After dangerously escaping inhumane conditions, people seeking asylum experience fear, hunger and violence, and are sometimes relocated to detention facilities in a poor country payed by a wealthy one [36]. Examples include Australia's offshore and Greek island detention centres [37]. Human rights violations are rampant, and children may be separated from their parents and detained for indefinite periods of time [38]. The lack of ethnographic and qualitative scientific studies in this area reminds us of the famous quote by Kurt Tucholsky attributed to Joseph Stalin: "The death of one man is a tragedy. The death of millions is a statistic." A case in point is that of the Iranian refugee Omid Masoumali, who set himself on fire in front of visiting UNHCR officials at the detention centre run by the Australian government on the Pacific island of Nauru in April 2016. Omid and his partner had arrived in Australia by boat and had been initially detained in Christmas Island, prior to detention in Nauru, and received refugee status in Nauru. The description of the suffering experienced by asylum seekers in Nauru as "burning hell" was prophetic of the series of self-immolations that ensued [39].

A week after Omid's self-immolation, Hodan, a 21-year-old Somali refugee, set herself on fire at Nauru, soon after she had been sent back to the detention centre after receiving treatment in Brisbane. Both Omid and Hodan succumbed to their injuries. NGO representatives described these incidents, documenting an epidemic of self-harm in Nauru. The Papua New Guinea (PNG) highest court ruled that detention of refugees on Manus Island was illegal and unconstitutional, and the centre's closure followed. The UNHCR (United Nation High Commissioner for Refugees) spokesperson in Canberra reiterated the consensus opinion amongst medical experts of the immense harm to the physical and mental health of the detainees from conditions in detention centres, requiring the urgent need to relocate them to more humane settings [40].

An asylum seeker trapped in a detention centre is multiply traumatised. Repeatedly failing in the immigration process, the trauma of displacement is perpetuated by further socio-political marginalisation. From a dialogical analytical perspective, self-immolation has been described as an act of communication, as an "attempt to restore intersubjectivity in the face of a loss of social recognition", and one where the audience is forced to not simply demonstrate "distant compassion" but are "encouraged to engage and self-reflect about local injustices and activism within their own vicinities [41].

7   Discussion and Analyses

Suicide by self-immolation in high-income countries varies widely. Beyond the literature review and description by country, this chapter explores a series of questions about the repeated "trues" taken for granted in this literature. It demonstrates that there are new forms of interpretation of this data, contributing to new knowledge in the field.

The classification of countries as high or low income based on their economic indicators is questionable as income may be a just one component of the cultural or social characteristics of countries and such classification may not reflect other similarities among them. The cultural differences between countries are remarkable, including language, relationship with work, human rights, social support and assistance, distribution of wealth and universal access to health care, educational opportunities and social services.

Most studies of suicide by self-immolation in high-income countries show that the majority of suicides are of nationals of the same country. Thus, self-immolation being more common among immigrants is a myth. Nevertheless, the mental and physical status of displaced individuals (asylum seekers and refugees) arriving in high-income country must be taken into account, and isolated cases that attract media attention forcefully convey mistreatment and xenophobic attitudes.

From a sociological perspective, people with deep existential questions and suffering are more likely to search for mental health care in high-income countries, since access to care is possible in these countries. Durkheim's observations and research findings showed that economic problems increase risk of suicide [42]. Together with relationship problems, these are the most frequent motivations found in the self-immolation studies in high-income countries.

Undeniably, there are high rates of a mental health illness and distress in the health history of persons who self-immolate. Mental and existential suffering precedes suicide by self-immolation and timely access to mental health treatment may prevent suicide.

8 Conclusions

All suicides are potentially avoidable deaths [22, 43]. The psychodynamic determinants of self-immolation may include the perception of unbearable social pressure and a complete lack of power to solve problems that destructively impact life and trigger affective states of hopelessness, rage, thwarted belongingness and perceived burdensomeness. These dynamics are also present in political or cultural suicides throughout the world, such as Tibetan monks who suicide against social injustices and political displacement, Afghan women against a system of misogyny and violence, or Italians and Germans against the financial system and economic domination. In all these instances, the social context, "the system", becomes an insurmountable barrier that is impossible for one person alone to overcome.

To a greater or lesser extent, in every country, lives are affected by a perception of overwhelming personal problems including fractured relationships and economic anxieties, especially in countries with poor or no social assistance and support. In addition, there is the unquestionable importance of the impact caused by mental disorders and distress. By calling attention to the sociological elements of the data, the authors are not denying the importance of psychiatric disorders in a substantial proportion of persons who suicide by self-immolation. Undoubtedly, accessing mental health care must be developed and encouraged in every country. However, mental health workers need to address the existential, moral and spiritual questions that are likely be raised during the process of providing care to these patients.

As Durkheim alerted, economic and social issues have a severe impact on the burden of each life. The different ways that countries address these questions, through their socio-political and institutional systems, in supporting or penalizing their people, can either help them navigate through a crisis or destabilize them. An interdisciplinary humanitarian approach grounded in ethics and science, and flexible enough to explore the existential and symbolic domains of an act like self-immolation, is needed to truly understand the predicaments of these individuals and make a therapeutic difference in their lives.

References

1. David C. Huguette Gaulin, soeur de feu. 13 février 2016. https://www.ledevoir.com/lire/462782/point-final-huguette-gaulin-soeur-de-feu. Accessed 9 Apr 2020.
2. Guy C. La parole des suicidés. 30 avril 2010. https://www.lapresse.ca/arts/chantal-guy/201004/30/01-4275715-la-parole-des-suicides.php. Accessed 9 Apr 2020.
3. Bank TW. World Bank country and lending groups. 2020. http://data.worldbank.org/about/country-and-lending-groups. Accessed 9 Apr 2020.
4. Bank TW. Country and lending groups. 2016. https://data.worldbank.org/indicator/si.pov.gini?end=2018&most_recent_value_desc=true&start=2015. Accessed 9 Apr 2020.
5. Mackenbach JP. Socioeconomic inequalities in health in high-income countries: the facts and the options. In: Detels R, Tan CC, editors. Oxford textbook of global public health. New York: Oxford University Press; 2015.
6. Crimmins EM, et al. Explaining divergent levels of longevity in high-income countries. Washington, DC: National Academies Press; 2011.
7. Woolf SH, Braveman P. Where health disparities begin: the role of social and economic determinants—and why current policies may make matters worse. Health Aff. 2011;30(10):1852–9.
8. Seoighe D, et al. Self-inflicted burns in the Irish national burns unit. Burns. 2011;37(7):1229–32.
9. Forster NA, et al. Attempted suicide by self-immolation is a powerful predictive variable for survival of burn injuries. J Burn Care Res. 2012;33(5):642–8.
10. Prosser D. Suicides by burning in England and Wales. Br J Psychiatry. 1996;168(2):175–82.
11. Biggs M. Dying for a cause—alone? Contexts. 2008;7(1):22–7.
12. Romm S, Combs H, Klein MB. Self-immolation: cause and culture. J Burn Care Res. 2008;29(6):988–93.
13. Wood R. Self-inflicted burn injuries in the Australian context. Australasian Psychiat. 2014;22(4):393–6.
14. Toppi J, Cleland H, Gabbe B. Severe burns in Australian and New Zealand adults: epidemiology and burn centre care. Burns. 2019;45(6):1456–61.
15. Shkrum M, Johnston K. Fire and suicide: a three-year study of self-immolation deaths. J Forensic Sci. 1992;37(1):208–21.
16. Caine P, et al. Self-inflicted burns: 10 year review and comparison to national guidelines. Burns. 2016;42(1):215–21.
17. Rothschild MA, Raatschen HJ, Schneider V. Suicide by self-immolation in Berlin from 1990 to 2000. Forensic Sci Int. 2001;124(2–3):163–6.
18. Franchitto N, et al. Self-inflicted burns: the value of collaboration between medicine and law -forensic aspects of self-inflicted burns. J Forensic Sci. 2011;56(3):638–42.
19. Amadasi A, et al. Observations on self-incineration characteristics in 24 years (1993–2016) of autopsies in the city of Milan. Med Sci Law. 2018;58(1):32–8.
20. Gauthier S, Reisch T, Bartsch C. Self-burning—a rare suicide method in Switzerland and other industrialised nations—a review. Burns. 2014;40(8):1720–6.
21. Modjarrad K, et al. The descriptive epidemiology of intentional burns in the United States: an analysis of the National Burn Repository. Burns. 2007;33(7):828–32.
22. Whiteford HA, et al. Global burden of disease attributable to mental and substance use disorders: findings from the Global Burden of Disease Study 2010. Lancet. 2013;382(9904):1575–86.
23. Laloë V. Patterns of deliberate self-burning in various parts of the world: a review. Burns. 2004;30(3):207–15.
24. Thombs BD, Bresnick MG. Mortality risk and length of stay associated with self-inflicted burn injury: evidence from a national sample of 30,382 adult patients. Crit Care Med. 2008;36(1):118–25.
25. Gray SJ. Suicide by self-immolation in Australia: characteristics, contributing factors & comparisons with other suicide methods. Victoria: Victoria University; 2014.
26. Cimino PJ, et al. Case series of completed suicides by burning over a 13-year period. J Forensic Sci. 2011;56:S109–11.

27. Raleigh VS, Balarajan R. Suicide and self-burning among Indians and West Indians in England and Wales. Br J Psychiatry. 1992;161(3):365–8.
28. Wiechman SA, et al. The management of self-inflicted burn injuries and disruptive behavior for patients with borderline personality disorder. J Burn Care Rehabilit. 2000;21(4):310–7.
29. Sonneborn CK, Vanstraelen PM. A retrospective study of self-inflicted burns. Gen Hosp Psychiatry. 1992;14(6):404–7.
30. Linehan MM. Cognitive-behavioral treatment of borderline personality disorder. New York: Guilford Press; 2018.
31. Rietschel CH, et al. Clinical and psychiatric characteristics of self-inflicted burn patients in the United States: comparison with a nonintentional burn group. J Burn Care Res. 2015;36(3):381–6.
32. Rashid A, Gowar JP. A review of the trends of self-inflicted burns. Burns. 2004;30(6):573–6.
33. Hahn AP, et al. Self-inflicted burns: a systematic review of the literature. J Burn Care Res. 2014;35(1):102–19.
34. Stoddard F, Pahlavan K, Cahners S. Suicide attempted by self-immolation during adolescence. I. Literature review, case reports, and personality precursors. Adolesc Psychiatry. 1985;12:251.
35. Gear AJ, et al. Self-inflicted burn injury. Am J Emerg Med. 1997;15(6):617–8.
36. Stevis-Gridneff M. Europe keeps asylum seekers at a distance, this time in Rwanda. S. Stevis-Gridneff, M. https://www.nytimes.com/2019/09/08/world/europe/migrants-africa-rwanda.html. Accessed 9 Apr 2020.
37. Kermeliotis T. Chios: Syrian refugee critical after self-immolation. 30 Mar 2017. https://www.aljazeera.com/news/2017/03/syrian-refugee-critical-immolation-chios-170330142455924.html. Accessed 9 Apr 2020.
38. Lind D. The horrifying conditions facing kids in border detention, explained. June 2019. https://www.vox.com/policy-and-politics/2019/6/25/18715725/children-border-detention-kids-cages-immigration. Accessed 9 Apr 2020.
39. Fiske L. Self-immolation incidents on Nauru are acts of 'hopeful despair'. May 2016. https://theconversation.com/self-immolation-incidents-on-nauru-are-acts-of-hopeful-despair-58791. Accessed 9 Apr 2020.
40. Doherty B, Davidson H (May 2, 2016). Somali refugee in critical condition after setting herself alight on Nauru. https://www.theguardian.com/australia-news/2016/may/03/somali-refugee-in-critical-condition-after-setting-herself-alight-on-nauru. Accessed 9 Apr 2020.
41. Womersley G, Kloetzer L. Being through doing: the self-immolation of an asylum seeker in Switzerland. Front Psychiatr. 2018;9:110.
42. Durkheim E. Suicide: a study in sociology (Spaulding JA, Simpson G, translators). Glencoe, IL: Free Press; 1951. (Original work published 1897).
43. Sisti DA, Joffe S. Implications of zero suicide for suicide prevention research. JAMA. 2018;320(16):1633–4.

Affective States in Suicide

David Choon Liang Teo, Constantine D. Della, Marco Christian Michael, and Andre Teck Sng Tay

1 Introduction

Each year, close to one million people worldwide die by suicide. Suicide accounts for about 1.5% of all mortality [1]. Since it is considered a psychiatric emergency, understanding predictive and protective factors is important in suicide prevention [2].

Identifying a suicide crisis is challenging because of the tendency of patients to withhold suicide intentions and plans from providers if not properly prompted, or deny suicide intent if questioning is inadequate [3]. Major precipitating life events may trigger the overwhelming mental pain that culminates in suicide [4]. However, even in the absence of a clear precipitating event, intense affects can drive a person to desperation, helplessness and suicide [5]. Recognizing high risk affective and

D. C. L. Teo (✉) · A. T. S. Tay
Department of Psychological Medicine, Changi General Hospital, Singapore

Duke-NUS Medical School, Singapore

Yong Loo Lin School of Medicine, National University of Singapore, Singapore
e-mail: david.teo.c.l@singhealth.com.sg; tay.teck.sng@singhealth.com.sg

C. D. Della
Section of Consultation-Liaison Psychiatry, Department of Psychiatry & Behavioral
Medicine, College of Medicine & Philippine General Hospital, University of the Philippines,
Manila, Philippines
e-mail: cddella@up.edu.ph

M. C. Michael
Department of Psychiatry and Behavioral Sciences, SUNY Downstate Health Sciences
University, New York, NY, USA
e-mail: marco.michael@downstate.edu

cognitive states is, therefore, a more reliable way of helping clinicians identify suicide crises independent of patients acknowledging suicide intentions [6].

This chapter will describe research and clinical findings that validate the association of specific affective states with suicide risk in general, and specifically comment on affective states present in suicides by self-immolation.

2 Negative Affective States and Suicide

Negative affects play an integral role in the development of suicidal thoughts and behaviour. Suicidal thoughts are commonly associated with affective states like depression and anxiety [7, 8]. Some individuals are more vulnerable than others, and personality types with a propensity for negative emotions, namely neuroticism, as well as psychological states such as impulsivity, aggression, depression, hopelessness, anxiety, self-consciousness and social disengagement increase suicide risk [8, 9]. Latent suicidogenic cognitive structures known as suicide schemas are present in some individuals [10]. Suicide schemas can be understood as a network of interconnected stimuli, response and emotional information relating to suicide [10]. These latent schemas are activated under stressful circumstances to induce suicidal thoughts as a way to escape from an overwhelming and intolerable emotional state or situation [11]. The theory of vulnerability to suicide caused by latent suicide schemas finds support in observations that individuals are seldom constantly suicidal. Instead, they experience spikes in suicidal thoughts and behaviours during crises [12].

Negative affective states can trigger dysfunctional thought patterns in at-risk individuals [11, 13]. Hopelessness, rage, guilt, feelings of abandonment, anxiety, feelings of loneliness, shame or humiliation and self-hatred are various affective and cognitive states linked with suicide [6, 14–19]. Intense affects are strong predictors of acute suicide risk [20]. Hendin and colleagues (2007), in a study comparing depressed patients who died by suicide with controls, reported that those who suicided had significantly more intense affects including desperation, hopelessness, feelings of abandonment, self-hatred, rage, anxiety and loneliness [6]. Desperation appears to be the strongest predictor of an acute suicide crisis. Central to the affective turmoil experienced by many of the patients who die by suicide is intolerable distress and desperation stemming from the belief that death is the only way to regain control and relief. Affective instability is also associated with increased risk of suicide [21]. In this section we will delineate affective states associated with suicide and present clinical case correlations. *In order to preserve confidentiality, the authors either disguised identifying information or obtained informed consent from patients or their next of kin.*

2.1 Hopelessness

Hopelessness is defined as a negative expectation of the future, as in giving up hope leading to a state of despair. Beck described hopelessness as the inability to tolerate one's suffering and difficulty finding solutions to problems [22]. While hopelessness is viewed as a state factor, it may also be a form of internalizing psychopathology with trait components [23].

Hopelessness is a strong predictor of suicidal behavior [9, 24]. It is the second most common risk factor for suicide besides prior suicide attempts [25]. In a seminal study, Kovacs and colleagues used hopelessness scores to predict 91% of suicides in a 10-year prospective study of hospitalized patients [14]. Hendin and colleagues found that depressed patients with suicidal ideation report hopelessness significantly more than non-suicidal depressed individuals [20]. Patients who die by suicide score higher in the Beck Hopelessness Scale, and those who attempt suicide experience hopelessness more than non-suicidal patients or those with suicidal ideation [25]. An acute increase in hopelessness, for example after death of a spouse, could increase the risk of suicide within hours or days. Consequently, it is clinically meaningful to measure level of hopelessness as a predictor of suicide [25].

2.2 Desperation

Desperation is a state of anguish or severe mental suffering accompanied by an urgent need for relief [20]. Patients experiencing desperation feel that they could no longer tolerate their present state of anguish. It often coexists with feelings of hopelessness; a hopeless person may find the current stressor intolerable and in desperation seek immediate relief through suicide. In contrast to hopelessness, desperation is usually acute and therefore can be a predictable marker of a suicide crisis. Desperation may be the final common pathway to suicide from other negative affective states, such as unrelieved rage, anxiety, and abandonment [6]. Maltsberger proposed that a person who is desperate experiences loss of control and fear of disintegration, and suicide symbolically becomes a way to achieve control [26]. Although most patients who experience desperation display affective consonance, some dissociate and portray a calm, quiet demeanour. It is therefore important to always inquire about affective distress in the presence of severe psychosocial stressors.

2.3 Anger

The emotional states of anger and rage (violently intense anger) strongly correlate with depression, especially in younger populations [27]. Adolescents with multiple suicide attempts have more severe depressive symptoms and affective expression of anger compared to those with just one suicide attempt [28]. Anger, combined with high impulsivity, significantly correlates with suicide risk in inpatient psychiatric units [29]. A cross-sectional study in a community sample found that anger is significantly associated with suicidal ideation regardless of age and after controlling for depression [30]. Suicide could be understood as a means of communicating rage or extinguishing anger [31]. Hawkins and colleagues studied the relationship between anger and suicide risk through the perspective of the interpersonal theory of suicide and found that anger is linked to suicidal behaviour via perceived burdensomeness-see Sect. 2.11 [32]. Anger may lead to suicide through painful and triggering events [32]. As such, identifying triggers and managing problematic anger may help decrease suicide risk.

2.4   Self-Hatred

Self-hatred is another negative affective state associated with suicide [20]. Self-hatred is a form of mental and physical self-abuse experienced by some suicidal people. It is a hateful attack by the self against itself, in addition to having a negative self-view, low self-esteem, self-anger, or lack of self-satisfaction [33]. Perhaps the easiest way to conceptualize self-hatred as an affective state relating to suicide is through the lens of people with borderline personality disorder (BPD), a mental disorder characterized by instability in self-identity, affective lability, chaotic interpersonal relationships and impulsive behaviour [34]. People with BPD have a high risk of self-harm and up to 10% die by suicide [35]. Suicidal individuals frequently provoke situations that result in losses, rejections, and subsequent self-hatred. In patients with BPD, self-inflicted injury could be understood as self-punishment stemming from extremely low self-evaluation coupled with expressed anger [36].

2.5   Anxiety

Anxiety is an emotion characterised by worrying thoughts in anticipation of a future concern, with associated feelings of tension, physical changes like increased heart rate and avoidance behaviour [37]. Anxiety and fear are closely related. Fear is an emotional reaction to an immediate threat that is associated with a fight or flight response [2]. Theories of anxiety include Freud's formulations emphasizing accumulation, repression and displacement of psychic tension; behavioural theories that suggest conditioning resulting in the development of phobias; cognitivism which focuses on anxiety arising from an 'appraisal' of a situation; as well as neurobiological theories highlighting the role of amygdala in fear reactions using neuroimaging [38].

Anxiety is a significant risk factor for suicide [39]. Joiner's interpersonal theory posits that for suicide to occur, individuals must develop high levels of acquired capability through repeated experiences with painful and provocative events [40]. Avoidance in states of anxiety may protect against the transition from suicidal ideation to death by suicide [41]. Conversely, affective states of anxiety (e.g. trait-like anxiety, future-oriented worry) with acute symptoms of anxiety and agitation (e.g. excessive motor and heightened mental arousal, severe panic attacks) are often present immediately prior to suicide [3, 42].

The experience of anxiety could result from underlying intrapsychic and interpersonal conflicts. When a person's defense mechanisms fail to contain anxiety, the distress caused by feeling overwhelmed may lead to acting out of suicidal thoughts or impulses. Intense affective states of anxiety, especially in depressed patients and persons experiencing posttraumatic and stressor related disorders, may signal a suicide crisis [6, 20]. Research shows a high association between anxiety and anguish and completed suicide [43].

Suicide could be conceptualized as the ultimate escape from aversive self-awareness and associated negative affect, which often includes anxiety [5]. Anxiety coupled with hopelessness heightens a person's urges to escape psychological pain and elevates suicide risk [44]. Recognizing anxiety and how it interacts with other affective states may help clinicians avert a suicide crisis in persons at risk.

2.6   Guilt

Guilt is a self-conscious emotion characterized by a painful appraisal of having done or not done (or thought about) something that is wrong, either in reality or in one's imagination, leading to real or imagined harm to others. Guilt normally brings about feelings of remorse, resulting in a sense of having to pay a debt (guilt derives from the German word "geld" which means money or debt), be punished or desire reparation in order to undo or mitigate this wrong [45].

In his structural model of the mind, Freud described guilt as arising from the superego expression of condemnation upon the ego, ultimately traceable to the Oedipal phase when one is supposed to learn to negotiate affection with caregivers with comfort [46]. Klein related guilt to the developing awareness that one's aggressive impulses might hurt loved ones—a phase of psychological development she termed "the depressive position" [47]. Winnicott later described this phase as the stage of concern, emphasising psychological achievement in reaching this level of awareness [48]. Thus, the capacity to feel guilt develops with a child's growing awareness that actions impact others. It represents the conscious or unconscious recognition of violating the internalized rules of right living acquired from caregivers.

Under intense guilt, especially in people with superego pathology, suicide may represent a form of self-punishment to atone for having engaged in sinful behaviour or unacceptable transgressions [49].

2.7 Humiliation and Shame

Humiliation involves feeling devalued in relation to others or to one's core sense of self, usually with an element of rejection or a sense of role failure that is brought upon one by others [50]. Humiliation involves abasement of honour and dignity and, with that, loss of status and standing. When humiliated, status claims cannot be easily recovered as one's authority to make public status claims is called into question.

Shame is a painful emotional state brought about by a negative self-evaluation that threatens family, social status and/or public image. It tends to occur with significant public failures, traumas (particularly physical violations), or when it involves a behaviour closely tied to a reduction in self-esteem. Shame is often harder to identify both for the sufferer and for the person trying to help [45]. The capacity to experience shame occurs with the development of self-consciousness where there is the realisation that the self can also be seen from the outside [51]. Shame also relates to a collapse of self-esteem or narcissistic wounds developmentally linked to a parent's failure to respond attentively and appreciatively to a vulnerable child [52].

Shame-proneness, the stable propensity to react with shame in various situations, relates to different expressions of psychopathology, such as depression, anxiety, anger, difficulties with interpersonal problem-solving, substance use, borderline personality, and suicide ideation [53–55]. Heightened shame sensitivity with feelings of humiliation may lead to disorders characterised by low self-esteem, such as introjective or atypical depressive states, which are associated with suicide. Many people with anxiety disorders, particularly social phobia, fear what others might see in them. This fear of exposure is usually related to a deep sense of shame. Individuals often develop avoidance strategies like social isolation, which in turn compound the problem [45]. Shame-proneness, which may trigger suicidality, is common in persons with borderline personality disorder [35, 56].

Suicide can be a consequence of shame, or function to avoid or attenuate shame. Some people with heightened shame sensitivity may experience disappointment that threatens self-esteem. Defensively and violently rebelling against the perceived aggressor may devolve into rageful homicide or suicide [57].

Illustrative Case Vignette 1
J was a 35-year-old Chinese gentleman who first presented to psychiatric services following his first suicide attempt. He reported feeling that life was worthless and meaningless after returning from an overseas training attachment a month earlier. He tried coming to terms with being gay during his leave but had great difficulty accepting his sexuality. Apart from feeling ashamed and guilty, he was afraid of how his family would view him if discovered. J had his first same-sex relationship during this overseas attachment.

Unfortunately, his boyfriend cheated, and the relationship collapsed, leaving J feeling abandoned and devastated in a foreign land. He had difficulty focusing on his training and had to return home prematurely with the burden of paying back his training fees.

J came from a conservative Chinese family where males carry on the family line. His paternal grandmother raised him after his mother died by suicide shortly after his birth. J, the youngest of three children, was the only son in the family. His father was mostly absent, distracted with work. Growing up in poverty, J learned that a good education results in professional and financial stability. His grandmother frequently shared her dreams of seeing him succeed with a family of his own. J worked hard and became the only person in his family to attain a university degree. He worked as an engineer and performed well enough to be awarded an overseas scholarship. He dated a woman for a short while, but the relationship did not work out. He was introverted and usually kept things to himself.

During his hospitalization, J did not display significant depressive symptoms. He occasionally mentioned that life was meaningless, and the future was bleak. He was guarded and appeared nonchalant. He declined medications but accepted psychotherapy. In view of his suicide risk, J received close follow-up after discharge. While he did not display significant depressive symptoms and denied being suicidal, he acknowledged feeling worthless and that life was meaningless.

J was subsequently found dead near a cemetery after ingesting poison. Conflicted about his sexuality, he experienced anxiety and extreme guilt, compounded by feelings of humiliation and shame. He also felt romantically abandoned, betrayed and rejected. These intense affective states were too overwhelming, resulting in losing the will to live and ending life to escape psychic pain.

2.8   Feelings of Abandonment

Feelings of abandonment include experiences of emotional deprivation, fearfulness related to self-doubt and insecurity, sadness and anger due to loss of support, as well as loneliness after being deserted or neglected. It is a type of grief involving the loss or perceived loss of a loved one, which leaves the person feeling isolated, devalued and helpless.

Feelings of abandonment can be excruciating, particularly for patients with borderline personality disorder, and suicide may be experienced as the only way to end psychic pain [35, 58]. Persons who had traumatic life experiences and describe feelings of abandonment have a higher suicide risk [59].

2.9 Loneliness

Loneliness is a feeling of aloneness coupled with the subjective experience of being socially disconnected or alienated from others [40, 60]. It is a facet of thwarted belongingness linked to negative mental and physical health outcomes. Chronic feelings of loneliness coexist with anxiety, anger, pessimism and fear of negative evaluation [61]. Loneliness involves disaffection towards interpersonal issues and it relates to depressive symptoms [62]. A German study found that loneliness correlates with depression, generalized anxiety, and suicidal ideation [63]. Persistent feelings of loneliness are linked to suicide although to a lesser degree than other negative affective states [20, 22, 62]. A Canadian population-wide study found that greater degree of loneliness correlates with increased prevalence of suicide ideation [18]. In vulnerable depressed older adults, loneliness and lower subjective social support correlate with suicidal ideation [64].

2.10 Thwarted Belongingness

Social isolation is one of the strongest and most reliable predictors of suicide across different age groups, populations and clinical settings [65]. Thwarted belongingness includes loneliness (feeling disconnected from others) and the absence of reciprocally caring relationships (not having anyone to turn to for support and care for in times of need) [40]. Persons innately need a sense of belonging [66], and a state of thwarted belongingness and desire for suicide develops when the fundamental need of belonging is unmet.

2.11 Perceived Burdensomeness

Perceived burdensomeness is related to feelings of expendability and comprises two dimensions of interpersonal functioning. First, the perception of the self is so defective that the person feels he or she is a liability to others. Second, the individual experiences affectively-charged thoughts of self-hatred, which may manifest as low self-esteem, guilt or self-blame and agitation [40]. Joiner and colleagues studied suicide notes and found that perceived burdensomeness is characteristic of the notes of those who die by suicide [67].

Illustrative Case Vignette 2

B is a 28-year-old Chinese woman who first presented to psychiatric services with severe depressive symptoms and social anxiety soon after quitting her job as a nurse. She was diagnosed with major depressive disorder, social anxiety disorder and borderline personality disorder. Despite ongoing treatment with medication and psychotherapy, she remained chronically unwell and was hospitalized on several occasions for suicide attempts triggered by crises at home.

B grew up in a traditional Chinese family. Her mother had a paranoid personality and constantly feared that B would be led astray by bad company. As a result, her mother exerted a lot of control over B's life. She did not permit B to socialize outside of school and imposed strict curfews. In order to maintain peace in the family, B's father, a timid and conflict-avoidant man, coaxed B to give in to her mother's demands even though he felt they were unreasonable. Despite experiencing these adverse psychosocial circumstances during formative years, B graduated with a nursing degree. However, overwhelmed by the level of social interaction her work demanded, she quit her job as a nurse after just 2 months. B continued to struggle with intense anxiety and feelings of hopelessness.

B wished to move out alone but could not as her mother would object and threaten to kill herself. In therapy, she acknowledged feelings of anger toward her mother for restricting her life. She also felt abandoned by her father for not standing up for her. Simultaneously, she struggled with guilt and self-blame for her mother's emotional distress. She felt lonely and isolated, trapped in a dysfunctional family setup.

B attempted to hang herself on her 28th birthday. Fortunately, her parents stopped her just in time. B was subsequently admitted to a psychiatric ward. When interviewed, B acknowledged feeling angry toward her mother for depriving her of the freedom and personal space she needed to individuate and launch her life in her adolescent and early adult years. Guilt at the unacceptable notion of anger and rage toward her mother for 'destroying her life' manifested as intense anxiety whenever her mother was present physically or in her mind. She also felt trapped, lonely and hopeless in her situation which she saw no escape from. The confluence of these intense affective states resulted in desperation that culminated in suicidal behaviour.

3 Affective States in Theories and Models of Suicide

The struggle against negative affects is common to various theories and models of suicide. Baumeister proposed the escape theory of suicide, viewing suicidal behaviour as an attempt to flee from negative emotions arising from awareness of one's inadequacies [5].

Joiner's interpersonal theory of suicide suggests that the desire for suicide develops when individuals simultaneously experience unmanageable feelings of perceived burdensomeness and thwarted belongingness. It further proposes that the capability to engage in suicidal behavior is separate from the desire to engage in it. When individuals lose hope in their capacity to manage thwarted belongingness and perceived burdensomeness, they experience an active desire to commit suicide. Suicidal behavior emerges when active suicidal desire (i.e., the convergence of thwarted belongingness, perceived burdensomeness, and the hopelessness about these states) interacts with an increased suicidal capability, which is in turn a result of repeated exposure to physically painful and/or frightening experiences [40, 68]. Self-reported loneliness, fear of negative evaluation, fewer friends, living alone, non-intact family, social withdrawal, and family conflict are components of the thwarted belongingness construct. The perceived burdensomeness construct, on the other hand, includes components such as perceptions of liability and self-hate [40, 68]. A meta-analysis of cross-national research found that the thwarted belongingness - perceived burdensomeness interaction is significantly associated with suicidal behavior [68]. Thwarted belongingness plays a greater role than perceived burdensomeness in contributing to suicidal capability, but perceived burdensomeness is a better longitudinal predictor of suicidal behavior.

O'Connor's integrated motivational-volitional model of suicide views suicide as a behaviour that develops through motivational and volitional phases. The motivational phase involves factors that determine the development of suicidal ideation and intent. The volitional phase describes factors that determine whether a person acts upon these. Feelings of defeat and entrapment drive the emergence of suicidal ideation and various volitional factors such as exposure to suicidal behaviour of others, impulsivity and access to means then mediate the shift to action [69].

Psychodynamic thinking similarly views suicidal people as experiencing a struggle against waves of negative emotions [26]. Freud proposed that suicide develops when destructive forces of the id and a harsh superego challenge the integrity of the ego [70]. Glover later highlighted the importance of ego regression that follows the superego attack against the self. This in turn generates intolerable affects culminating in suicidal behaviour [71]. Bibring theorized that helplessness of the ego in the face of crushing forces engenders depression [72]. When helplessness persists, it gives way to hopelessness, a well-known indicator of suicidal states [73]. Bibring viewed suicide as a form of self-attack in which aggression against the self results from a breakdown of self-esteem [72]. Maltsberger proposed four aspects of suicidal collapse as the ego disintegrates. Affect deluge, the first aspect, is akin to flooding and described as being overwhelmed with a torrent of intolerable painful feelings. The second aspect, efforts to master affective flooding, involves a struggle to contain feelings. The person stays afloat and sinks alternately. When this fails, he or she has a sensation of drowning, loss of control and desperation. This is the third aspect, loss of control and disintegration. The fourth aspect, grandiose survival and body jettison, occurs when the patient identifies the body as a source of emotional pain. The patient experiences the body as an enemy that needs to be annihilated in an act of self-defense [26].

4 Suicide Contagion, Identification with Victims and Related Affective States

Suicide contagion is the direct or indirect transmission of suicidal behaviour from one person to another, in the manner of an infectious disease [74]. It may be transmitted unconsciously, interpersonally or intergenerationally through a pattern of imitation [75]. Cheng and colleagues noted that a mechanism called contagion-as-imitation "provides the greatest heuristic utility for examining whether and how suicide and suicidal behaviours may spread among persons at both individual and population levels." Contagion-as-imitation involves a stimulus-response process where interpersonal, group, and mass media communications play a significant role. When suicides are highly publicized, they are essentially rewarded and, in effect, imitated. In vulnerable individuals, the notoriety of published suicides may serve to overcome internal constraints. Contagion-as-imitation, therefore, involves dynamic processes that reflect sociological, psychological, medical, and public health perspectives [76]. Blood and Pirkis identified social learning theory as a framework to understand suicide contagion. A suicidal person may become disinhibited and triggered by similar actions of others. Contagion mediation may be vertical (with an admired person) or horizontal (with someone like oneself) [77]. The element of contagion is of importance in self-immolators. When persons in distress encounter social, political or religiously endorsed attitudes encouraging suicide, both horizontal and vertical contagion may take place. In times of distress, vulnerable persons who identify with the circumstances and intense affective states of others who self-immolated, may resort to self-immolation as a means of escape. Media guidelines could play an important role in mitigating the risk of contagion of suicide by self-immolation [78].

Illustrative Case Vignette 3

C, a 29-year-old Caucasian woman with a psychiatric diagnosis of bipolar disorder, entered a partial hospitalization program after being hospitalized for a suicide attempt by self-immolation. She stopped taking her mood stabilizing medications weeks prior to her suicide attempt. She reported feeling miserable, misunderstood, and was tired of being treated with contempt by family and friends. She had frequent thoughts of being dismissed by others and discriminated with hatred because of her mental illness. These negative cognitions resulted in feelings of shame, loneliness and a sense of thwarted belongingness. Furthermore, she had fluctuating mood states, affective dissonance and difficulty expressing emotions. On the day of her suicide attempt by self-immolation, C was on her way to see her psychiatrist and impulsively decided to take her own life. She went to a shop to buy lighter fluid and hailed a cab to the city's downtown.

When she arrived in front of a subway station, she doused herself and set herself on fire. Recounting what was going through her mind at that moment, she said "I thought about it, just like this, and in a snap, I decided to burn myself". She denied any premeditated plan to self-immolate. C later recounted that as she was engulfed in fire, feeling her skin burning and intense pain, she regretted what she had done. She rolled on the floor in order to extinguish the fire engulfing her body. She recalls "As I was trying to put the fire out, I saw bystanders nearby recording me with their phones. It was horrible". She was admitted to the burns unit and subsequently transferred to an inpatient psychiatric unit. After stabilization, she was discharged to a partial hospitalization program.

In the program she received group and individual psychotherapy. She was able to contract for safety and did not report suicidal thoughts. She developed better insight into her illness and agreed to switch to a long acting injectable form of medication. She responded well to interpersonal therapy working on identifying intense emotional states predominantly triggered by her low self-esteem, feelings of alienation, shame, and stigma. She was successfully transferred to outpatient psychiatric care.

5   Affective States in Suicide by Self-Immolation

Suicide by self-immolation is a strikingly dramatic way of ending one's life. It is a complex and riveting act that captivates the thoughts of witnesses and survivors and stirs up powerful emotions because of its shocking, gruesome and visceral nature. An unfathomable confluence of intense affects shrouds the decision to end one's life in such an excruciating and sensational way. As such, one can only tentatively postulate what emotions a person may be experiencing when he or she self-immolates.

Self-immolation could be an ultimate expression of self-hatred. Psychodynamic theory considers that suicide results from self-directed aggression, pathological grief to object loss, disrupted ego functioning and pathological interpersonal relations [79]. In object relations theory, people identify with their good self and punish the bad self [80]. In extreme mental anguish, one may split off the bad self and seek to punish or destroy it [26]. Subjecting one's body to be engulfed by fire may be viewed symbolically as being ultimately consumed by intolerable rage against oneself.

Self-immolation may also symbolize unassuaged guilt. Consumed by overwhelming guilt and need for atonement, self-immolators engage in extreme self-punishment. Self-immolation could also be viewed as an expression of extreme anger and rage towards others. Suicide can be a form of control exerted by people who feel torn apart by rage or experiencing vengeful fantasies towards chronic aggressors. The horrific image of burning flesh will remain etched in the minds of witnesses long after the person is dead, suicide in this fashion serving as a lasting act of revenge.

Whereas psychoanalytic theory views suicide as anger or self-directed aggression, other psychological theories underscore the importance of desperation and hopelessness [19]. Hope involves an expectation that one can influence and be satisfied in the world. It relates to one's ability to live happily in an interconnected way. Acts of self-immolation such as that of Jan Palach and Thich Qung Duc were motivated by despair and hopelessness at their nation's or religious community's subjugation. More than 80% of reported self-immolations occur in low-and-middle-income countries [81]. Many of these countries are plagued by war, political instability and poverty. Women, being more vulnerable, bear the brunt of oppression and abuse. Such dire circumstances have a propensity to evoke feelings of hopelessness and despair.

6 Conclusion

Intense negative affective states are an important driver for suicidal behavior, and perhaps even more so in cases of self-immolation, which are often associated with oppression and persecution. Recognition of high risk affective and cognitive states can help mental health professionals to more reliably identify suicide crises in clinical populations and thereby play an important role in secondary and tertiary suicide prevention. Suicide prevention efforts should seek ways to address social factors such as disconnectedness and alienation of vulnerable or marginalized populations who experience affective states that heighten suicide risk.

References

1. O'Connor RC, Nock MK. The psychology of suicidal behaviour. Lancet Psychiatry. 2014;1(1):73–85.
2. Rudd MD, Berman AL, Joiner TE, Nock MK, Silverman MM, Mandrusiak M, et al. Warning signs for suicide: theory, research, and clinical applications. Suicide Life-Threaten Behav. 2006;36(3):255–62.
3. Busch KA, Fawcett J, Jacobs DG. Clinical correlates of inpatient suicide. J Clin Psychiatry. 2003;64(1):14–9.
4. Maltsberger JT, Hendin H, Haas AP, Lipschitz A. Determination of precipitating events in the suicide of psychiatric patients. Suicide Life-Threaten Behav. 2003;33(2):111–9.
5. Baumeister RF. Suicide as escape from self. Psychol Rev. 1990;97(1):90.
6. Hendin H, Maltsberger JT, Szanto K. The role of intense affective states in signaling a suicide crisis. J Nerv Ment Dis. 2007;195(5):363–8.
7. Pinto A, Whisman MA. Negative affect and cognitive biases in suicidal and nonsuicidal hospitalized adolescents. J Am Acad Child Adolesc Psychiatry. 1996;35(2):158–65.

8. Conner KR, Duberstein PR, Conwell Y, Seidlitz L, Caine ED. Psychological vulnerability to completed suicide: a review of empirical studies. Suicide Life-Threaten Behav. 2001;31(4):367–85.
9. Brezo J, Paris J, Turecki G. Personality traits as correlates of suicidal ideation, suicide attempts, and suicide completions: a systematic review. Acta Psychiatr Scand. 2006;113(3):180–206.
10. Pratt D, Gooding P, Johnson J, Taylor P, Tarrier N. Suicide schemas in non-affective psychosis: an empirical investigation. Behav Res Ther. 2010;48(12):1211–20.
11. Bower GH. Mood and memory. Am Psychologist. 1981;36(2):129.
12. Joiner TE Jr, Rudd MD. Intensity and duration of suicidal crises vary as a function of previous suicide attempts and negative life events. J Consult Clin Psychol. 2000;68(5):909.
13. Fresco DM, Heimberg RG, Abramowitz A, Bertram TL. The effect of a negative mood priming challenge on dysfunctional attitudes, explanatory style, and explanatory flexibility. Br J Clin Psychol. 2006;45(2):167–83.
14. Kovacs M, Garrison B. Hopelessness and eventual suicide: a 10-year prospective study of patients hospitalized with suicidal ideation. Am J Psychiatry. 1985;1(42):559–63.
15. Weissman M, Fox K, Klerman GL. Hostility and depression associated with suicide attempts. Am J Psychiatry. 1973;130(4):450–5.
16. Fawcett J, Clark DC, Busch KA. Assessing and treating the patient at risk for suicide. Psychiatr Ann. 1993;23(5):244–55.
17. Heikkinen ME, Isometsä E, Henriksson M, Marttunen M, Aro HM, Lönnqvist J. Psychosocial factors and completed suicide in personality disorders. Acta Psychiatr Scand. 1997;95(1):49–57.
18. Stravynski A, Boyer R. Loneliness in relation to suicide ideation and parasuicide: a population-wide study. Suicide Life Threat Behav. 2001;31(1):32–40.
19. Shneidman ES. The psychological pain assessment scale. Suicide Life-Threaten Behav. 1999;29(4):287.
20. Hendin H, Maltsberger JT, Haas AP, Szanto K, Rabinowicz H. Desperation and other affective states in suicidal patients. Suicide Life-Threaten Behav. 2004;34(4):386–94.
21. Bowen R, Balbuena L, Peters EM, Leuschen-Mewis C, Baetz M. The relationship between mood instability and suicidal thoughts. Arch Suicide Res. 2015;19(2):161–71.
22. Beck AT. Thinking and depression: I. Idiosyncratic content and cognitive distortions. Arch Gen Psychiatry. 1963;9(4):324–33.
23. Young MA, Fogg LF, Scheftner W, Fawcett J, Akiskal H, Maser J. Stable trait components of hopelessness: baseline and sensitivity to depression. J Abnorm Psychol. 1996;105(2):155.
24. Beevers CG, Miller IW. Perfectionism, cognitive bias, and hopelessness as prospective predictors of suicidal ideation. Suicide Life-Threaten Behav. 2004;34(2):126–37.
25. Franklin JC, Ribeiro JD, Fox KR, Bentley KH, Kleiman EM, Huang X, et al. Risk factors for suicidal thoughts and behaviors: a meta-analysis of 50 years of research. Psychol Bull. 2017;143(2):187.
26. Maltsberger JT. The descent into suicide. Int J Psychoanalysis. 2004;85(3):653–68.
27. Goldney R, Winefield A, Saebel J, Winefield H, Tiggeman M. Anger, suicidal ideation, and attempted suicide: a prospective study. Compr Psychiatry. 1997;38(5):264–8.
28. Esposito C, Spirito A, Boergers J, Donaldson D. Affective, behavioral, and cognitive functioning in adolescents with multiple suicide attempts. Suicide Life-Threaten Behav. 2003;33(4):389–99.
29. Horesh N, Rolnick T, Iancu I, Dannon P, Lepkifker E, Apter A, et al. Anger, impulsivity and suicide risk. Psychother Psychosom. 1997;66(2):92–6.
30. Jang J-M, Park J-I, Oh K-Y, Lee K-H, Kim MS, Yoon M-S, et al. Predictors of suicidal ideation in a community sample: roles of anger, self-esteem, and depression. Psychiatry Res. 2014;216(1):74–81.
31. McCandless FD. Suicide and the communication of rage: a cross-cultural case study. Am J Psychiatry. 1968;125(2):197–205.
32. Hawkins KA, Hames JL, Ribeiro JD, Silva C, Joiner TE, Cougle JR. An examination of the relationship between anger and suicide risk through the lens of the interpersonal theory of suicide. J Psychiatr Res. 2014;50:59–65.

33. Orbach I. Therapeutic empathy with the suicidal wish: principles of therapy with suicidal individuals. Am J Psychother. 2001;55(2):166–84.
34. Association AP. Diagnostic and statistical manual of mental disorders (DSM-5®). New York: American Psychiatric Pub; 2013.
35. Pompili M, Girardi P, Ruberto A, Tatarelli R. Suicide in borderline personality disorder: a meta-analysis. Nordic J Psychiatry. 2005;59(5):319–24.
36. Brown MZ, Comtois KA, Linehan MM. Reasons for suicide attempts and nonsuicidal self-injury in women with borderline personality disorder. J Abnorm Psychol. 2002;111(1):198.
37. American Psychological Association. Anxiety. 2020. https://www.apa.org/topics/anxiety/.
38. Freeman D, Freeman J. Anxiety: a very short introduction. Oxford: OUP; 2012.
39. Khan A, Leventhal RM, Khan S, Brown WA. Suicide risk in patients with anxiety disorders: a meta-analysis of the FDA database. J Affect Disord. 2002;68(2-3):183–90.
40. Van Orden KA, Witte TK, Cukrowicz KC, Braithwaite SR, Selby EA, Joiner TE. The interpersonal theory of suicide. Psychol Rev. 2010;117(2):575–600.
41. Bentley KH, Franklin JC, Ribeiro JD, Kleiman EM, Fox KR, Nock MK. Anxiety and its disorders as risk factors for suicidal thoughts and behaviors: a meta-analytic review. Clin Psychol Rev. 2016;43:30–46.
42. Ribeiro JD, Bender TW, Buchman JM, Nock MK, Rudd MD, Bryan CJ, et al. An investigation of the interactive effects of the capability for suicide and acute agitation on suicidality in a military sample. Depress Anxiety. 2015;32(1):25–31.
43. Fawcett J. Treating impulsivity and anxiety in the suicidal patient. Ann N Y Acad Sci. 2001;932(1):94–105.
44. Riskind JH, Long DG, Williams NL, White JC. Desperate acts for desperate times: looming vulnerability and suicide. Suicide science. New York: Springer; 2002. p. 105–15.
45. Clark A. Working with guilt and shame. Adv Psychiatr Treat. 2012;18(2):137–43.
46. Freud S. The ego and the id. The Standard Edition of the Complete Psychological Works of Sigmund Freud, Volume XIX (1923-1925): The Ego and the Id and Other Works. 1961. pp. 1–66.
47. Klein M. A contribution to the psychogenesis of manic-depressive states. Int J Psycho-Anal. 1935;16:145–74.
48. Pedder JR. Failure to mourn, and melancholia. Br J Psychiatry. 1982;141(4):329–37.
49. Hughes JM. Guilt and its vicissitudes: psychoanalytic reflections on morality. London: Routledge; 2007.
50. Kendler KS, Hettema JM, Butera F, Gardner CO, Prescott CA. Life event dimensions of loss, humiliation, entrapment, and danger in the prediction of onsets of major depression and generalized anxiety. Arch Gen Psychiatry. 2003;60(8):789–96.
51. Jacoby M. Shame and the origins of self-esteem: a Jungian approach. London: Taylor & Francis; 2016.
52. Kohut H. The analysis of the self. New York: Int. Univ. Press; 1971.
53. Tangney JP, Wagner P, Gramzow R. Proneness to shame, proneness to guilt, and psychopathology. J Abnorm Psychol. 1992;101(3):469.
54. Lester D. The association of shame and guilt with suicidality. J Soc Psychol. 1998;138(4):535–6.
55. Brown MZ, Linehan MM, Comtois KA, Murray A, Chapman AL. Shame as a prospective predictor of self-inflicted injury in borderline personality disorder: a multi-modal analysis. Behav Res Therapy. 2009;47(10):815–22.
56. Rüsch N, Lieb K, Göttler I, Hermann C, Schramm E, Richter H, et al. Shame and implicit self-concept in women with borderline personality disorder. Am J Psychiatry. 2007;164(3):500–8.
57. Torres WJ, Bergner RM. Severe public humiliation: its nature, consequences, and clinical treatment. Psychotherapy. 2012;49(4):492.
58. Lieb K, Zanarini MC, Schmahl C, Linehan MM, Bohus M. Borderline personality disorder. Lancet. 2004;364(9432):453–61.
59. Blaauw E, Arensman E, Kraaij V, Winkel FW, Bout R. Traumatic life events and suicide risk among jail inmates: the influence of types of events, time period and significant others. J Trauma Stress. 2002;15(1):9–16.

60. Mushtaq R, Shoib S, Shah T, Mushtaq S. Relationship between loneliness, psychiatric disorders and physical health? A review on the psychological aspects of loneliness. J Clin Diagn Res. 2014;8(9):WE01.
61. Cacioppo JT, Hawkley LC, Ernst JM, Burleson M, Berntson GG, Nouriani B, et al. Loneliness within a nomological net: an evolutionary perspective. J Res Pers. 2006;40(6):1054–85.
62. Lasgaard M, Goossens L, Elklit A. Loneliness, depressive symptomatology, and suicide ideation in adolescence: cross-sectional and longitudinal analyses. J Abnorm Child Psychol. 2011;39(1):137–50.
63. Beutel ME, Klein EM, Brähler E, Reiner I, Jünger C, Michal M, et al. Loneliness in the general population: prevalence, determinants and relations to mental health. BMC Psychiatry. 2017;17(1):97.
64. Bogers IC, Zuidersma M, Boshuisen ML, Comijs HC, Voshaar RCO. Determinants of thoughts of death or suicide in depressed older persons. Int Psychogeriatr. 2013;25(11):1775–82.
65. Trout DL. The role of social isolation in suicide. Suicide Life-Threaten Behav. 1980;10(1):10–23.
66. Baumeister RF, Leary MR. The need to belong: desire for interpersonal attachments as a fundamental human motivation. Psychol Bull. 1995;117(3):497.
67. Joiner TE, Pettit JW, Walker RL, Voelz ZR, Cruz J, Rudd MD, et al. Perceived burdensomeness and suicidality: two studies on the suicide notes of those attempting and those completing suicide. J Soc Clin Psychol. 2002;21(5):531–45.
68. Chu C, Buchman-Schmitt JM, Stanley IH, Hom MA, Tucker RP, Hagan CR, et al. The interpersonal theory of suicide: a systematic review and meta-analysis of a decade of cross-national research. Psychol Bull. 2017;143(12):1313.
69. O'Connor RC. Towards an integrated motivational–volitional model of suicidal behaviour. Int Handbook Suicide Prevent. 2011;1:181–98.
70. Freud S. Mourning and melancholia. The Standard Edition of the Complete Psychological Works of Sigmund Freud, Volume XIV (1914–1916): On the History of the Psycho-Analytic Movement, Papers on Metapsychology and Other Works. 1957. pp. 237–58.
71. Glover E. Grades of ego-differentiation. Int J Psycho-Anal. 1930;11:1–11.
72. Bibring E. The mechanism of depression. 1953.
73. Beck AT, Steer RA, Beck JS, Newman CF. Hopelessness, depression, suicidal ideation, and clinical diagnosis of depression. Suicide Life-Threaten Behav. 1993;23(2):139–45.
74. Gould MS. Suicide clusters and media exposure. 1990.
75. Zemishlany Z, Weinberger A, Ben-Bassat M, Mell H. An epidemic of suicide attempts by burning in a psychiatric hospital. Br J Psychiatry. 1987;150(5):704–6.
76. Cheng Q, Li H, Silenzio V, Caine ED. Suicide contagion: a systematic review of definitions and research utility. PLoS One. 2014;9(9):e108724.
77. Blood RW, Pirkis J. Suicide and the media: Part III. Theoretical issues. Crisis. 2001;22(4):163.
78. Pirkis J, Nordentoft M. Media influences on suicide and attempted suicide. In: International handbook of suicide prevention: research, policy and practice. Hoboken: Wiley-Blackwell; 2011. p. 531–44.
79. Kaslow NJ, Reviere SL, Chance SE, Rogers JH, Hatcher CA, Wasserman F, et al. An empirical study of the psychodynamics of suicide. J Am Psychoanal Assoc. 1998;46(3):777–96.
80. Kernberg OF. Borderline conditions and pathological narcissism. Lanham: Rowman & Littlefield; 1985.
81. Laloë V. Patterns of deliberate self-burning in various parts of the world: a review. Burns. 2004;30(3):207–15.

Early-Life Adversity, Suicide Risk and Epigenetics of Trauma

César A. Alfonso and Thomas G. Schulze

1 Introduction

Suicide results from an interaction of biological and environmental factors. This chapter summarizes five decades of research dedicated to understanding the neurobiology of suicide, including distinct neurochemical and neuroendocrine pathways, genetics, epigenetics, and the relationship between trauma, specifically early life adverse events and adult retraumatization, and suicidality. Understanding the neurobiology of suicide, in particular gene-environment interactions, could be relevant in the clinical assessment of suicide risk and prevention. The authors are aware that there are no studies examining the neurobiology of suicide by self-immolation. However, general findings from suicide research may prove relevant in the care of persons at risk for self-immolation, in particular persons in low-and-middle income countries who experienced adverse early life events and women experiencing the intergenerational transmission of trauma.

C. A. Alfonso (✉)
World Psychiatric Association Psychotherapy Section, Geneva, Switzerland

Columbia University Medical Center, New York, NY, USA

Universitas Indonesia, Jakarta, Indonesia

National University of Malaysia, Kuala Lumpur, Malaysia
e-mail: cesaralfonso@mac.com, caa2105@cumc.columbia.edu

T. G. Schulze
World Psychiatric Association Secretary for Scientific Sections, Geneva, Switzerland

Institute of Psychiatric Phenomics and Genomics (IPPG), University Hospital, LMU, Munich, Germany

Department of Psychiatry and Behavioral Sciences, SUNY Upstate Medical University, Syracuse, NY, USA
e-mail: thomas.schulze@med.uni-muenchen.de

Since one-third to one-half of suicides are genetically mediated [1] and about 50% of the risk for suicide attempts is heritable [2], understanding the neurobiology and pathophysiology of suicide is of essence to clinical practitioners caring for individuals with depressive and trauma and stressor-related disorders at risk for self-immolation.

2   Neurobiology of Suicide

This chapter section will first review correlates of neurochemistry and neurotransmission with heightened suicide. We will summarize study findings of neuropathological changes in brains of those who died by suicide, including MRI and functional imaging studies of persons with suicidal behavior. We will then examine the correlation of inflammatory biomarkers and lipid levels with suicide, and lastly, review the association of neuroendocrine changes in the hypothalamic-pituitary-adrenal (HPA) axis with impulsivity, aggression and suicide.

2.1   Neurotransmitters and Suicide

Studies looking at the association between serotonin neurotransmission and suicide date back to the 1970s. Low levels of the serotonin metabolite 5-hydroxyindoleacetic acid (HIAA) in the cerebrospinal (CSF) fluid correlates with suicidal behavior [3], and also with extreme violence and fire setting [4]. Furthermore, low CSF 5-HIAA levels are predictive of future death by suicide [5].

Decreased activity in the brainstem serotonin pathways correlates with suicide, a finding that seems to be transdiagnostic [6]. The prefrontal cortex in persons who suicide shows a decrease in pre-synaptic serotonin transporter binding on nerve terminals and increases in post-synaptic serotonin$_{1A}$ and serotonin$_{2A}$ receptors [7, 8]. Using quantitative autoradiography to study post-mortem brains of over 200 patients, Underwood [9] and colleagues found that childhood trauma affects the serotonin system and contributes to a higher suicide risk in persons who experienced adverse childhood events who later develop major depression and alcoholism.

While the role of the serotonin system positively relates to suicidal behaviors, studies of other neurotransmitter pathways such as the dopaminergic system yield inconclusive findings. Studies of the noradrenergic system, similarly, show conflicting results while searching with specific biomarkers or correlates of suicide [10]. Low 3-methoxy-4-hydroxy-phenylglycol (MHPG) levels in the CSF of persons with major depression seem to correlate with lethality of suicidal behavior [2].

Increased glutamate signaling between cells in the brain is associated with suicide, with decreased expression of glutamate transporters by astrocytes in the locus

Table 1 Brain structural changes of suicidal patients documented by MRI studies[a]

Affected area of the brain	Clinical disorder
Subcortical grey matter hyperintensities	Major depression [12]
Periventricular white matter hyperintensities	Major depression [13]
Lower volume of bilateral orbitofrontal cortex	Major depression [14]
Lower volume of right amygdala	Major depression [14]
Smaller putamen	Major depression [15]
Smaller posterior third of corpus callosum	Major depression [16]
Smaller bilateral globus pallidus	Adjustment disorder [17]
Smaller right caudate	Adjustment disorder [17]

[a]Adapted from van Heeringen and Mann [2]

coeruleus and upregulated expression of N-methyl-D-aspartate (NMDA) receptors. Suicidal persons have measurably increased levels of quinolinic acid in the CSF, suggesting a connection between inflammation and glutamatergic pathways [11].

2.2 Structural and Functional Changes in the Brain and Suicide

Imaging studies are able to measure brain structural and functional changes in suicidal persons. Table 1 summarizes study findings of brain structural changes seen in magnetic resonance imaging (MRI) of suicidal persons.

Functional Positron Emission Tomography (PET) neuroimaging study findings show that prefrontal localized hypofunction is proportional to the lethality of suicide attempts [18]. Also, there is decreased connectivity between the anterior cingulate and posterior insula, and increased connectivity in the striatal motor-sensory network [2]. Brain areas generally involved in depressive disorders and suicide include the brainstem monoaminergic system, prefrontal cortex, anterior cingulate cortex, amygdala and hippocampus [11].

2.3 Inflammatory Biomarkers and Suicide

There is a well-established relationship between inflammation and depression, and emerging research findings suggest the same with suicidal behavior. Reduction in the density and soma size of astrocytes and oligodendrocytes in the subgenual anterior cingulate cortex and amygdala seem to correlate with suicidal behavior [19]. Astrocytes, as other glial cells, have a key role in modulating immunity and inflammatory processes. Low level inflammation altering glial cell functioning occurs in depressed and suicidal persons in the white matter of the prefrontal cortex and dorsal anterior cingulate cortex.

Pro-inflammatory cytokines, such as tumor necrosis factor, interleukin-6 (IL-6), IL-2, IL-8 and IL-1β, are inflammatory markers associated with depressive disorders. Higher levels of IL-6 and lower levels of IL-2 seem to correlate with suicidality. Other potential biomarkers for suicide include increased CSF levels of quinolinic acid and kynurenic acid [11].

2.4   Lipids and Suicidal Behavior

While some studies show an association between hypocholesterolemia and suicide [20], other investigators found no correlation [21, 22]. It could be that total serum cholesterol is not a precise or consistent biomarker for suicidal behavior, while CSF and brain measurements are more reliable. Moreover, there is some evidence that cholesterol may influence neurotransmitter signaling and that polyunsaturated fatty acids impact DNA methylation, therefore mediating gene-environment interactions that could result in suicidal behavior [11].

2.5   HPA Axis Dysregulation in Suicide, Impulsivity and Aggression

The hypothalamic-pituitary-adrenal (HPA) axis is the neuroendocrine system that intermediates our reactions to environmental stress. A blunted cortisol response in the dexamethasone suppression test significantly correlates with major depression but equivocally with suicidal behavior. Suicidal persons have elevated levels of cortisol in the urine and CSF, and these measurements are predictive of death by suicide [23]. As will be clarified later, life adversity may trigger DNA methylation and other epigenetic mechanisms causing HPA axis abnormalities as a possible pathway in the pathophysiology of suicide. Additionally, the HPA axis plays a role in impulsivity and aggression, and investigators that used a standardized laboratory social stress paradigm showed that stress responsivity differs in subtypes of suicidal individuals. Those who are highly impulsive and aggressive show a consistent hyperactive cortisol response [24].

3   Familial History of Suicide and Heightened Risk

An important risk factor for suicide is a family history of suicide, and all clinicians should ask patients at risk pertinent questions about family members who died by suicide or had known psychiatric illness with comorbid suicidal behavior. Those with a family history of suicide have twice the risk of suicide after controlling for family psychiatric history [1].

Consensual validation among clinicians and researchers suggest that when there is a positive family history of suicide heightened risk results from a combination of factors, including modeling and imitation, contagion, the transmission of an impulsive aggression phenotype, early child rearing styles and concomitant environmental stressors, and a shared genetic makeup and biological predisposition [25, 26].

Although close to 50% of the familial transmission of suicide could be attributed to genes, predisposing factors for suicide include the familial transmission of impulsivity, aggression and the intergenerational transmission of trauma [26]. Epigenetic changes triggered by life stressors during critical and sensitive periods of development may alter gene expression, at least partially explaining how familial suicides heighten risk in future generations.

4   Early Life Trauma and Health Outcomes

Research studies of large population samples during the late 1990s found a definitive association between negative life experiences in childhood and poor health outcomes in adulthood [27]. The original ACE (adverse childhood experiences) studies in the United States coded *emotional, physical, and sexual abuse, witnessing domestic violence, and witnessing drug use* as traumatic life experiences. As expected, ACE correlate with adult mental health disturbances such as depressive disorders, anxiety disorders, and drug dependence. A surprising finding from the earlier studies was the additional association with obesity, hypersexuality and sleep disturbance. Later studies found that ACE correlate with PTSD, and increase prevalence of stroke, heart disease, HIV infection and other sexually transmitted diseases, and suicide. [27–30].

Data from 2015–2017 from 27/50 states in the United States based on clinical interviews of close to 150,000 subjects, and follow up systematic reviews and meta-analysis [28–30] found that:

- 2/3 Adults experienced at least one type of ACE traumatic event.
- 1/6 Adults experienced four or more types of trauma.
- Adults with the highest level of ACE exposure have higher prevalence of chronic health conditions and die younger.
- ACE increases the risk of harmful use of alcohol by a factor of 1.9
- ACE increases the risk of anxiety disorders by a factor of 2.5
- ACE increases the risk of major depression by a factor of 2.7
- ACE increases the risk of harmful use of illicit drugs by a factor of 3.5
- ACE increases the risk of PTSD by a factor of 4.4
- ACE correlates with poverty, lower educational attainment, lack of health insurance, and unemployment.
- ACE increases the risk of suicide and violence.

Although these study findings are clinically intuitive, an important contribution to the way mental health workers and caregivers conceptualize trauma is that the cumulative effect of trauma seems to be more important than the qualitative effect. Another important finding that informed research in epigenetics is that there is a sensitive period of development and traumatic experiences during this period may have a lasting impact on the brain, affecting the pathogenesis of illness.

Katz and colleagues [31] propose that psychodynamic and biopsychosocial formulations should incorporate the concept of allostasis as a way to understand the link between traumatic life events and negative health outcomes. Allostasis is defined as maintaining homeostasis through changes in the environment over time. Dysregulation of allostasis, referred to as *allostatic overload*, represents the physiological erosion caused by stressors on the brain circuitry involved in the stress response, or the multisystem response to stress. *Allostatic overload* could be mediated by epigenetic, inflammatory and neuroendocrine changes triggered by environmental factors that include traumatic life experiences. [31, 32].

Physiological alterations and structural changes caused by chronic stressors include neuronal loss in the hippocampus, development of atherosclerotic plaques, left ventricular hypertrophy, increased oxidative stress, and a prolonged inflammatory response. Currently, biomarkers such as cortisol, dehydroepiandrosterone, aldosterone, interleukin-6, tumor necrosis factor-alpha, c-reactive protein, insulin-like growth factor-1, high density lipoprotein, low density lipoprotein, total cholesterol, glycosylated hemoglobin, creatinine, variations in blood pressure and heart rate measurements, waist to hip ratio and body mass index are being assessed to create algorithms in order to quantify *allostatic overload* and an allostatic composite score. The allostatic composite score may provide an assessment of inflammatory, neuroendocrine and immune function when faced with adversity to be able to objectively measure the health protective effects of psychosocial interventions. [31, 32].

5   Trauma and Suicide

ACE and a chaotic early family environment increase suicide risk. It is important for clinicians when working with suicidal patients to identify the following early life adverse events as risk factors for suicide [33], especially when in combination with psychiatric symptoms, recent stressors and retraumatization:

- History of death of a parent
- Emotional abuse
- Physical abuse
- Sexual abuse
- Witnessing family violence
- Witnessing use of substances in the household
- Relocation and changing homes
- Separation from caregivers

A functional imaging study of suicidal individuals [34] found hypoconnectivity in the frontoparietal network of the brain in persons with major depressive disorder with a history of childhood trauma. The study investigators proposed that the scar of trauma is reflected in functional dysconnectivity decades after the occurrence of trauma. [34].

It is important to realize that early life adversity and adult retraumatization may or may not cause posttraumatic stress disorder (PTSD). Nevertheless, traumatic life experiences during the vulnerable period of development in early childhood cause long-lasting biological changes that affect coping skills when faced with stressors later in life. ACE increase suicide risk, even if diagnostic criteria for PTSD are not met. Subsyndromal or subthreshold PTSD carries significant morbidity, which includes heightened risk for suicide [35].

6 Gene-Environment Interactions and Epigenetics of Suicide

The relationship between early trauma and the pathogenesis of suicide is multifactorial, including allostatic overload, inflammatory changes, the body's response to stress mediated by HPA axis shifts, and epigenetic changes.

Epigenetic changes result in the alteration of gene activity without changes in DNA nucleotide sequence or structure. These changes can be triggered by the environment, hence the proposed paradigm of gene-by-environment interactions as a new way to reframe the biopsychosocial model of health and illness [36]. Epigenetic changes are triggered by toxins, pollutants, bacteria, viruses, radiation exposure, nutritional changes, hormonal exposure, changes *in utero,* and psychosocial stressors. Trauma, in particular during the sensitive period of brain development, may trigger enduring epigenetic changes.

Studies show that epigenetics may be an important underlying mechanism for all neuroscience and behavior [37]. Epigenetic processes occur through different means, including *DNA methylation, histone modifications* and non-coding *RNA interference* and silencing [38]. Of these, DNA methylation—the addition of methyl groups to cytosines in the DNA sequence—is the most widely studied epigenetic mechanism. DNA methylation can alter gene expression, a process by which gene by environment interactions could affect biological responses. Epigenetic changes may be permanent, reversible, and are heritable by offspring, perhaps explaining the intergenerational transmission of trauma. Additionally, study findings suggest that epigenetics plays an important role in the neurobiology and pathogenesis of suicide. [9, 10, 23].

While the heritability of suicide remains unclear, epigenetic mechanisms may regulate gene expression in suicidal behavior [39]. Table 2 summarizes study findings of epigenetic mechanisms associated with suicide.

The interactions between acute trauma, enduring stressors, emotions, hormonal and peptide surges, up and down regulation of receptors and neurotransmission cause epigenetic changes in the brain with associated changes in endocrine and

Table 2 Epigenetic mechanisms in suicide

DNA methylation
Ribosomal RNA promoter hypermethylation in the hippocampus [40]
Hypermethylation in the HTR2A promoter region in the frontal lobe [41]
Hypermethylation of the BDNF promoter (exon IV) in the Wernicke area [42]
Hypermethylation in the promoter region of GABAA receptor subunit alpha 1 in the frontal cortex [43]
Histone modification
H3K27 (Histone 3 Lysine 27) hypermethylation and decreased TrkB.T1 (Tropomyosin- related kinase B) expression in the orbitofrontal cortex [44]
Increased levels of H3K4me3 (transcriptional active chromatin biomarker) in the promoter region upregulating the activity of OAZ1 (ornithine decarboxylase antizyme 1) [45]
RNA interference
Increase in Hsa-miR-185 expression in the frontal cortex [46]

immune systems and inflammatory response. It is clinically important to recognize that although epigenetic changes may remain stable through life, they may be altered and reversible trough psychotherapy, psychosocial and environmental interventions.

There seems to be a sensitive period of development where epigenetic changes occur and "adversity leaves behind biological memories that persistently alter genome function and increase susceptibility to illnesses". [47] The effect of adversity on DNA methylation depends primarily on the developmental timing of exposure to traumatic events. Exposure in very early childhood is associated with widespread epigenetic changes. If exposure to adverse events occurs in middle childhood changes in DNA methylation can be detected when there is severe sexual or physical abuse, but not consistently for other types of trauma [47].

A systematic review by Jiménez and colleagues from the Universidad de Chile and Luyten and colleagues from the University College of London [48] found that a variety of psychosocial interventions reverse epigenetic changes that correlate with psychopathology and suicide risk. These include brief manualized interventions such as prolonged exposure therapy for PTSD, cognitive behavioral therapy for anxiety disorders, cognitive behavioral therapy in combination with medication for depressive disorders, and dialectical behavioral therapy for borderline personality disorder. Psychotherapies serve to recalibrate the individual's sensitivity to the social environment. Further studies are needed to clarify if the biological changes achieved with these brief interventions endure through time and to compare study results with psychotherapeutic interventions of longer duration.

7 Conclusion

The neurobiology and pathogenesis of suicide is complex and involves multiple neurotransmitter systems (serotonergic, noradrenergic, dopaminergic, glutamatergic) and different regions of the brain (brainstem, prefrontal cortex, anterior cingulate cortex, amygdala and hippocampus). Although there are no clinically practical biomarkers of suicide that could be presently used for screening patients at risk, research is underway testing the sensitivity and specificity of levels of pro-inflammatory cytokines, quinolinic acid and kynurenic acid, among others, to assess their potential use in suicide screening and prevention.

Gene-environment interactions and epigenetic processes may mediate heightened risk of suicide in vulnerable populations. Even though there are no studies to date looking at the neurobiology of suicide by self-immolation, it is plausible that factors such as the intergenerational transmission of trauma, early life adversity and violent retraumatization during young adulthood could cause epigenetic changes that place individuals at suicide risk. Nevertheless, research on epigenetics and suicide, although seemingly promising, is in its infancy. Sample sizes for the studies reviewed in this chapter are quite small, and while the combination of study results clearly show a pattern, they still do not constitute hard evidence and findings need to be replicated in larger cohorts and diverse settings before asserting correlation and causality.

There is some data showing that psychosocial interventions, including brief psychotherapy interventions, could reverse epigenetic changes associated major depression, PTSD and stressor related disorders, decreasing suicide risk. Since these disorders are present in most persons who self-immolate, brief psychotherapies, an integral part of suicide prevention strategies, could have long lasting benefits.

References

1. Joiner TE, Brown JS, Wingate LR. The psychology and neurobiology of suicidal behavior. Annu Rev Psychol. 2005;56:287–314.
2. Van Heeringen K, Mann JJ. The neurobiology of suicide. Lancet Psychiatry. 2014;1(1):63–72. https://doi.org/10.1016/S2215-0366(14)70220-2.
3. Asberg M, Traskman L, Thoren P. 5-HIAA in the cerebrospinal fluid: a biochemical suicide predictor? Arch Gen Psychiatry. 1976;33:1193–7.
4. Virkkunen M, Rawlings R, Tokola R, Poland RE. CSF biochemistries, glucose metabolism, and diurnal activity rhythms in alcoholic, violent offenders, fire setters, and healthy volunteers. Arch Gen Psychiatry. 1994;51:20–7.
5. Mann JJ, Malone KM, Sweeney JA, et al. Attempted suicide characteristics and cerebrospinal fluid amine metabolites in depressed inpatient. Neuropsychopharmacology. 1996;15:576–86.
6. Mann JJ, Arango V, Marzuk PM, et al. Evidence for the 5-HT hypothesis of suicide: a review of post-mortem studies. Br J Psychiatry. 1989;155:7–14.
7. Arango V, Underwood M, Mann JJ. Biological alterations in the brainstem of suicides. In: Mann JJ, editor. Suicide, psychiatric clinics of North America. Philadelphia: WB Saunders; 1997.
8. Underwood MD, Mann JJ, Arango V. Serotonergic and noradrenergic neurobiology of alcoholic suicide. Alcohol Clin Exp Res. 2004;28:57s–69s.
9. Underwood MD, Kassir SA, Bakalian MJ, Galfalvy H, Dwork AJ, Mann JJ, Arango V. Serotonin receptors and suicide, major depression, alcohol use disorder and reported early life adversity. Transl Psychiatry. 2018;8:279.
10. Currier M, Mann JJ. Stress, genes and the biology of suicidal behavior. Psychiatr Clin North Am. 2008;31(2):247–69. https://doi.org/10.1016/j.psc.2008.01.005.

11. Lutz PE, Mechawar N, Turecki G. Neuropathology of suicide: recent findings and future directions. Mol Psychiatry. 2017;22:1395–412.
12. Ehrlich S, Breeze JL, Hesdorff er DC, et al. White matter hyperintensities and their association with suicidality in depressed young adults. J Affect Disord. 2005;86:281–7.
13. Pompili M, Innamorati M, Mann JJ, et al. Periventricular white matter hyperintensities as predictors of suicide attempts in bipolar disorders and unipolar depression. Prog Neuro-Psychopharmacol Biol Psychiatry. 2008;32:1501–7.
14. Monkul ES, Hatch JP, Nicoletti MA, et al. Fronto-limbic brain structures in suicidal and non-suicidal female patients with major depressive disorder. Mol Psychiatry. 2007;12:360–6.
15. Dombrovski AY, Siegle GJ, Szanto K, Clark L, Reynolds CF, Aizenstein H. The temptation of suicide: striatal gray matter, discounting of delayed rewards, and suicide attempts in late-life depression. Psychol Med. 2012;42:1203–15.
16. Cyprien F, Courtet P, Malafosse A, et al. Suicidal behavior is associated with reduced corpus callosum area. Biol Psychiatry. 2011;70:320–6.
17. Vang FJ, Ryding E, Trskman-Bendz L, van Westen D, Lindstrom MB. Size of basal ganglia in suicide attempters, and its association with temperament and serotonin transporter density. Psychiatry Res. 2010;183:177–9.
18. Oquendo MA, Placidi GP, Malone KM, et al. Positron emission tomography of regional brain metabolic responses to a serotonergic challenge and lethality of suicide attempts in major depression. Arch Gen Psychiatry. 2003;60:14–22.
19. Steiner J, Bielau H, Brisch R, Danos P, Ullrich O, Mawrin C, et al. Immunological aspects in the neurobiology of suicide: elevated microglial density in schizophrenia and depression is associated with suicide. J Psychiatr Res. 2008;42:151–7.
20. Wu S, Ding Y, Wu F, Xie G, Hou J, Mao P. Serum lipid levels and suicidality: a meta-analysis of 65 epidemiological studies. J Psychiatry Neurosci. 2016;41:56–69.
21. Deisenhammer EA, Kramer-Reinstadler K, Liensberger D, Kemmler G, Hinterhuber H, Fleischhacker WW. No evidence for an association between serum cholesterol and the course of depression and suicidality. Psychiatry Res. 2004;121:253–61.
22. Roy A, Roy M. No relationship between serum cholesterol and suicidal ideation and depression in African American diabetics. Arch Suicide Res. 2006;10:11–4.
23. Mann JJ. Neurobiology of suicidal behavior. Nat Rev Neurosci. 2003;4:819–28.
24. Stanley B, Michel CA, Galfalvy HC, Kelp JG, Rizk MM, Richardson-Vejlgaard R, Oquendo MA, Mann JJ. Suicidal subtypes, stress responsivity and impulsive aggression. Psychiatry Res. 2019;280:112486. https://doi.org/10.1016/j.psychres.2019.112486.
25. Mann JJ. A current perspective of suicide and attempted suicide. Ann Intern Med. 2002;136:302–11.
26. Brent DA, Melhem N. Familial Transmission of Suicidal Behavior. Psychiatr Clin North Am. 2008;31(2):157–77.
27. Felitti VJ, Anda RF, Nordenberg D, et al. Relationship of childhood abuse and household dysfunction to many of the leading causes of death in adults: the adverse childhood experiences (ACE) study. Am J Prev Med. 1998;14:245–58.
28. Merrick MT, Ford DC, Ports KA, et al. Vital signs: estimated Proportion of Adult Health Problems Attributable to Adverse Childhood Experiences and Implications for Prevention—25 States, 2015–2017. MMWR Morb Mortal Wkly Rep. 2019;68:999–1005.
29. Slopen N, Koenen KC, Kubzansky LD. Cumulative adversity in childhood and emergent risk factors for long-term health. J Pediatr. 2014;164:631–8.
30. Hughes K, Bellis MA, Hardcastle KA, et al. The effect of multiple adverse childhood experiences on health: a systematic review and meta-analysis. Lancet Public Health. 2017;2:e356–66.
31. Katz DA, Sprang G, Cooke C. The cost of chronic stress in childhood: understanding and applying the concept of allostatic load. Psychodyn Psychiatry. 2012;40(3):469–80.
32. Alfonso CA, Friedman RC, Downey JI. Advances in psychodynamic psychiatry. New York: Guilford Press; 2018.

33. Lagomasino IT, Stern TA. The suicidal patient. In: MGH guide to primary care psychiatry. New York: McGraw-Hill; 2004.
34. Yu M, Linna KA, Shinohara RT, Oathes DJ, Cook PA, Duprata R, Mooree TM, Oquendo MA, Phillips ML, McInnis M, Fava M, Trivedi MH, McGrath P, Parseyk R, Weissman MM, Sheline YI. Childhood trauma history is linked to abnormal brain connectivity in major depression. PNAS. 2019;116(17):8582–90.
35. Marshall RD, Olfson M, Hellman F, Blanco C, Guardiano M, Struering EL. Comorbidity, impairment, and suicidality in subthreshold PTSD. Am J Psychiatry. 2001;158:1467–73.
36. Plakun EM. What psychotherapists should understand about DNA methylation. J Psychiatr Pract. 2019;25(3):212–4.
37. Chambers J. The neurobiology of attachment: from infancy to clinical outcomes. Psychodyn Psychiatr. 2017;45(4):542–63.
38. Labonte B, Turecki G. The epigenetics of suicide: explaining the biological effects of early life environmental adversity. Archiv Suicide Res. 2010;14:291–310.
39. Bani-Fatemi A, Howe S, De Luca V. Epigenetic studies of suicidal behavior. Neurocase. 2015;21(2):134–43. https://doi.org/10.1080/13554794.2013.826679.
40. McGowan PO, Sasaki A, Huang TC, Unterberger A, Suderman M, Ernst C, Szyf M. Promoter wide hypermethylation of the ribosomal RNA gene promoter in the suicide brain. PLoS One. 2008;3(5):e2085.
41. Abdolmaleky HM, Yaqubi S, Papageorgis P, Lambert AW, Ozturk S, Sivaraman V, Thiagalingam S. Epigenetic dysregulation of 5-HTR2A in the brain of patients with schizophrenia and bipolar disorder. Schizophr Res. 2011;129(2–3):183–90.
42. Keller S, Sarchiapone M, Zarrilli F, Videtic A, Ferraro A, Carli V, Chiariotti L. Increased BDNF promoter methylation in the Wernicke area of suicide subjects. Archiv Gen Psychiatr. 2010;67(3):258–67.
43. Poulter MO, et al. GABAA receptor promoter hypermethylation in suicide brain: implications for the involvement of epigenetic processes. Biol Psychiatry. 2008;64(8):645–52.
44. Ernst C, Chen ES, Turecki G. Histone methylation and decreased expression of TrkB.T1 in orbital frontal cortex of suicide completers. Molecul Psychiatr. 2009;14(9):830–2.
45. Fiori LM, Turecki G. Genetic and epigenetic influences on expression of spermine synthase and spermine oxidase in suicide completers. Int J Neuropsychopharmacol. 2010;13(6):725–36.
46. Maussion G, Yang J, Yerko V, Barker P, Mechawar N, Ernst C, Turecki G. Regulation of a truncated form of tropomyosin-related kinase B (TrkB) by Hsa-miR-185* in frontal cortex of suicide completers. PLoS One. 2012;7(6):e39301.
47. Dunn EC, et al. Sensitive periods for the effect of childhood adversity on DNA methylation: results from a prospective, longitudinal study. Biol Psychiatry. 2019;85:838–49.
48. Jiménez JP, Botto A, Herrera L, Leighton C, Rossi JL, Quevedo Y, Luyten P. Psychotherapy and genetic neuroscience: an emerging dialog. Front Genet. 2018;9(257):1–19.

Social Sciences, Suicide and Self-Immolation

Renato Antunes dos Santos, Bipin Ravindran, Newton Duarte Molon, and Eduardo Chachamovich

1 Introduction

Suicide is an intriguing, controversial, highly stigmatized and taboo subject. Suicide is unlike other causes of death as it is the only one where a person purposefully strives to move towards rather than away from death, and where questions of purpose, resolve and meaning potently permeate the narrative of existence and mortality.

Throughout time, the power relationship between different disciplines concerning suicide shifted dominance, from religion to philosophy and from law to the social sciences and medicine. Additionally, political determinism is omnipresent, in particular when societal inequities trickle down from the sphere of government to

R. A. dos Santos (✉)
Department of Psychiatry, The University of Toronto, Waypoint Centre for Mental Health Care, Toronto, ON, Canada
e-mail: renato.psiquiatria@gmail.com

B. Ravindran
Hunter New England Mental Health Service, Newcastle, NSW, Australia

School of Medicine and Public Health, The University of Newcastle, Callaghan, NSW, Australia
e-mail: Bipin.Ravindran@health.nsw.gov.au

N. Duarte Molon
Institute of Psychology, Social Psychology of Work and Organizations, University of Brasília, Brasília, Brazil
e-mail: ndmolon@gmail.com

E. Chachamovich
Department of Psychiatry, McGill University, Montreal, QC, Canada

Northern Mental Health Program, McGill Group for Suicide Studies (MGSS), Douglas Mental Health University Institute, Montreal, QC, Canada
e-mail: eduardo.chachamovich@mcgill.ca

© The Author(s), under exclusive license to Springer Nature Switzerland AG 2021
C. A. Alfonso et al. (eds.), *Suicide by Self-Immolation*,
https://doi.org/10.1007/978-3-030-62613-6_13

the individual at risk for suicide. Social scientists enlighten efforts to understand motivations, explain vulnerabilities, search for causative or enabling circumstances, and prevent deaths from suicide.

Social sciences and philosophy are complex fields with multiple frameworks that provide an opportunity to explore the phenomenology of suicide. This chapter presents sociological and philosophical perspectives on suicide highlighting the contributions of seminal thinkers and researchers. We will examine how culture, gender, conflict, politics, religion, and inequities relate to suicide. We will describe existential standpoints of human life and death and develop from a sociological perspective an understanding of suicide in general and self-immolation in particular.

2   Life, Death and Existence

"I think, therefore I am" (*Je pense, donc je suis*), often quoted from the *Discourse on the Method of Rightly Conducting One's Reason and of Seeking Truth in the Sciences* by René Descartes, emphasizes the conscience of existence [1]. Beyond the concreteness of the animal body that allows us to biologically exist, humans delight themselves with the abstract experience of living. What is the conscience of existence? Or in Paul Gauguin words, personified in the title of his 1897 enigmatic painting *"Where do we come from? What are we? Where are we going?"*

These unsolved questions repeatedly lead us to the separation of σῶμα (*soma*, body) and ψυχή (*psyche*, breath, essence of the mind, or soul). The Pythagorean philosophers postulated that the body is the "prison of the soul", expressed in the wordplay *soma-sema*: σῶμα (*soma*, body) and σῆμα (*sema*, a sign by which a grave is known). If the body serves as container of the soul, life must remain in the body until (the) God(s) determine(s) otherwise [2].

In order to protect the soul, Socrates advocated for the body to be preserved in pure form, through self-care and avoiding distractions such as alcohol, ornaments or sex. Nevertheless, he questioned the interpretation of suicide as unscrupulous or aberrant and challenged its prohibition [2, 3]. Classical Greek philosophers made a distinction between "honorable" and "cowardly" suicides. They recognized that suicide could be a response to societal pressure, fear of shame, honor, or altruistic self-sacrifice [4, 5].

Stoics of the Roman Imperial period argued that the soul is not inside the body, but the soul is the body itself. This affirmation resonates with the contemporary biological understanding of the mind, thus interchangeably capturing the soul and mind within the ψυχή (*psyche*) [6]. Sigmund Freud's aphorism that "the ego is first and foremost a bodily ego"[7] similarly revisits the mind-body problem placing mind and body as interrelated and indivisible.

A notable contribution of the Stoic philosophers addresses the rationality of suicide as a way to unburden inescapable misfortune. For example, the suffering caused by intractable health problems, according to Seneca, would allow for suicide as a dignified way to die when faced with extraordinary adversity [8].

3   To Whom Does Life Belong? When Society Fails the Individual

Over the years, the study of suicide evolved, framed interchangeably as a fundamental philosophical problem [9] and classified as a sin, crime or pathology [10], representing the tragic outcome of irremediable social suffering [11]. Although stigmatized in distinct ways in different cultural groups, an unfortunate transcultural bias that still troubles us is the belief that suicide constitutes a failure on the part of the individual, either in terms of faith, morality or defective health. This perspective prevents society from assuming responsibility, constructing suicide as arising solely from the conscious decision of a person to take her/his own life. This conflict uncovers another problematic dialectic: the duty of the individual versus the responsibility of society over one's life [12].

The attitude of organized religion toward suicide, since time immemorial, is punitive and controlling, with the general tendency to take ownership over a person's life as a possession of God. By the late nineteenth century, however, an approach that researched "moral statistics" (empirical data looking and social pathology) transformed the study of suicide from a paradigm dominated by religion, dogma and law to a subject of scientific inquiry through the disciplines of psychology and psychiatry. When the ψυχή (*psyche*) fields crossed over to suicide studies, the search for predisposing, enabling and protective factors began to gain in importance. Nevertheless, this dominance and scientific inquiry side-tracked important sociological research that took place during the latter part of the nineteenth century. A cross-disciplinary power dispute, unfortunately, prevented multidisciplinary or transdisciplinary collaborations to be an option until much later in the twentieth century. It is our opinion that the key to heightened prevention may be through a respectful and thorough consideration of multidimensional perspectives.

Suicide can be seen as a negative outcome arising from interactions of social or contextual factors and personal or psychological factors [13], but may also extend far beyond these factors to incorporate collective and individual past experiences that are culturally determined. It can be understood as a social act in itself, shaping the world through the making and breaking of relationships and challenging rigid social constraints placed on individuals by the forces of society, so much so that "we live by suicide as much as we might die by suicide"[14]. Suicide may be the end result of a society that fails to protect the individual. It is the aim of this book to address suicide in a complementary fashion through collaborative efforts. Understanding the place of the individual in society and the responsibility of society to protect and nurture wellbeing is key to suicide prevention.

4   Contributions of Durkheim

Durkheim conducted empirical social research to investigate causative factors linked to suicidal behaviors within societies. [15, 16]. His pioneering work analyzing aggregate statistics suggested that causative factors are situated within societal variables. Although his work overgeneralized findings that could not be replicated transculturally, his approach focusing on sociological determinants is meaningful and relevant to this day.

Durkheim found differences in suicide rates among Protestant, Catholic and Jewish communities. He described the impact of familial, political and societal factors on the individual, resulting in behaviors within the spectrum of meaningful and satisfactory interrelatedness to perceived burdensomeness and suicide.

Durkheim observed changes in suicide rates across time. He identified that societal bonds can be strengthened during historical periods like wars, with purposeful nationalism and pride over meritorious causes serving as suicide protective. He also recognized that economic changes and inequities impact suicide rates. Additionally, he stated, there are extra-social determinants of suicide. Heredity, for instance, rarely can be isolated from the several other existing intra-familial and interpersonal factors. Recent work on the intergenerational transmission of trauma and epigenetics bridges the gene-environment divide. Durkheim also recognized imitation as a factor for suicide, as in the *Werther effect*. However, he thought that the association was insufficient to significantly impact suicide rates. He adamantly opposed the causation hypothesis doubting that presence of a mental disorder by itself could lead to a suicide act. Nevertheless, he recognized that mental disorders may predispose individuals to suicide, while highlighting that it is not a sufficient cause to explain society's oscillations in suicide rates. Durkheim asserted that suicide rates reflect the moral constitution of a society. Suicide results from insufficient or excessive degree of integration or regulation of egoism, altruism, anomie and fatalism.

4.1   Egoistic Suicide

Egoistic suicide commonly occurs in highly individualistic societies where separation and individuation are valued over interdependence. In these societies, the importance of the collective group disintegrates weakening the bonds that maintain and sustain the life of the individual. This concept recognizes human beings as a social species requiring social interaction and support rather than merely the satisfaction of individual biological needs [6].

4.2   Altruistic Suicide

Altruistic suicide results when the group places unreasonable pressures and responsibilities on the individual. In societies capable of destroying individuality, a sense of self that is separate from the social self becomes incompatible and undue pressure is placed on the individual convincing the person that suicide can lead to common benefits for all. Self-immolation suicides motivated by political conflicts and some protest suicides are examples of altruistic suicides.

4.3 Anomic Suicide

A state of societal breakdown and the absence of social norms and values increase suicide rates. The anomic suicide may be triggered by financial crises, economic disparities or excessive gains. Durkheim observed that moral dysregulation and aimlessness often follow drastic economic changes. Fulfillment of individuals' aspirations and needs must occur for human beings to experience joy and satisfaction. The descent into an underserved class of society might destroy hope to meet expectations, but the lack of constraints on meeting needs might also cause a loss of interest in life.

4.4 Fatalistic Suicide

When societal conditions are barely compatible with sustaining life, persons may resort to suicide rather than succumbing to constant aggression or deprivation. Fatalistic suicides are common in low-and-middle-income regions and countries with a high prevalence of suicide among disenfranchised individuals, and among marginalized groups subjected to human rights violations.

5 Contributions of Foucault, Hobbes, Hume and Frank

In 1976, in *La Volonté de Savoir*, Foucault introduces the concept of bio-power or the power over life that targets populations at large rather than individuals. In the final section of *La Volonté de Savoir*, he offers comments about suicide in the essay *"Right of death and power over life"*[17]. Akin to the notion of a collective super-ego, bio-power is based on a juridical-medical composite and does not rely on threats and punishments, but rather in control and regulations driven by the desire to positively influence life. The supremacy of the state over life or death has repercussions on how societies experience suicide.

Foucault's concept of governmentality, or governmental rationality, originates from the tension between mercantilism and liberalism. In the mercantilist logic, which is protectionist and self-aggrandizing, a country amasses wealth through unfair trade practices. Regulating and controlling the population is an essential task of the mercantilist state. Suicide, considered a crime by the state and religion, was punished in mercantilist states through the confiscation of the victim's properties by the sovereign and the denial of a religious burial [18].

Liberalism focused on less intervention by the state and deconstructed the idea of culpability and punishment towards suicide. The British empiricist Hobbes was one of the first to reject the idea of the state punishing the suicidal individual and considered suicide as resulting from inner torment with a compromised perception of reality, making the individual unfit to be criminalized.

Hume, in his unpublished 1783 essay *"Of Suicide"*, critiqued God and state's ownership of life, describing suicide as morally permissible and a right of the individual, being intentional more so than consequential, and giving an opportunity to evade inescapable misfortune or intractable illness. Montesquieu, Rousseau and Voltaire similarly advocated against punishment of suicidal persons.

Within the German deontological philosophical tradition, Kant condemned suicide as debasing of one's humanity. Johann Peter Frank, a pioneer in social medicine and public health, considered it an act of insanity not liable to punishment. He advocated that suicide was a right, but unlike Hume and Voltaire, he considered suicide detrimental to the community [6].

Frank, an advocate of sound health and hygiene, suggested that the community should invest in better education, promoting culture and moral values, and care for melancholic persons to prevent suicide. He also worried about the impact of fictional glorification of suicide in novels, such as in Goethe's *The Sorrows of Young Werther* [19]. Frank posited that several behaviors could lead to the "silent insanity" that results in suicide, including lacking a moral compass, idleness, and debauchery [6].

6 Contributions of Marx and Peuchet

During several periods in his life, Karl Marx studied suicide, a distinguished work being the annotated translation of the work of Jacques Peuchet [20]. Peuchet started his scholarly work as a monarchist and later became pro-French revolution. He worked as a police administrator engaged in describing and discussing the movements of culture and society. Familiarized with statistical methods, he initially used its knowledge to enhance the power of the state, later shifting his political position to correcting inequality in society. His vision of society's impact on causes of suicide went beyond stressing the importance of economic factors and social bonds to encompass the whole of culture [6].

Marx and Peuchet observed that European society was based on a culture of aggression, with prisons, physical punishments and instruments of death leaving an astonishing number of people in misery. They highlighted how governments manipulated the masses with strategies that subjugated individuals, creating a state of oppression without exit. Peuchet postulated that poverty was the main social actor in increasing suicide rates but was also interested in the private lives of people and the mistreatments they endured through the vicissitudes of everyday life. On suicide he concluded that "the primary cause was the maltreatment, injustices, secret punishments that these people received at the hands of harsh parents and superiors, upon whom they were dependent" [20]. Rejecting the traditional judgment of people who suicide as being criminals, sinners, or insane, Peuchet believed that individuals faced with inequality and tragic circumstances chose death to escape from a dismal existence [6, 20]. Marx found nobility in these persons, in that they could have chosen to inflict violence on members of the wealthier classes, but decided to kill themselves instead [6].

7   Suicide and Religions

The dominant monotheistic religions condemn suicide with vehement convictions and prohibitions against it [21]. Judaism considers suicide a serious transgression, since the preservation of life is a duty to God. Maimonides declared that those who die by suicide are guilty of murder and shall be judged in celestial court [22]. Christianity finds suicide unjustifiable. Fundamentalist Christian dogma may lead to excessive guilt, shame and feelings of abandonment [22]. Islam considers suicide a more serious offense than murder, including punishment in some parts of the world of family members through dishonor and marginalization [23]. Chapter 14 discusses the aforementioned religious traditions plus Hinduism and Buddhism and explores in more detail how religion and spirituality may protect against or predispose persons to suicide. Although religion provides guiding precepts that are prosocial and can be suicide protective, states of religious alienation and disillusionment may lead to distress. Fanaticism may incentivize suicide through cognitive distortions and violent radicalization.

8   Meaningfulness and Social Construction of Suicide

In societies where gender imbalance and historical injustices and marginalization silence the voices of women, suicide serves as a powerful but covert method of communication to alter the power imbalance. Guzder proposes that if social defeat and social defiance are two tropes of agency for historically marginalized women, then suicide functions like a "swinging bridge" between them, allowing for identification as either an "assaulted victim" or a triumphant and defiant "fighter against injustice" [24].

Andriolo suggests that all suicides contain within their webs of meanings an inherent "strand of protest". Seen in its most symbolic sense, with the body used as a medium to convey simultaneously the angst of the individual and marginalized society, suicide is a form of "dying with a message, for a message, and of a message"[25].

The traditional debate on causes of suicide centers on social determinism and individual agency. But seen within modern Japanese society, the emergence of internet suicide pacts serves as a counterpoint to this debate. Rather than being situated differently, individual existential suffering needs to be seen against the background of the transformative social changes and collective traumas within modern Japanese society, mediated further by factors like cultural aestheticization. Ozawa-de writes that a true understanding of suicide within Japanese society necessitates going beyond the pure categories of Durkheim, and needs to incorporate cosmological theories and to understand how the meanings of life and death are made through the socio-historical construction of ideas [26].

Seen through a developmental life span perspective, while the loss and weakening of social bonds can have a significant negative impact on individuals across the duration of life, they may be particularly potent triggers for suicide in people in young adulthood and mid-life, with an amplification of the sense of loss and personal failure [13].

9 Traditional and Indigenous Communities

Colonization, institutional racism and structural violence heighten suicide risk in cultural groups like the Innuit communities in Nunavut, Canada [27], Aboriginal youth in rural Australia [28], the Mayan-Chol in Southern Mexico, and the Kaiowa in Brazil [29].

Kral described that for suicide reduction interventions to be effective in the Nunavut, it is important to examine the ways in which the role of traditional institutions in the lives of young people have been eroded by Western cultural systems, and how the youth cope with these challenges in their own culturally specific way [30].

Similarly, to properly understand suicides in Aboriginal communities in rural Australia it is important to consider how biopsychosocial, political and historical factors interact to disrupt their life narrative and disconnect the "individual from the earth, the universe and the spiritual realm" and respect the "life-affirming stories that are central to cultural resilience and continuity"[31].

Societies like the Mayan-Chol indigenous people of Southern Mexico underwent significant collective transformation through state interventions affecting education and transport, exposure to consumerism and economic migration. These changes shifted the folkloric anthropological explanatory models of suicide involving attribution to external influences from supernatural beings to incorporate more social explanations like family conflicts, socioeconomic disparities and responses to debilitating illness [14]. Hundreds of Guarani-Kaiowa in Brazil, when stripped of their land and livelihood in what has been described as a genocide, succumb to alcoholism and suicide, as their land is closely linked to identity, a sense of belonging and social purpose [30].

10   Suicide in Zones of Conflict

While war, conflict and forced displacement put extraordinary strain on individuals and families, post-conflict social and cultural changes could play a major role in precipitating suicide. Some of these changes include the impact of forces of modernization, change in gender roles and expectations, and dissonance between family values and community expectations.

Zonal conflicts affect suicide rates in different ways. During the Palestinian Intifadas, suicide rates remained low reflecting the impact of social unification during this period of war against a common enemy, and following the conflict the rise in suicide rates indicated the likely influence of the various social, cultural and political upheaval in the life of ordinary Palestinians [14, 32]. Suicide rates in women rose dramatically in the years following civil conflict in Sri Lanka and Bangladesh, exposing the links between vulnerability of women to suicide and large-scale conflicts. The partition of the Indian subcontinent resulted in terrible loss of life, women bearing the brunt of the violence. Violence and rupture were inscribed on the bodies of these women like layers of intergenerational and historical trauma [24, 33].

In conflict and post conflict situations, a common factor driving suicide in individuals appears to be the lack of the very agency that could be used to manage the extraordinary social and cultural upheavals and injustices. Yet, suicide can be seen as an active choice in such settings, especially for women, reclaiming an agency they had lost to deeply entrenched patriarchal systems, abuse and marginalization. Rasool and Payton describe how the method of self-immolation called *xo sûtandn* among women in Kurdish Iraq, emerged as a "symbol of women's responses to subordination within a male and kinship dominated society"[34].

11   Gender and Suicide

Young South Asian women have a high suicide risk, especially those from rural backgrounds with gendered expectations about the position of women within familial and societal hierarchies and restraints on their modes of communication. Within the rural South Asian context, stressors for women include poverty, intimate partner conflict and violence. In addition, with changes brought about by economic advancement, women facing these stressors may become dislocated from their socially meaningful sources of identity and resilience, their suffering leading an unending cycle of marginalization and trauma [24].

Gender imbalance is a major contributory factor in the significant number of women who attempt suicide by self-immolation in Central Asia. In Tajik society, the role of women is constricted by patriarchal attitudes leading to lower levels of education, employment and social involvement of women. Self-immolation in this context can be understood as a form of protest against systemic alienation and marginalization [35].

In countries with a low Human Development Index (HDI), self-immolation can be seen as a "gendered form of self-harm"[34]. In a study of self-immolation of Iraqi Kurdish women, the authors describe how the institution of marriage can be used to control female sexuality, stunting a young woman's sense of identity, which is aptly described by the Kurdish proverb *'Bume bûk, bume pepûk'*: 'I became a bride; I became miserable' [34]. In the context of the patriarchal Kurdish society, being young and female confers a double disadvantage for women, increasing their vulnerability to suicide.

12   Self-Immolation

More than other forms of suicide, self-immolation tragically and powerfully expresses failure of empowerment and agency. The sovereignty of life is deeply disembodied in self-immolation. Suicide by self-immolation defies reductionist biological theories or those based solely on social determinants or mental disorders. At times it is a direct and aggressive act against forms of sociopolitical or economic oppression by the state. In denouncing the misery of private life and relationships, self-immolation is a synthesis of how challenges in interpersonal relationships or difficult societal problems enable suicide [36]. It is a particularly violent form of suicide, where the pain inflicted on the victim makes witnesses to the act participants [37]. During self-immolation, the body as receptacle of the essence of being physically disintegrates proxemic boundaries creating a continuum between the suicidal person and witnesses to the lugubrious spectacle.

Self-immolation as a rhetorical stratagem is a powerful response by a marginalized individual to the body–politic and a protest against the state's attempt to control the narrative of their bodies. In the case of protest suicides, this rhetoric is effective only when the actions and underlying motives strongly resonate with the cultural values of the population it attempts to address, and where suicide is seen as justifiable due to a perceived crisis by a majority of the public. The effectiveness of the act is modulated by the power of the state to control the dissemination and meaningfulness of the message [38].

Self-immolation of young Afghan women is a performative form of protest that serves a powerful communicative function, and through defiance, challenges the traditional gendered narrative of a fragile female prone to self-harm [39]. The hermeneutics of suicide location also highlights the performative nature, with the majority of female self-immolations studied in Kurdish Iraq happening at home, a location where domesticity and abuse coexist, and suicide involves the family as the audience and participant-observers [34].

Sociological studies on self-immolation among Kurdish women in Iraq show that a significant majority are married women, thus challenging the simplistic notion of risks and vulnerabilities related to social isolation. These studies also show how self-immolation as a suicide method has a pattern of cultural transmission parallel-ing the movement of population subgroups. Examples include increased prevalence of self-immolation in Afghanistan following the return of Afghan refugees from Iran, and similar transmissions across the borders of various central Asian countries [34]. In Afghanistan, suicide stories among Afghan women serve as powerful com-municative "narratives of dramatic social change"[14].

In the psychological assessment of patients who self-immolate, researchers emphasize the importance of assessing if there could be a religious motive behind suicide, and spiritual or religious considerations should inform culturally sensitive clinical interventions [40]. A study of self-immolation in burn centers in the United States, conducted by chaplains, sought to understand how patients imagined and understood God and their understanding of how God would respond to their actions. They found that the patient's individual beliefs and their world view, rather than the formal expression of those beliefs through an "organized worshipping community" are associated with self-immolation. Also, a rigidly held image of God as punishing is common in those who self-immolate. Consequently, chaplains and spiritual advi-sors may help suicidal persons as they reflect on themes of atonement, sin and God to deflect away from rigid stances that could place them at risk [41].

Andreasen and Noyes' study of patients who self-immolated in the United States describes a significant proportion as having a strong religious background, with some feeling they deserved punishment for their sins or being abandoned by God, and one patient reporting command auditory hallucinations attributed to a divine source [41, 42]. Stoddard's study of adolescents who self-immolated found signifi-cance in high religiosity, a more literal and fundamentalist scriptural interpretation, the experience of significant guilt for sins committed, and having a strict concept of punishment. More fundamentalist religious traditions in families with rigid forms of scriptural interpretation, along with incorporation of strong feelings of deserving punishment and guilt for wrongdoings can also be contributory factors for self-immolation in young individuals [36, 39].

Hahn and colleagues elaborate on the significance of taking culture into account when exploring, treating and researching suicide by self-immolation and describe how cultural factors can influence the experience, diagnosis and documentation of mental disorders. They succinctly state that "fire can convey a number of meanings in various cultures including purification, sacrifice, and punishment, as well as more contemporary images associated with war, political protest, and nuclear destruction"[40].

13   Conclusion

Humans beings are social beings. Since the beginning of the cognitive revolution, our success as a species depends on our collective capacity, language and sociability [43]. The good functioning of our biological unit-our body is as important as our collective functioning-our society. A disruptive society might fail to be inclusive, leaving people jettisoned and feeling expendable, and possibly causing death by suicide.

For centuries, philosophers pondered about suicide and sociologists studied determinants and protective factors. Religion, law, economy, politics, culture and gender may play a role in increasing the burden of society over the individual.

In some extreme situations, human rights are constantly compromised and challenged. Life in conflict zones, indigenous people in western societies, and refugees escaping from traumatic circumstances are examples of situations where society fails to protect individuals.

Suicide by self-immolation forcefully expresses failure of empowerment and agency. It commonly affects disenfranchised and vulnerable groups. Suicide prevention efforts must include interventions that effect change in social, economic, educational, spiritual and political dimensions.

References

1. Descartes R. Discours de la méthode. Bibliotheque: Nationale de France; 1879.
2. Miles M. Plato on Suicide ("Phaedo" 60C–63C). Phoenix. 2001:55, 244–258.
3. Plato (trans. by C.J. Emlyn-Jones, and W. Preddy). Euthyphro: Apology; Crito; Phaedo. Cambridge, MA: Harvard University Press; 2017.
4. Garrison EP. Attitudes toward suicide in ancient Greece. Trans Am Philol Assoc. 1991;121:1–34.
5. Strachan JCG. Who did forbid suicide at Phaedo 62b? Class Q. 1970;20(2):216–20.
6. Tierney TF. The governmentality of suicide: Peuchet, Marx, Durkheim, and Foucault. J Class Sociol. 2010;10(4):357–89.
7. Freud S. The ego and the id (1923). TACD J. 1989;17(1):5–22.
8. Ramos BS. Enfermar, envejecer y morir en los tiempos de Tito a Trajano/To fall ill, to age and to die by the time between Titus and Trajanus. Cuadernos de Filología Clásica. Estudios Latinos. 2007;27(1):87.
9. Camus A. The myth of Sisyphus and other essays (J. O'Brien, Trans.). New York: Vintage International; 1955.
10. Marsh I. Suicide: foucault, history and truth. Cambridge: Cambridge University Press; 2010.
11. Cheikh IB, Rousseau C, Mekki-Berrada A. Suicide as protest against social suffering in the Arab world. Br J Psychiatry. 2011;198(6):494–5.
12. Douglas JD. Social meanings of suicide. Princeton: Princeton University Press; 2015.
13. Shiner M, et al. When things fall apart: gender and suicide across the life-course. Soc Sci Med. 2009;69(5):738–46.
14. Staples J, Widger T. Situating suicide as an anthropological problem: ethnographic approaches to understanding self-harm and self-inflicted death. Cult Med Psychiatry. 2012;36(2):183–203.
15. Jones RA. Emile Durkheim: an introduction to four major works. Thousand Oaks: Sage Publications, Inc; 1986.
16. Durkheim E. Suicide: a study in sociology (JA Spaulding & G. Simpson, trans.). Glencoe, IL: Free Press; 1951. (Original work published 1897)
17. Foucault M. Histoire de la sexualité, tome I: la volonté de savoir. Paris: Gallimard; 1994.
18. Foucault M, Rabinow P, Faubion JD. The essential works of Foucault, 1954–1984. New York: New Press; 1997.
19. Frank J. In: Lesky E, editor. A system of complete medical police. Baltimore: Johns Hopkins University Press; 1976.

20. Marx K. Marx on suicide. Evanston: Northwestern University Press; 1999.
21. Hellern V, Notaker H, Gaarder J. O livro das religiões. São Paulo: Companhia das Letras; 2000.
22. Dias ML. Suicídio: testemunhas de adeus. Sao Paulo: Brasiliense; 1991.
23. Añón F. Aproximación teológico-ética y filosofica a la problemática del suicidio. La Problemática del Suicidio en el Uruguay de Hoy. 1992;1:71–92.
24. Guzder J. Women who jump into wells: reflections on suicidality in women from conflict regions of the Indian subcontinent. Transcultural Psychiatry. 2011;48(5):585–603.
25. Andriolo K. The twice-killed: imagining protest suicide. Am Anthropol. 2006;108(1):100–13.
26. Ozawa-de SC. Too lonely to die alone: internet suicide pacts and existential suffering in Japan. Cult Med Psychiatry. 2008;32(4):516–51.
27. Chachamovich E, et al. Suicide among Inuit: results from a large, epidemiologically representative follow-back study in Nunavut. Can J Psychiatr. 2015;60(6):268–75.
28. Stacey K, et al. Promoting mental health and well-being in Aboriginal contexts: successful elements of suicide prevention work. Health Promot J Austr. 2007;18(3):247–54.
29. Ferreira MEV, Matsuo T. d. Souza RKT. Aspectos demográficos e mortalidade de populações indígenas do Estado do Mato Grosso do Sul, Brasil. Cadernos de Saúde Pública. 2011;27:2327–39.
30. Kral MJ, et al. Unikkaartuit: meanings of well-being, unhappiness, health, and community change among Inuit in Nunavut, Canada. Am J Community Psychol. 2011;48(3–4):426–38.
31. Hunter E, Milroy H. Aboriginal and Torres Strait Islander suicide in context. Archiv Suicide Res. 2006;10(2):141–57.
32. Dabbagh N. Behind the statistics: the ethnography of suicide in Palestine. Cult Med Psychiatry. 2012;36(2):286–305.
33. Das V, Nandy A. Violence, victimhood, and the language of silence. Contribut Indian Sociol. 1985;19(1):177–95.
34. Rasool IA. PaytonJL. Tongues of fire: women's suicide and self-injury by burns in the Kurdistan Region of Iraq. Sociol Rev. 2014;62(2):237–54.
35. Khushkadamova KO. Women's self-immolation as a social phenomenon. Sociol Res. 2010;49(1):75–91.
36. Rezaeian M. Why it is so important to prevent self-immolation around the globe? Burns. 2013;39(6):1322–3.
37. Prosser D. Suicides by burning in England and Wales. Br J Psychiatry. 1996;168(2):175–82.
38. Neville-Shepard MD. Fire, sacrifice, and social change: the rhetoric of self-immolation. Kansas: University of Kansas; 2014.
39. Billaud J. Suicidal performances: voicing discontent in a girls' dormitory in Kabul. Cult Med Psychiatry. 2012;36(2):264–85.
40. Hahn AP, et al. Self-inflicted burns: a systematic review of the literature. J Burn Care Res. 2014;35(1):102–19.
41. Grossoehme D, Springer L. Images of God used by self-injurious burn patients. Burns. 1999;25(5):443–8.
42. Andreasen NC, Noyes R. Suicide attempted by self-immolation. Am J Psychiatry. 1975;132(5):554–6.
43. Harari YN. Sapiens: a brief history of humankind. New York: Random House; 2014.

Religion, Spirituality, Belief Systems and Suicide

David Choon Liang Teo, Katerina Duchonova, Samaneh Kariman, and Jared Ng

1 Introduction

In parallel with remarkable advances in science and technology, religion and spiritual practices remain an integral part of many individuals and communities. Today, an estimated 90% of the world's population is involved in some form of religious or spiritual practice [1]. Religion is a powerful coping resource that helps people make sense of suffering, fosters a sense of control in the face of life's stressors, and promotes social constructs that facilitate communal living, collaboration and mutual support [2]. All world religions are identical in this respect but differ in their cultural expression.

Suicide occurs in all nations often in the context of many religious traditions. Attitudes concerning suicide are diverse and complex [3], and the experience of

D. C. L. Teo (✉)
Department of Psychological Medicine, Changi General Hospital, Singapore

Duke-NUS Medical School, Singapore

Yong Loo Lin School of Medicine, National University of Singapore, Singapore
e-mail: david.teo.c.l@singhealth.com.sg

K. Duchonova
Department of Psychiatry, Military University Hospital, Prague, Czech Republic
e-mail: katerinaduchonova@seznam.cz

S. Kariman
WPA Psychotherapy Section, Geneva, Switzerland
e-mail: samanekariman@yahoo.com

J. Ng
Emergency & Crisis Services, Institute of Mental Health, Singapore
e-mail: jared_ng@imh.com.sg

spiritual and religious thoughts and feelings is part of everyday life. Religiosity and spirituality provide a framework for adapting to the vicissitudes of life. Religion and spirituality have a profound impact on social perceptions of suicide.

Suicide by self-immolation frequently has religious undertones. For example, Judeo-Christian traditions associate fire with the act of cleansing and purification; Islamic tradition considers fire the harshest form of punishment; the ritualistic *Sati* is closely connected with Hindu beliefs; and Buddhists may self-immolate as a form of social protest and altruistic act of self-sacrifice [4]. This chapter reviews the complex relationship between spirituality, religion, and suicide, and examines suicide and self-immolation through the lens of the world's leading religions.

2 Spirituality, Religion, Belief Systems and Suicide

Spirituality is difficult to define. It is universal, yet unique to everyone. It is personal and self-defined; free of the rules and regulations associated with religion [2]. It is concerned with the transcendent and an individuals' connection to a larger reality or context of meaning [5]. Whether it is reflected in religious practice or something else such as artistic expression, spirituality serves to shape values and purpose in life [6]. It is an integrating force for other aspects of human life: biological, psychological and social [7]. Religion is the form that spirituality takes in certain traditions arising from a group of people with common beliefs and practices encompassing the mystical, supernatural or God, or the Ultimate Truth [2].

We exist in an environment of beliefs that shapes who we become, evokes and supports the ways in which we view and experience the world, influences our behaviour and the choices we make, and fosters a sense of purpose and meaning [8]. Spirituality and belief systems may deeply influence views of suffering, and this in turn may influence suicide risk. For example, youth suicide is linked to a spiritual vacuum and inability to find meaning or truth in life [9]. In some contexts, suicide is viewed as heroic or an act of martyrdom, self-sacrifice or self-denial. Socrates thought that life without room for critical thinking was not worth living and his beliefs about the blessedness of death inspired the suicides of others [10]. Transculturally, suicide becomes an honourable act in the face of unjust governmental oppression to avoid subjugation [3].

3 Sociological Aspects of Religion and Suicide

Durkheim's ground-breaking work on suicide laid the foundation for more than a century of research on religion and suicide. He posited that spiritual commitment may promote emotional well-being as it provides a source of meaning and order in the world [11]. He noted that Catholics had lower suicide rates compared to Protestants and proposed that this was because of Catholicism explicitly prohibiting suicide as opposed to Protestantism permitting free inquiry and diverse beliefs [12].

Judaism, while valuing freedom of thought, had an even stronger protective effect against suicide than Catholicism, theorizing that this was because of the strong communal spirit within Jewish traditions and strict prohibitions against suicide [12].

Durkheim regarded religion as a reflection of society and viewed suicide from a social rather than individual perspective. He emphasized the role of external factors in a person's decision to die by suicide and proposed that various states disrupt the equilibrium between the individual and community. Altruism can result when the bond between the two is strong. Conversely, too weak a bond can result in egoism and anomie [10]. Notwithstanding methodological limitations, Durkheim's seminal work established that suicide could be understood from a sociological perspective with religion serving regulative and integrative functions [13].

Other researchers purported the religious commitment theory where religion decreases suicide risk regardless of denomination [14]. Stack suggested that devotion to a few core religious beliefs, such as the afterlife, a responsive God, or that suffering has purpose protect against suicide [15]. Pescosolido and Georgianna emphasized the role that the religious community, participation in rituals, and network contacts play in suicide prevention. They noted how the relationship between religion and suicide evolved and changed with the sociohistorical trends of secularization, ecumenicalism and evangelism [16].

4   Research on Religion and Suicide

Research data on the relationship between religion and suicide largely draws from non-clinical samples, with mixed findings underscoring the complex nature of the relationship. Most studies suggest that greater religiosity is protective against suicide [13]. However, research in this area is complicated by factors including affiliation, degree of participation, doctrine, and the cultural and socio-political context. Similarly, research on suicide is heterogenous with different studies examining a range of suicidal behaviours. The prevailing culture of the setting also influences suicide reporting. Whalen concluded that religion may function as the source of the suicidal agent, as a suicide-genic agent, a suicide-static agent, or as a protective agent against suicide [17]. Additionally, there is a nuanced relationship between specific religions and suicide in different cultural contexts. For example, among Indian adolescents suicide ideation and attempts are higher among Hindus [18]. In Taiwan, Christians have higher rates of suicide compared to Buddhists [19]. In Israel, Jews were more likely than Muslims to be suicidal [20].

4.1   Religion as Protective Against Suicide

Ecological studies suggest that suicide rates in countries with strong religious traditions are significantly lower than that in secular ones [21]. Greater intensity of religious commitment is also associated with lower suicidal behaviours [22]. Gender differences exist in the relationship between religiosity and suicide. In males, higher suicide rates correlate with lower levels of religious beliefs and religious attendance, while this is not the case with females [23].

Positive religious coping methods such as spiritual support, religious reframing of stressors, and spiritual connectedness correlate with better mental health and may be protective against suicide [24]. Almost all religions promote optimism about the future and encourage resilience, which are qualities antithetical to suicide [25]. Religions also assuage human suffering and socioeconomic disappointments providing comfort and meaning in the face of adversity [26].

Religion protects against suicide in part through doctrines that forbid suicide [27]. Most religions like Islam and Judaism have strong sanctions and teachings against suicide. One study suggests that in addition to religious teachings the strength of the clergy's condemnation is suicide protective, especially when religious leaders perceive suicide as unpardonable, unforgivable and unthinkable [28].

Durkheim theorized that religion is a source of social integration [11]. Involvement in an organized religion through a supportive community provides opportunities to develop a network that extends beyond the family and into the congregation. This level of integration becomes a protective factor against suicide [29].

Prohibition of substance and alcohol use in many religions could also have an indirect effect of reducing suicide rates, as many suicides are related to impulsivity [30]. Religion may also protect against suicide by lowering aggression and hostility [31].

4.2   Religion as a Risk Factor for Suicide

Some studies show that religion has no effect on suicidality and some find that religiosity triggers an increased risk [32]. Varying definitions of religiosity may be a confounding factor. Moreover, negative studies do not imply causality. Nevertheless, negative religious coping, defined by Pargament as "a maladaptive pattern that may include deferring all responsibility to God, feeling abandoned by God, blaming God for difficulties, experiencing spiritual tension or doubt, or experiencing conflict and struggle with God", correlates with greater frequency and intensity of suicidal ideation [33].

Distress related to religious or spiritual concerns also correlates with suicidal ideation [34]. Negative or punitive images of God can also turn religion from a resource into a cause of spiritual struggle. The belief of having committed a sin of unforgivable magnitude is associated with suicidal thoughts [34]. While increased religion and spirituality can promote social connectedness, it can conversely present opportunities for misunderstanding and negative interpersonal interactions. Feelings of religious alienation and disillusionment may lead to distress.

For some, religion may play a role in incentivizing suicide. Religious fanaticism can lead to radicalization and a distortion or misinterpretation of doctrine and scriptures [35]. In the era of the Internet and vast social media networks, rhetoric propagated by self-proclaimed preachers can influence large numbers of people, sometimes with devastating consequences that exploit the dynamics of social contagion and tragically result in suicide and violence. From a psychopathological perspective, religious delusions in severe mental illness, perhaps rooted in intrapsychic conflicts, can have a profound influence on a person's behaviour and at times precipitate suicide [36].

5 Christianity

Christianity is the world's largest religion with about 2.3 billion adherents [37]. Central to Christian tradition are the four Gospels which record the birth, life, ministry, suffering, death and resurrection of Jesus of Nazareth. Following the Great Schism of 1054, the Christian Church divided into the Eastern (Orthodox) and Western (Catholic) branches. Following the sixteenth Century Reformation, Western Christianity further split into Protestant and Catholic Divisions [38].

While Christianity today is practiced in diverse ways, its central tenet is belief in Jesus as the Son of God, Messiah, and God incarnate. Christians believe that through the acceptance of the death and resurrection of Jesus, those who sin can be forgiven, reconciled with God, gain salvation and the promise of eternal life [39].

Hebrew Scriptures form the Old Testament of the Christian Bible. These include the Torah (Law), books detailing the history of the Israelites, "Wisdom books" addressing questions of good and evil in the world, and books of biblical prophets cautioning the consequences of turning away from God. Christian scriptures (The New Testament) include the Gospels, which record the birth, life, ministry and resurrection of Jesus, an account of the early Church history (The Acts of the Apostles), letters written by the apostles, and a prophetic book (The Revelation of John) [6].

5.1 Christianity and Suicide

Christianity's view on suicide is much debated. Early Christians viewed suicide as a sin. In modern times, some churches reject this teaching while others continue to espouse this view.

While the word 'suicide' does not appear in the Bible, several recorded examples of suicide include the deaths of Samson, King Saul and Judas [40]. The Bible neither condemns nor condones these suicides. St. Augustine contended in the fifth century that suicide is a violation of the sixth commandment, "Thou shall not kill". He argued that God's prohibition against murder applies to one's life as well and all life should be preserved [40]. In the thirteenth century, St. Thomas Aquinas stated that suicide goes against nature's inclination to preserve life, damages social community, and that only God, the giver of life, has the right to decide when a person will live or die [41]. These views influenced the early Church's official stance against suicide and strong condemnation of suicide as a sin by the Church throughout the Middle Ages influenced the criminalization of suicide in the West. Other influential clerics, such as John Donne, did not view suicide as always sinful but deserving of compassion [6].

Catholicism has a condemnatory attitude toward suicide, which is classified as a mortal sin that prevents salvation of the soul. Suicide is stigmatised by practices such as bans against the burial of those who die by suicide [14].

Many Protestants also consider suicide sinful. However, Protestantism lacks the concept of a mortal sin and thus does not outrightly prohibit suicide. Since the age of the Enlightenment, the Church adopted a more compassionate stance seeking to understand why people die by suicide. The Biblical teaching to love thy neighbour fosters greater emphasis on suicide prevention through caring for those in suicide crises [10].

The Christian doctrine of inherent sin can potentially lead to auto-accusations and feelings of failure in life. In a fundamentalist environment, feelings of inadequacy and guilt may arise when one falls short of complete adherence to religious commandments. Suicide risk increases when religion leaves a person feeling guilty, distant from God, or abandoned by the religious community [9].

5.2   Christianity and Self-Immolation

In some denominations, Christianity honours self-sacrifice and martyrdom by some Catholic or Orthodox Saints, extolling how they imitated Christ's suffering during the crucifixion. Around AD 300, Christians persecuted by Diocletian in Nicomedia participated in a mass act of self-immolation to protest the Roman persecution of Christians [42]. In the seventeenth century, faced by government-ordered reforms to the Orthodox Church, thousands of followers of the ascetic Kapiton locked themselves in churches and self-immolated. They saw the Tsar as the Antichrist and his interference with their worship as a sign of the end times [42].

The Self-Immolation of Jan Palach
"Palach's self-immolation is impalpable, substandard. It defies common ethical evaluation. It evokes great emotions, many questions, debates and often opposing assessments. He is both condemned and glorified." (Jindřich Šrajer, Catholic priest and theologian, 2009)

Jan Palach was born in Prague in 1948 and grew up in Všetaty. His father was a Czech National Socialist and mother a member of the Evangelical Church of Czech Brethren. When Palach studied philosophy at Charles University he experienced the Prague Spring. This caused his fledgling interest in public affairs to grow. He later witnessed the August 1968 occupation of Prague by the Warsaw Pact troops and his nation's demoralization and acceptance of its occupation. In protest of the Soviet invasion, Palach set him-self on fire in Wenceslas Square on 16 January 1969. He died in a hospital 3 days later. His stated goal was to galvanize the Czech public to protest the occupation of their country by the Soviets. Although his act was soon dishon-oured and downplayed by the authorities of the totalitarian regime of Czechoslovakia, his legacy lived in many people beyond the solitary act and inspired them to fight against the regime.

Palach was probably inspired by the protest self-immolation acts of Buddhist monks in Southern Vietnam a few years earlier. He came from a patriotic and Christian environment and within the Church his self-immolation sparked controversy. After the fall of the totalitarian communist regime of Czechoslovakia, it was idealized as an act of self-sacrifice in pursuit of higher social values. Palach's suicide was also a reflection of the demoralization and societal discontent experienced by his contemporaries [43].

6   Islam

Islam is the world's second largest and fastest growing religion with more than 1.8 billion followers [37]. Muslims may soon exceed Christians. Apart from being a religion, Islam is also a socio-political system that offers a holistic approach to solving mankind's spiritual, intellectual and day-to-day problems.

Islam derives from the Semitic word for peace (*shalom*), which means submission to God [6]. While it shares the Abrahamic traditions of Judaism and Christianity, it emphasizes the ministry of the Prophet Muhammad. Islamic tradition recognizes a series of revelations made to Muhammad through the archangel Gabriel, which he wrote down and collated as the Holy Quran [6]. The Sunnah and Hadith constitute the teachings and examples of Muhammad [13]. Like other Abrahamic religions, Islam teaches that there will be a final judgment with the righteous being given a place in paradise while the unrighteous punished with condemnation [6].

There two major branches in Islam—Sunni and Shi'ite. The key difference stems from beliefs about who should have been the rightful successor to Muhammad. Sunni Muslims make up about 85% of Muslims around the world [6].

The Five Pillars of Islam form the framework for Muslim spiritual beliefs and practices [13]. These include:

1. Declaration of faith (Al-shahadah): "To bear witness that there is no one worthy of God (Allah), and that Muhammad is His final servant and messenger."
2. Prayer (Al-salah) five times a day
3. Alms-giving (Al-Zakah)
4. Obligatory fasting during Ramadan (Al-Sawm)
5. Pilgrimage to Mecca (Al-Hajj)

Islam teaches that Allah is the absolute creator and master of everything. Hence, complete submission to His will and trust in His mercy brings peace. Illness and suffering are considered Allah's tests for mankind and enduring these tests with fortitude and faithfulness elevates one's standing in His eyes [13].

6.1 Islam and Suicide

Islam strongly condemns suicide. In Islam, the body is considered sacred. Intentionally damaging one's body is considered sinful. The Quranic verse: "The lit candle should burn until daybreak", is often interpreted as a prohibition against the wilful termination of life. Islam teaches that people who commit suicide will be deprived of Allah's blessings and mercy in the afterlife [6]. The Quran and Hadith explicitly instruct: "Do not kill yourselves. Surely Allah is ever compassionate to you." (Quran 4:29).

Limited research shows that suicide rates are lower in Islamic countries compared to other countries [44]. However, it is noteworthy that Islamic countries may under report suicide. Islamic law criminalizes suicide in many Arab League countries [45]. Surviving family members are often shunned and stigmatized in Muslim communities. As suicide is considered *haram* (forbidden death), Muslim graveyards are often reluctant to bury individuals who die by suicide [45].

6.2 Islam and Self-Immolation

Self-immolation is a common method of suicide among women in certain parts of the world, such as Iran, Iraq and Afghanistan. In Iran 83% of women who die by suicide do so via self-immolation [46]. Additionally, the proportion of women who commit suicide by self-immolation increased over the years [47].

Socio-cultural influences appear to mediate the effect of Islamic faith on self-immolations. Even today, many traditional Islamic societies regard women as inferior to men. Women are accorded lesser rights, resulting in their marginalization and oppression by men [48]. Many women who self-immolate live in poverty, have low education, are forced into arranged marriages at a very young age, or suffered male domination and degradation in the family [46]. Self-immolations by women in these communities are a form of protest against abuse and lack of basic human rights [48]. Furthermore, the taboo of divorce may drive women suffering abusive marriages to desperation and believe that suicide is the only escape. These women often self-immolate in the presence of their oppressors ostensibly to induce feelings of guilt and symbolically defend themselves. Self-immolations may also serve the purpose of avoiding honor killings [48].

The Self-Immolation of "Bemani"

Based on true stories, the Iranian film "Bemani", by acclaimed Iranian film director Dariush Mehrjouei, depicts the tragic lives of three girls from Ilam—a western province of Iran with the highest incidence of self-immolation in the country.

Bemani, one of the girls, was a high school girl from a poor family living in a crowded home. Her father, a sweeper, arranged for her to marry their landlord in exchange for 3 years' rent. She rebelled and ran away from home to live with her aunt. Her father and brother, however, pursued and brought her home, forcing her to marry the rich old landlord. The landlord was very disrespectful and treated her like a maid. Bemani rebelled against her oppressive husband and ultimately escaped, returning to her own family. Facing criticism from them, she suicided by dousing herself with gasoline and setting herself on fire.

7 Hinduism

Hinduism is one of the oldest religions in the world, calling itself the "eternal religion" (*Sanātana dharma*). The diversity of Hinduism is vast and its history long and complex. Its earliest scripture, the *Veda*, dates to approximately 1500 BC; some features, such as goddess worship, might go back to the Indus Valley Civilization, around 2500 BC [49].

There are approximately 1.1 billion Hindus in the world, with the majority living in India [37]. The rest reside in communities in neighbouring states (such as Nepal and Mauritius), and in places such as Bali, South-West Africa and the Caribbean. The four largest denominations of Hinduism are the Vaishnavism, Shaivism, Shaktism and Smartism [50].

Describing Hinduism is challenging because of its wide range of traditions and ideas. It does not have a single historical founder and accepts a multiplicity of divine forms, with many Hindus considering the deities to be aspects or manifestations of a single impersonal absolute or ultimate reality or God, while other maintain that a specific deity represents the supreme being and various deities are lower manifestations of this supreme being [51]. Hinduism is described as a religion, a religious tradition, a set of religious beliefs, and a way of life [52].

In Hinduism, the *Vedas,* which consist of hymns, incantations and rituals, serve as the scriptures for a universal Hindu framework. The *Bhagavad Gita* and the *Upanishads* are the main integrative scriptures [53]. Hindu practices include rituals such as worship (*puja*) and recitations, meditative repetition of a mantra (*japa*), meditation, family-oriented rites of passage, annual festivals, and pilgrimages. Some Hindus may leave their social world and material possessions to engage in lifelong monastic practices (*Sannyasa*) [54].

Hinduism is often characterised by the belief in reincarnation (*Saṃsāra*) determined by the law that all actions have effects (*karma*), and that salvation is freedom from this cycle (*Moksha*). Essentially, Hindus believe that all beings can reach enlightenment through actions in their lives and progression through cycles of rebirth. Beings can transcend many lives and undergo numerous experiences before merging with the divine. In death, there is a disconnection between the physical body and the mind; while in rebirth, the body and mind return to Earth. It is important to note that Hindu doctrine accepts that suffering in life is inevitable.

7.1 Hinduism and Suicide

Hinduism generally perceives suicide as an act against humanity and reprehensible [53]. However, unlike some other dominant world religions, Hindu scriptures are less resolute on the issue of suicide as strictly unacceptable [55]. There are scholars who believe that the "reincarnation tenet" is tolerant of suicide [56], as life does not end with death; rather, death leads to rebirth. Research studies suggest a higher suicide rate of Hindus compared to Muslims and those practicing other religions [55].

Hinduism seems to endorse some suicides [57]. For example, *Prayopavesha* is a practice where the person voluntarily fasts to death as a mean of deliberate spiritual enlightenment. Individuals must not have any desires, ambitions and responsibilities left, and the decision to fast to death must be declared publicly in advance. The *Matsya Purana* compiled in the fifth to thirteenth century, approvingly describes Hindu ritual suicide by drowning. The Chinese pilgrim Xuanzang, who travelled to India in the seventh century, wrote about the *Prayag Kumbha Mela* (the sacred rivers confluence festival). Xuanzang claimed seeing ascetics clinging to tall posts embedded in the river, staring at the sun until they were blinded, then jumping into the water to drown themselves. We describe the practice of *Sati* in the next section.

7.2 Hinduism and Self-Immolation

In India, forms of suicide by self-immolation included *Jauhar*, the act of mass self-immolation by women and sometimes their children, "to avoid capture, enslavement and rape by foreign invaders, when facing certain defeat during a war" [58]. The Rajput clan in medieval India practiced *Jauhar* [59], considered an act of heroism as the death of women and children would free their male fighters from worry and also save women from the shame of rape by enemy forces [60].

The practice of *Sati* is the self-immolation of a widow on the funeral pyre of her husband so that their destinies will converge. The word is derived from the Sanskrit word "*sat*" which means "truth". *Sati*, he first wife of *Shiva* (one of the supreme beings) self-immolated to protest that *Shiva* was not invited to a holy ritual. In frenzied anger, Shiva bore the corpse of *Sati* on his shoulder and threatened to destroy the universe [59].

There are numerous variants of the *Sati* ritual. In some, women sit or lie on the funeral pyre beside the deceased husband. Other accounts describe women walking or jumping into the flames [61]. The Mahābhārata, compiled between third century BCE and third century, is the first scripture to mention *Sati* self-immolations, as in the case of Madri, wife of Pandu. The first inscriptional evidence of the practice took place in Nepal in 464 CE, and then India in 510 CE [62]. The practice of *Sati* spread together with Hindu migrants to regions in Southeast Asia, such as Sumatra, Java and Bali, though it remained rare outside of India.

Some report *Sati* as possibly stemming from severe bereavement [63]. Harlan explained the process of Sati in three main stages: being a *pativrata* (dutiful wife) during the husband's life; making a solemn vow at the husband's deathbed, gaining status as a *sativrata* (transitional stage between the living and the dead); and enduring being burnt alive, achieving status as a *satimata* (a spiritual embodiment of goodness) [60].

Sati was outlawed in December 1829 after the British passed the "XVII Prevention of *Sati* Act" declaring Sati illegal and punishable by courts [64]. Although rare, the ritual continues to be practiced in some rural areas in India [65]. In September 1987, a woman named Roopkuvarba Kanwar self-immolated in Rajasthan, India. She was 18-year-old at the time and married for a few months. The adulation from some quarters of society eventually led to a public outcry and propelled debates about women's choice to practice *Sati*. In 1988, the Commission of Sati (Prevention) Act passed prohibiting the glorification of *Sati* in any form [66].

8 Buddhism

Buddhism is considered a philosophy and code of ethics [67]. Its teachings offer a set of beliefs about reality, insight about the human mind and behaviour, and recommendations for appropriate conduct. Practiced by an estimated 350 million people worldwide [68], it currently comprises two major sects with their unique communities, teachings and practices—Theravada and Mahayana. Theravada Buddhism is a major religion in India, Sri Lanka, Thailand, Cambodia, Myanmar and Laos. Mahayana Buddhism has a significant following in China, Japan, Korea, Taiwan, Tibet, Nepal, Mongolia and Vietnam.

Buddhist doctrine teaches that life and death are part of an unending cycle until a person reaches *Nirvana*—a state devoid of desire and suffering epitomized by bliss and peace. Unless one achieves *Nirvana*, death is merely the start of another cycle of pain and suffering [69]. *Dukkha* is the inability to be satisfied, translated by some as suffering. It is inevitable and results from seeking happiness in impermanent things or states.

The Four Noble Truths form the basic orientation of Buddhism:

1. Impermanence and suffering are universal and inevitable.
2. Suffering is created by our mind and attitudes when attaching to objects or states that are impermanent.
3. Suffering only ceases and gives way to peace and contentment when desire for impermanent things is eradicated.
4. The Eightfold Noble Path is the only means to this cessation and end to a dissatisfactory life, a process by which individuals are empowered to master control of their mind, wants and desires [70].

Both Theravada and Mahayana Buddhism teach that suffering and happiness arise from the mind. Craving and desire result in unskilful acts (those lacking in compassion toward other living things) and produce more suffering and misery [69]. At the same time, skilful acts based on contentment bring happiness. The teaching of *karma* exhorts one to live with fortitude through unavoidable suffering that results from past acts while concurrently refraining from unskilful acts to reduce future suffering [71]. Buddhist teachings on *dukkha* also help people take suffering less personally and reframe their experiences of personal pain into a larger context.

8.1   Buddhism and Suicide

Buddhist teachings mandate non-violence and abstinence from the destruction of life. As suicide involves killing a living being (the self), it is an action that will result in more suffering. Buddhism condemns suicide as an expression of desire (*tanha*) and delusion (*moha*). Desire for non-existence characterizes an unenlightened person, and delusion because one who commits suicide is gravely mistaken that suicide is the solution to one's problems. Therefore, if a person tries to end suffering through suicide instead of purifying the mind through meditation and following the Eightfold Noble Path, as part of karmic retribution for violating the most important Buddhist moral precept of not taking life, the consequence is rebirth into a lower level of existence and further suffering [72].

8.2   Buddhism and Self-Immolation

Notwithstanding the general condemnation of suicide in Buddhism, two forms of elective death are celebrated in Buddhist tradition. These are firstly, self-sacrifice or sacrificing one's life for the benefit of others, and secondly, taking one's life as a ritual offering in an act of devotion [72].

Buddhist texts (*jatakas*) recounting the past life stories of the Buddha contain stories of the Bodhisattva repeatedly sacrificing life and limb on behalf of the others in successive rebirths. For example, in the Buddha's birth as Prince Mahasattva, he allows himself to be eaten by a starving tigress to prevent her from devouring her own cubs. It is important to note that self-sacrifice in these stories is motivated by compassion for other beings rather than for personal spiritual advancement [73].

Self-immolation is celebrated and commended in Mahayana Buddhist texts. A well-known example is depicted in the "Medicine King" chapter of the Lotus Sutra. In this account, the Bodhisattva sets his body ablaze as a devotional offering to the Buddha. In his ensuing rebirth, he burns his forearms for 72,000 years as a ritual offering. In the absence of any 'fields of merit', the Bodhisattva displayed his benevolence in the particularly extreme form of self-burning [72]. Hubert and Mauss note that every sacrifice is a sacrifice of oneself, and therefore every ritual offering is in fact an offering of oneself [74]. However, in modern day religious practice, one typically employs a substitute such as a ritual offering that symbolizes oneself. Buddhist self-immolators can thus be thought of as repaying the debt of gratitude owed to the Buddha for making substitutionary offerings possible by making themselves the direct sacrifice.

In Chinese traditions, self-immolation is a means to the spiritual attainment of immortality [75]. Self-immolations, such as Ning Fengzi's, are portrayed as performed for the greater good [75]. In China, acts of self-immolation carry a variety of meanings and motivations. In addition to spiritual implications, such acts were symbolically purposeful to bring rain during droughts and end wars [76]. Likewise, in more recent times, public self-immolations carried out in protest by Buddhist monks are motivated by compassion and altruistic desire to relieve the suffering of others by drawing attention to injustices and perceived oppression [73].

The self-immolation of Thich Quang Duc in 1963, a Vietnamese Buddhist monk who burned himself at death at busy traffic intersection outside the Cambodian embassy in Saigon, generated international awareness of self-immolation as a form of political protest [77]. The self-immolation took place in the face of persecution of Buddhists in Vietnam by the oppressive regime of a dictatorial President, Ngo Dihn Diem. In response to a petition for religious equality that Thich Quang Duc made before his self-immolation, President Diem made a conciliatory statement. However, media reports of the incident sparked further Buddhist self-immolations and protests. This intensified international pressure on Diem's regime and eventually led to its collapse. In the aftermath of this incident, the Vietnamese regarded Thich Quang Doc as a Bodhisattva because he sacrificed his life for his religion and the benefit of others. His self-immolation left a lasting influence in many countries around the world [78].

9 Religion and Suicide Prevention

Suicide prevention demands a multi-sectoral approach, involving not only health care professionals but also representatives from other disciplines. In many communities, religious leaders are key stakeholders in suicide prevention [79]. A study in

Singapore showed that amongst people with mental illnesses, 12% spoke to a religious or spiritual healer before seeking any medical help [80]. Having ties to the community, social support and religious networks are additional protective factors against suicide [81]. Religious leaders are frequently approached by persons in distress, including those harbouring thoughts of ending their lives. However, they are often not trained to identify and assess suicide risk. Obstacles include lack of financial resources, time, and training opportunities. Even though it seems intuitive that collaboration between religious leaders and mental health professionals is essential for suicide prevention, efforts in this direction are minimal in many parts of the world.

Clinicians often neglect to explore the relationship between the individual's spirituality or religiosity and suicidality. Given the potential protective effect religious commitment and affiliation may have against suicide risk, we recommend that mental health professionals routinely inquire about religious identity and beliefs in clinical and risk assessments. It is helpful to delve deeper into the actual role that religion plays in a person's life, including the level of religious participation and support from the faith community. This may help to identify potential interventions that may enhance life-affirming and preserving beliefs, values and hopes. At the same time, it is also important to identify negative religious coping and distress related to religious or spiritual concerns, which may elevate suicide risk in other individuals. Maladaptive coping or distress as such should be addressed by helping the person find ways to minimize these harmful effects.

10   Conclusion

Most religions either condemn or discourage suicide. However, some have a qualified acceptance of suicide in certain socio-cultural contexts including altruistic motivations and self-immolation as a form of protest leading to martyrdom.

Different social, political, economic and ideological implications of religious affiliation influence suicidality. Therefore, sensitivity to a person's life narrative and how they experience being a member of a religious body is essential to understand the complex link between religion and suicide [82]. To gain better insight into the complex and nuanced relationship between religion, spirituality and suicide, we need to understand what it means to an individual to identify with a religious or spiritual group, the level of involvement, internal and external beliefs and experiences as the person interacts with society within their cultural context.

Religious and political motivations framed within certain socio-cultural contexts at times drive suicide by self-immolation as a powerful proclamation of one's beliefs and values. Dramatic acts of self-immolation may be performed in defence of one's honour, protest and against persecution and injustice, or in affirmation of one's beliefs in the face of persecution, oppression or marginalization.

As a strong spiritual orientation is protective against suicide, collaborative efforts between mental health professionals and religious leaders to support a person's spirituality may be key to preventing suicide and self-immolation.

References

1. Barrett D, Johnson T. World Christian database: atheists/nonreligious by country. World Christian trends [Internet] [place unknown]. Pasadena: William Carey Library; 2001.
2. Koenig HG. Research on religion, spirituality, and mental health: a review. Can J Psychiatr. 2009;54(5):283–91.
3. Koslow SH, Ruiz P, Nemeroff CB. A concise guide to understanding suicide: epidemiology, pathophysiology and prevention. Cambridge: Cambridge University Press; 2014.
4. Grossoehme D, Springer L. Images of God used by self-injurious burn patients. Burns. 1999;25(5):443–8.
5. Josephson AM, Peteet JR. Handbook of spirituality and worldview in clinical practice. New York: American Psychiatric Pub; 2008.
6. Cook CC, Powell A, Sims A. Spirituality and psychiatry. London: RCPsych Publications; 2009.
7. Culliford L. Spiritual care and psychiatric treatment: an introduction. Adv Psychiatr Treat. 2002;8(4):249–58.
8. Cobb M, Puchalski C, Rumbold B. Oxford textbook of spirituality in healthcare. Oxford: OUP; 2012.
9. Tacey D. The spirituality revolution: the emergence of contemporary spirituality. London: Routledge; 2004.
10. Bille-Brahe U. Sociology and Suicidal Behaviour. In: The international handbook of suicide and attempted suicide, vol. 193. Hoboken: Wiley; 2000.
11. Durkheim E. Suicide. 1951.
12. Morselli E. Il suicidio: saggio di statistica morale comparata. Milano: Fratelli Dumolard; 1879.
13. Koenig H, Koenig HG, King D, Carson VB. Handbook of religion and health. New York: OUP; 2012.
14. Stark R, Doyle DP, Rushing JL. Beyond Durkheim: religion and suicide. J Sci Study Relig. 1983;22:120–31.
15. Stack S. Religiosity, depression, and suicide. Religion mental health. New York: Oxford University Press; 1992. p. 87–97.
16. Pescosolido BA, Georgianna S. Durkheim, suicide, and religion: toward a network theory of suicide. Am Sociol Rev. 1989;54:33–48.
17. Whalen EA. Religion and suicide. Rev Relig Res. 1964;5(2):91–110.
18. Sidhartha T, Jena S. Suicidal behaviors in adolescents. Indian J Pediatr. 2006;73(9):783–8.
19. Fang C-K, Lu H-C, Liu S-I, Sun Y-W. Religious beliefs along the suicidal path in northern Taiwan. OMEGA J Death Dying. 2011;63(3):255–69.
20. Gal G, Goldberger N, Kabaha A, Haklai Z, Geraisy N, Gross R, et al. Suicidal behavior among muslim Arabs in Israel. Soc Psychiatry Psychiatr Epidemiol. 2012;47(1):11–7.
21. Dervic K, Oquendo MA, Grunebaum MF, Ellis S, Burke AK, Mann JJ. Religious affiliation and suicide attempt. Am J Psychiatry. 2004;161(12):2303–8.
22. Nelson FL. Religiosity and self-destructive crises in the institutionalized elderly. Suicide Life-Threaten Behav. 1977;7(2):67–74.
23. Neeleman J, Halpern D, Leon D, Lewis G. Tolerance of suicide, religion and suicide rates: an ecological and individual study in 19 Western countries. Psychol Med. 1997;27(5):1165–71.
24. Olson MM, Trevino DB, Geske JA, Vanderpool H. Religious coping and mental health outcomes: an exploratory study of socioeconomically disadvantaged patients. Exp Dermatol. 2012;8(3):172–6.

25. Stack S. The effect of religious commitment on suicide: a cross-national analysis. J Health Soc Behav. 1983;24:362–74.
26. Greening L, Stoppelbein L. Religiosity, attributional style, and social support as psychosocial buffers for African American and White adolescents' perceived risk for suicide. Suicide Life-Threaten Behav. 2002;32(4):404–17.
27. Van Tubergen F, Te Grotenhuis M, Ultee W. Denomination, religious context, and suicide: neo-Durkheimian multilevel explanations tested with individual and contextual data. Am J Sociol. 2005;111(3):797–823.
28. Early KE. Religion and suicide in the African-American community. Westport: Greenwood Publishing Group; 1992.
29. Cheng AT, Chen TH, Chen C-C, Jenkins R. Psychosocial and psychiatric risk factors for suicide: case-control psychological autopsy study. Br J Psychiatry. 2000;177(4):360–5.
30. Hilton SC, Fellingham GW, Lyon JL. Suicide rates and religious commitment in young adult males in Utah. Am J Epidemiol. 2002;155(5):413–9.
31. Gearing RE, Lizardi D. Religion and suicide. J Relig Health. 2009;48(3):332–41.
32. Zhao J, Yang X, Xiao R, Zhang X, Aguilera D, Zhao J. Belief system, meaningfulness, and psychopathology associated with suicidality among Chinese college students: a cross-sectional survey. BMC Public Health. 2012;12(1):668.
33. Rosmarin DH, Bigda-Peyton JS, Öngur D, Pargament KI, Björgvinsson T. Religious coping among psychotic patients: relevance to suicidality and treatment outcomes. Psychiatry Res. 2013;210(1):182–7.
34. Exline JJ, Yali AM, Sanderson WC. Guilt, discord, and alienation: the role of religious strain in depression and suicidality. J Clin Psychol. 2000;56(12):1481–96.
35. Kubacki Z. The question of salvation and faith-based radicalism. Faith based radicalism Christianity, Islam and Judaism: between constructive activism and destructive fanaticism. Brussel: PIE Peter Lang; 2007. p. 131–8.
36. Grover S, Davuluri T, Chakrabarti S. Religion, spirituality, and schizophrenia: a review. Indian J Psychol Med. 2014;36(2):119.
37. Hackett C, McClendon D. Christians remain world's largest religious group, but they are declining in Europe. Pew Research Center. 2017.
38. Rhodes R. The complete guide to Christian denominations. Irvine: Harvest House Publishers; 2015.
39. Metzger BM, Coogan MD. The Oxford companion to the Bible. Oxford: Oxford University Press; 1993.
40. Phipps W. Christian perspectives on suicide. Christian Century. 1985;30:970–2.
41. Alvarez A. The savage god: a study of suicide. London: A&C Black; 2002.
42. Verini J. A terrible act of reason: when did self-immolation become the paramount form of protest. New Yorker. May 16, 2012.
43. Jan Palach Charles University Multimedia Project. Jan Palach. http://www.janpalach.cz/en/default/jan-palach.
44. Abdel-Khalek AM. Neither altruistic suicide, nor terrorism but martyrdom: a muslim perspective. Arch Suicide Res. 2004;8(1):99–113.
45. Sarfraz MA, Castle D. A muslim suicide. Australasian Psychiatr. 2002;10(1):48–50.
46. Aliverdinia A, Pridemore WA. Women's fatalistic suicide in Iran. Violence Against Women. 2009;15(3):307–20.
47. Toobaei S, Loghmani A, Yoosefian R. Suicidal causes among 15 to 30-year olds in Shiraz, Southern Iran. Iran J Med Sci. 1999;24:14–9.
48. Campbell E, Guiao I. Muslim culture and female self-immolation: implications for Global Women's Health Research and Practice. Health Care Women Int. 2004;25(9):782–93.
49. Smith D. Hinduism, Religions in the Modern World. London: Routledge; 2016. p. 57–88.
50. Lipner J. Hindus: their religious beliefs and practices. London: Routledge; 2012.

51. Flood GD, Flood GDF. An introduction to Hinduism. Cambridge: Cambridge University Press; 1996.
52. Sharma A. The study of Hinduism. Columbia: University of South Carolina Press; 2003.
53. Lakhan SE. Hinduism: life and death. BMJ. 2008;337:0809310.
54. Ellinger H. Hinduism. London: Bloomsbury Publishing; 1996.
55. Ineichen B. The influence of religion on the suicide rate: Islam and Hinduism compared. Ment Health Relig Cult. 1998;1(1):31–6.
56. Gearing RE, Alonzo D. Religion and suicide: new findings. J Relig Health. 2018;57(6):2478–99.
57. Hendin H. Suicide and suicide prevention in Asia. Geneva: WHO; 2008.
58. Hawley JS. Sati, the blessing and the curse: the burning of wives in India. Demand: Oxford University Press; 1994.
59. Lal M. SATI/JAUHAR (SATĪ/JAUHAR). Keywords for India: a conceptual lexicon for the 21st Century. 2020:70.
60. Harlan L. Religion and Rajput women: the ethic of protection in contemporary narratives. Berkeley: University of California Press; 1992.
61. Kamat J. The Tradition of Sati in India. 1997. Accessed 24 Feb 2004.
62. Michaels A. Hinduism: past and present. Princeton: Princeton University Press; 2004.
63. Bhugra D. Sati: a type of nonpsychiatric suicide. Crisis. 2005;26(2):73–7.
64. Sharma I, Pandit B, Pathak A, Sharma R. Hinduism, marriage and mental illness. Indian J Psychiatry. 2013;55(Suppl 2):S243.
65. Roye S. Suttee Sainthood through selflessness: pain of repression or power of devotion? South Asia Res. 2011;31(3):281–99.
66. Ahmad N. Sati tradition-widow burning in India: a socio-legal examination. Web J Curr Legal Issues. 2009;2(1):4.
67. Bodhi B. A comprehensive manual of Abhidhamma: the philosophical psychology of Buddhism. Onalaska, WA: Buddhist Publication Society Pariyatti Editions; 2000.
68. Maoz Z, Henderson EA. The World religion dataset, 1945–2010: logic, estimates, and trends. Int Interact. 2013;39(3):265–91.
69. Chamlong Disayavanish M, Primprao Disayavanish M, Tala Thammaroj M, Surut Jianmongkol M, Kimaporn Kamanarong M, Somjit Prueksaritanond M, et al. A Buddhist approach to suicide prevention. J Med Assoc Thail. 2007;90(8):1680–8.
70. Keown D. Suicide, assisted suicide and euthanasia: a Buddhist perspective. J Law Religion. 1998;13(2):385–405.
71. Harvey P. An introduction to Buddhist ethics: foundations, values and issues. Cambridge: Cambridge University Press; 2000.
72. Ohnuma R, Kitts M. To extract the essence from this essenceless body: self-sacrifice and self-immolation in Indian Buddhism. In: Martyrdom, self-sacrifice, and self-immolation: religious perspectives on suicide. Oxford: OUP; 2018. p. 241–65.
73. Kelly BD. Self-immolation, suicide and self-harm in Buddhist and Western traditions. Transcult Psychiatry. 2011;48(3):299–317.
74. Hubert H, Mauss M. Sacrifice: its nature and functions. Chicago: University of Chicago Press; 1981.
75. Yu J, Kitts M. Reflections on self-immolation in chinese buddhist and daoist traditions. In: Martyrdom, self-sacrifice, and self-immolation: religious perspectives on suicide. Oxford: OUP; 2018. p. 264–79.
76. Benn JA. Burning for the Buddha: self-immolation in Chinese Buddhism. Honolulu: University of Hawaii Press; 2007.
77. Halberstam D. The making of a quagmire: America and Vietnam during the Kennedy era. Lanham: Rowman & Littlefield; 2008.
78. Biggs M. Dying without killing: self-immolations, 1963–2002. In: Making sense of suicide missions. Oxford: OUP; 2005. p. 173–208.
79. WHO. Public health action for the prevention of suicide: a framework. Geneva: WHO; 2012.

80. Picco L, Abdin E, Chong SA, Pang S, Vaingankar JA, Sagayadevan V, et al. Beliefs about help seeking for mental disorders: findings from a mental health literacy study in Singapore. Psychiatr Serv. 2016;67(11):1246–53.
81. Chance SE, Kaslow NJ, Summerville MB, Wood K. Suicidal behavior in African American individuals: current status and future directions. Cult Divers Ment Health. 1998;4(1):19.
82. Lawrence RE, Brent D, Mann JJ, Burke AK, Grunebaum MF, Galfalvy HC, et al. Religion as a risk factor for suicide attempt and suicide ideation among depressed patients. J Nerv Ment Dis. 2016;204(11):845–50.

Caring for the Suicidal Person

Alma Lucindo Jimenez, Constantine D. Della, Angeline Monica A. Arcenas, and Katrina Therese R. Esling

1 Introduction

A sweeping glance at the World Health Organization (WHO) suicide epidemiologic data shows a global health problem, with an estimated 804,000 suicide deaths worldwide, representing a global age-standardized suicide rate of 11.4 per 100,000 population [1–3]. However, differential analysis of these suicide rates and methods demonstrates variations when looking at economic level, sex, age, religion, and geography (see Table 1). Consequently, care of the suicidal person varies within diverse biological, social, and cultural contexts.

Average suicide rates are slightly higher in high-income countries (12.7) compared to low-and-middle-income countries (LAMICs) (11.2). The suicide rate among men is three times higher than that of women in high-income countries but this ratio decreases to 1.5 to 1 in LAMICs [2]. Conversely, suicide rates are higher in women in Afghanistan, Bangladesh, Iran, Iraqi Kurdistan, Pakistan, Turkey, Western Pacific countries, and prior to 2006, China [2, 3].

A. L. Jimenez (✉) · C. D. Della
Department of Psychiatry and Behavioral Medicine, College of Medicine, University of the Philippines—Philippine General Hospital, Manila, Philippines
e-mail: amljimenez@yahoo.com, aljimenez2@up.edu.ph; cddella@up.edu.ph

A. M. A. Arcenas
Medical Center Manila, Manila, Philippines
e-mail: am.arcenas@gmail.com

K. T. R. Esling
Department of Psychiatry and Behavioral Medicine, University of the Philippines—Philippine General Hospital, Manila, Philippines
e-mail: katrinaesling@gmail.com

© The Author(s), under exclusive license to Springer Nature Switzerland AG 2021
C. A. Alfonso et al. (eds.), *Suicide by Self-Immolation*,
https://doi.org/10.1007/978-3-030-62613-6_15

Table 1 WHO estimated suicide rates by region of the world, 2012 [2]

Region	% of global population	Number of suicides, (thousands)	% of global suicides	Age-standardized[a] suicide rates (Per 100,000)			Male: Female ratio
				Both sexes	Females	Males	
Global[b]	100.0	804	100.0	11.4	8.0	15.0	1.9
HICs	17.9	192	23.9	12.7	5.7	19.9	3.5
LAMICs	81.7	607	75.5	11.2	8.7	13.7	1.6
LAMICs-Africa	12.6	61	7.6	10.0	5.8	14.4	2.5
LAMICs-Americas	8.2	35	4.3	6.1	2.7	9.8	3.6
LAMICs-Mediterranean	8.0	30	3.7	6.4	5.2	7.5	1.4
LAMICs-Europe	3.8	35	4.3	12.0	4.9	20.0	4.1
LAMICs-South East Asia	25.9	314	39.1	17.7	13.9	21.6	1.6
LAMICs-Western Pacific	23.1	131	16.3	7.5	7.9	7.2	0.9

Abbreviations: *HICs* high-income countries, *LAMICs* low-and-middle-income countries
[a]Rates are standardized to the WHO World Standard Population, adjusted for differences in age structure, facilitating comparisons between regions and over time
[b]Includes data for three territories that are not WHO Member States

Suicide rates are lowest in children less than 15 years old and highest among the elderly [3]. Worldwide, among the 15–29 age group, suicide ranks as the second leading cause of death, but stratified into country income level, it ranks highest in the same demographic in high-income countries and some LAMICs in Southeast Asia [2].

Suicide rates are lower in some countries where suicide is forbidden by religion [4]. Bertolote and Fleisichmman observed that areas dominated by Islam, Hinduism or Christianity reported lower rates while Buddhism-dominated Japan and atheism-dominated China showed higher rates, up to 17.9% and 25.6% [4].

Suicide rates are higher in minority groups such as indigenous peoples, refugees, immigrants, and gender-diverse communities [3, 5, 6]. Native Americans in the US, First Nations and Inuits in Canada, Aboriginal and Torres Strait Islander peoples in Australia, and Māori in New Zealand report more suicides compared to the general population of their respective countries [2, 7, 8]. In the United States, the suicide rate of Mexican immigrants is greater than that of native Mexicans after acculturation and assimilation takes place [9]. Haas and colleagues and Virupaksha and colleagues report that the prevalence of suicide attempts among gender-diverse individuals reaches 30–50% in some countries [4].

Inferences about the impact of certain variables on suicidality should be tempered with caution, as under-reporting of suicides could be explained by gender norms, religious practices, cultural perceptions, and legal impediments [3]. In

Table 2 Common methods of suicide per region

Continent	Suicide method
Africa	Hanging, pesticide poisoning, self-immolation [4]
Americas	Firearm use, overdose, poisoning, hanging [4, 15]
Asia	Poisoning, hanging, jumping, self-immolation [2, 4, 15]
Europe	Hanging, firearms, overdose, poisoning, jumping [4]
Australia and New Zealand	Hanging, overdose, poisoning [4, 7]

Muslim societies, Canetto suggests that suicide could be under-reported because Islam strongly reproaches suicide, more so in women than in men, while noting that it can be over-reported to disguise homicides [3]. Indian statistics may under-report suicides of married women in part because a husband or his family are deemed legally responsible for the wife's suicide within the first 7 years of marriage [10].

Like suicide rates, methods vary within and across regions along economic, social, and cultural strata [4, 11–15]. Worldwide statistics on suicide methods rank hanging, pesticide ingestion, and firearm use as the most common methods employed [15] (see Table 2). However, Canetto reports local variations in the choice of method and attributes them to differences in terms of access to means, acceptability of suicide, and meaning conveyed by suicide.

2 A Conceptual Framework for the Care of the Suicidal Person

The WHO Mental Health Action Plan 2013–2020 targeted reduction of country suicide rates by 10% by 2020 [16]. To this end, WHO proposed a public health model for suicide prevention, with four focal areas:

1. Surveillance
2. Identification of risk and protective factors
3. Development and testing of interventions
4. Implementation [2].

Mrazek et al. and Gordon [2] categorized evidence-based suicide prevention interventions into *universal*, *selective* or *indicated*:

Universal interventions generally target health systems and society, and focus on preventing suicide, strengthening protective factors, and limiting risk factors.

Selective interventions mainly address communities at risk and focus on early detection.

Indicated interventions tackle specific vulnerable individual and relational concerns and use pharmacological and psychosocial interventions.

A meta-analysis of therapeutic interventions for self-harm reduction [17] and the National Action Alliance for Suicide Prevention (Action Alliance) framework for suicide prevention [18] both support this model of care. Notwithstanding general acceptance of the WHO framework, Barnes and colleagues [19] advocate sensitivity to the local community structures and systems of suicide care.

3 Suicide Risk Assessment

Suicide risk assessment consists of core WHO-recommended components of any national prevention program: enhanced surveillance, identification of vulnerable groups, assessment of suicidal behavior, and promotion of protective factors [2]. It represents a composite of degree of suicidality and risk and protective factors.

The magnitude of past suicidality, gauged by frequency, lethality, intentionality, and medical consequences of past attempts, serves as the foremost indicator of present suicidality. Since suicidality is described in terms of the individual's choices of method, its cultural motivators and messages usually go unrecognized. Risk factor assessment, described on systemic, societal, community and individual levels provide a multicultural view of a person's predisposition to suicide [2, 4].

Common individual risk factors for suicide include previous self-harm, psychiatric disorders, substance use disorders, job or financial loss, relationship failures, hopelessness, co-morbid medical conditions, and family history of suicidal behaviors [2, 3]. Community risks comprise war, disaster, acculturation, discrimination, isolation, abuse, violence and conflictual relationships [2, 3]. The U.S. Office of the Surgeon General, the Action Alliance, and the American Psychiatric Association list membership to a minority group as a risk factor [3, 5, 6]. Health system and societal risk factors include access to means, limited access to care, inappropriate media reporting and social media use, and stigma [2, 3].

Suicide protective factors include effective clinical screening and diagnosis, easy access to a variety of clinical interventions, support for on-going medical and mental health care relationships, family and community support, cultural and religious beliefs, and skills in problem-solving and conflict resolution [20].

Some factors shift between being protective to conferring risk across cultures [3]. For example, the married civil status protects women in high-income countries, but confers suicidal risk to women in many countries including Afghanistan, Bangladesh, Iran, and the Kurdistan region of Iraq, Pakistan, India, and China [3]. Religion generally protects a person from suicide as it provides access to supportive communities and limits alcohol use, but puts the person at risk when it stigmatizes suicide as immoral and consequently discourages help-seeking, or encourages self-immolation [2, 3].

The traditional biomedical model of illness regards suicide as a consequence of psychiatric disorders and therefore, concentrates research on quantifiable risk factors [3]. However, risk factors poorly predict suicide attempts and deaths [3, 21] as time-invariant and non-specific [21]. Thus, other investigators like Hjelmeland [3] advocate for contextualizing people's life with particular attention to oppression, marginalization, racism, unemployment, and stigmatization [3]. This contextualization explains most suicides by self-immolation.

Most suicide risk assessment instruments suffer from unsatisfactory diagnostic accuracy [22] and therefore, should not replace clinical evaluation nor serve as the sole basis for treatment or aftercare [5, 7]. However, when used appropriately and in combination with triage protocols they may reduce burden on limited mental health services [7, 22, 23].

Commonly utilized risk assessment tools include the following:

- Patient Health Questionnaire (PHQ-9)
- Columbia Suicide Severity Rating Scale (C-SSRS)
- Beck Depression Inventory (BDI)
- Scale for Suicide Ideation–Current (SSI-C)
- Scale for Suicide Ideation–Worst (SSI-W)
- Beck's Suicide Intent Scale
- Ask Suicide-Screening Questions (ASQ)
- Risk of Suicide Questionnaire (RSQ)
- Patient Safety Screener (PSS)
- Suicide Affect-Behavior-Cognition Scare (SABCS)
- ReACT Self-Harm Rule

For a more exhaustive list of screening tools and their respective sensitivities and specificities, the reader is referred to the cited references [22, 23].

Chu and colleagues identified cultural suicide risk factors and developed the *Cultural Assessment of Risk for Suicide (CARS) measure*, adding to much needed research in this area [24]. Furthermore, Kreuze and Lamis expanded on the neglected research component of diverse representation and need for cultural and linguistic sensitivity [25].

4   Suicide Prevention Interventions

4.1   Indicated Interventions—Biological

The biological treatment of suicidal behaviour, consisting of pharmacological and somatic treatments, is based on the Western model that suicidality is caused by underlying disease and is therefore focused on treating the underlying psychiatric diagnoses [3]. However, since these treatments have not drastically decreased suicide rates, psychopharmacotherapy has shifted its focus from treating disorders to reducing suicidal behaviour and suicide deaths [26].

Pharmacological approaches to reduce suicidal behaviour commonly include the following drugs: antidepressants, mood stabilizers (particularly lithium), antipsychotics, and anxiolytic agents [5]. For specific mechanisms of action, dosing, potential adverse effects, and drug interactions, the reader is advised to refer to standard pharmacological textbooks.

Among these agents, clozapine is solely and specifically indicated by the United States Food and Drug Administration as an anti-suicide agent [26]. However, with the potentially life-threatening risk of its adverse effect of agranulocytosis, its clinical application is limited. Antidepressants constitute the main agents for the treatment of depression, anxiety, and substance use but their efficacy in reducing rates of suicide remain inadequately demonstrated [5]. Lithium's strong and consistent evidence for major reduction in suicide rates [5, 26] is theorized as an indirect effect of impulsivity mitigation [26] or a functional outcome of improved mood [27]. Anxiolytics such as benzodiazepines mitigate anxiety, panics attacks, and sleep disturbances but show limited evidence of direct anti-suicide effect [5].

Somatic therapies such as electroconvulsive therapy (ECT), transcranial magnetic stimulation (TMS) demonstrate effectivity in reducing suicidality, albeit hampered by various limitations. Consensus shows ECT as effective but costly and not readily accessible. It is stigmatizing, with unclear long-term impact [26]. TMS shows limited effect on depressive symptoms, including suicidal behavior [26].

Ketamine, lacking official accreditation and established safety profile, nevertheless, reduces depression, anxiety, and suicidality. Additional research is necessary to address its risk/benefit ratio [28, 29].

The use of psychotropic medications in the treatment of mental disorders is standardized in widely accepted Clinical Practice Guidelines (CPG). Challenging this 'one size fits all' approach, Ng and Bousman assert that pharmacokinetics and pharmacodynamics of drugs differ across cultures, affecting response to treatment [30, 31].

Pharmacogenetics and socio-cultural factors such as cultural practices and environmental factors, attitudes towards medications, treatment adherence, and placebo and nocebo effects account for the ethnocultural differences in psychopharmacology.

Genetic polymorphisms in metabolic enzyme systems, notably, CYP450 isoenzymes, CYP2D6 and CYP2C19 result in phenotypic differences in the ability to metabolize psychotropics [30]. These metabolic phenotypes vary across different ethnic populations, causing variations in dosage requirements, response and tolerability [31]. Poor metabolizers tend to experience more adverse effects and lower efficacy of the drug, while fast metabolizers may require higher doses to achieve efficacy [31].

CYP2D6 genotyping studies show that 5–10% of Caucasians and 1–2% of Asians are poor metabolizers [32]. Overall, Asians show lower CYP2D6 activity [33] while ultra-rapid metabolizers among Caucasians demonstrate 1–2%, Mediterranean population, 7–10%, Arabs, 19% and East African populations, with a 29% metabolic activity [34]. Since most SSRIs and antipsychotics are metabolized by CYP2D6, patients with African or Middle Eastern background need higher doses of these medications [31]. The genotyping studies of CYP2C19, important in SSRI metabolism, shows further ethnic differences which are possibly attributed to variant allele groups that create other metabolic phenotypes [35, 36]. Ethnic variations in allelic frequencies associated with transporters also contribute to variations in drug response such as observed by Lin et al. [37] that majority of Asians are fast acetylators, and therefore, fast metabolizers of clonazepam. Serotonin transporter–linked polymorphic region (5-HTTLPR) polymorphisms have likewise shown ethnic-dependent SSRI efficacy. [38, 39]

Socio-cultural practices, including dietary practices, recreational substance use, agricultural practices regulating exposure to toxins and pollutants, and traditional medication use may also affect pharmacokinetics of psychotropics. Ng and Bousman [30] suggest that CYP3A4 metabolism is decreased by flavinoid-rich diets, citrus juices grapefruit juice and red wine, causing an increase in the frequency and side effects of CYP3A4 substrates like clozapine, risperidone, sertraline, venlafaxine, diazepam and zaleplon. Earlier studies [30] reported that CYP1A2 induction results from its interaction with smoking, and certain foods like brussel sprouts, cabbage, broccoli, cauliflower, and high-protein sources, thereby increasing the metabolism of clozapine, olanzapine and fluvoxamine. This interaction seems to be reversed by CYP1A2 inhibitors, such as foods common in South Asian diets, like cumin, coriander, and grapefruit [40].

Cultural beliefs and explanatory models of psychiatric disorders and treatment affect psychotropic use [30]. In many non-Western settings, the usual patient expects fast relief with no regard for monitoring or education about drug effects and rejects side effects and standardized doses [30]. African-American and Latino-American patients challenge antidepressant efficacy and prefer 'watchful waiting' over active treatment, perhaps due to the nocebo effect and negative attitudes to medications [41]. Cultural dissonance on medication values, beliefs, and practices contributes to variations in treatment adherence and therapeutic outcomes [30].

The role of the placebo response in producing or enhancing clinical effects in pharmacotherapy is largely underestimated and neglected in clinical trials. The fact that it seems to be higher in non-Caucasians [30] has not been factored into cultural variations in psychopharmacological practice.

4.2 Indicated Interventions-Psychosocial

Psychosocial interventions, mainstays of suicide management as per CPGs, hinge on the relationship between a patient and a professional who recognizes the patient's compromised coping ability and prioritizes his or her safety in the therapeutic plan [5, 7, 42, 43]. Psychotherapies, including cognitive behavioral therapy (CBT), dialectical behavior therapy (DBT), interpersonal therapy (IPT), family therapy, psychodynamic psychotherapy (PP), mentalization-based psychotherapy (MBT), and other therapeutic strategies like bibliotherapy, mindfulness-based treatment and digital technologically-formatted approaches and safety planning present themselves as options to treat suicidal individuals and those at risk [43–54].

In general, these therapies, aside from a few exceptions, [43, 55] are structured, short-term, manualized, present-oriented, centered on a person's internal experience, emotional regulation, dysfunctional thinking, mindfulness, as well as on the development of skills [43–46, 49–52].

These therapies measure outcomes by changes in the frequency of suicidal thoughts, non-suicidal self-injury, and suicidal behaviors [47, 48, 50–54, 56]. DBT, CBT, PP and IPT have been shown to be effective in reducing suicidal risk [5, 57, 58]. DBT demonstrates an ability to reduce the incidence of self-induced violence but does not significantly affect suicidal ideation [53]. However, it does reduce the rate of repeat self-harm [51] as observed in a meta-analysis of psychotherapies for adolescents with Borderline Personality Disorder [54]. CBT reduces the frequency of self-harm and severity of suicidal ideation [53, 54].

Jerome Frank lists the features of effective psychotherapies as an emotionally charged, confiding relationship with a helping person, a healing setting, a rationale, conceptual scheme or myth and a ritual [59]. Following this notion, as the rational, conceptual scheme of myth on suicide differs across cultures, so do the foci of the psychosocial interventions.

Descriptions of suicide in non-Western cultures challenge the account that suicide is "closely connected to, even caused by, mental disorder" [3]. These narratives depict suicide as a reaction to social stresses from changing gender roles and responsibilities, family problems in an oppressive, poverty-stricken and post-colonialization milieu. [60, 61].

In the northern Ugandan context, changes in gender roles associated with reversals in economic responsibilities precipitate suicide in young men and women [3]. On the other hand, Hjelmeland [3] also cited several studies in Ghana, South Africa Ireland, and Australia that found that the constraints of traditional roles and accountabilities of masculinity drive suicide in men. Simultaneously, protest against the very same traditional male role triggers suicide in women [62]. Studies on suicide of disenfranchised women [3] narrate that inescapable family problems in the context of poverty put women at risk. In the Inuit of Arctic Canada, the high suicide rate is attributed in part to the colonial changes introduced by the Canadian government in the 1950s and 1960s [63].

Among suicidal aboriginal people in Canada, Mehl-Madrona determined that common themes and purposes of suicide attempts and beliefs about death revolved around disruptions in social status involving relationship breakups, public humiliation, and 'chronic life stress with relative isolation' [64].

4.3   Selective and Universal Interventions

Selective and universal interventions, in the form of community-based and national suicide prevention programs succeed when they display the following features:

- Holistic
- Multisectoral
- Empowering
- Integrated into primary care
- Structured

- Evidence-based
- Standardized

A holistic multisectoral approach to suicide prevention consisting of programs to heighten knowledge, reduce stigma, and promote help-seeking behavior started 20 years ago under the leadership of Norway, Finland, Sweden, and Australia [65]. General practitioners, youth workers, teachers, police, paramedics, armed forces, security services, non-government organizations, human resource professionals, and employers, were empowered to do risk assessment and assist patients to access appropriate services [7]. A study comparing these countries with four control countries (Canada, Austria, Switzerland and Denmark) suggests that this implementation approach is an effective tool in suicide prevention [65].

The integration of suicide prevention programs into primary care pushed for increased primary health workers' capability building for risk assessment and management of suicide [66]. The fact that 91.7% of patients who died by suicide had some type of past-year health care contact prior to death (of which 25.3% had non-mental healthcare contact) justifies this primary healthcare approach [67].

Highly structured, evidence-based suicide prevention programs have been integrated into primary care in the United States. The National Action Alliance for Suicide Prevention introduced the Zero Suicide (ZS) Model that utilizes a multilevel approach in applying evidence-based practices [1], combining carer clinical and administrative skills. Brodsky and colleagues enhanced this program's incorporation into primary care using the Assess, Intervene and Monitor for Suicide Prevention model (AIM-SP), integrating a ten-step suicide risk assessment interview into standard clinical practice screening [1].

Hegerl and colleagues described an initiative to optimize and standardize the implementation of suicide prevention programs in Europe (OSPI-Europe), specifically in Ireland, Portugal, Hungary, and Germany [68]. This program facilitated the transfer of the multilevel, evidence-based, efficient suicide prevention program to European Union-member states. In evaluating this intervention, the authors found that the decrease in suicide rates reflected local circumstances in each of the countries, highlighting the significance of considering culture-specific factors when interpreting findings from studies on complex community based multilevel interventions [68]. They argued that evaluations of interventions of this nature 'do not allow a straightforward interpretation of cause and effect' [68].

5   Research on the Care of the Suicidal Person

Translational research on suicide care derives its data from clinical and non-clinical community-based studies through a deliberate process of stakeholder collaboration, monitoring and data dissemination [69].

LAMICs, at varying stages of development of national strategy, are exhorted by WHO to take steps to engage stakeholders in public fora on stigma, needs of vulnerable groups, local research priorities, and public and media awareness. Such community-oriented initiatives place importance on communities and their ways of caring for the suicidal person [2, 69].

Community stakeholder consultations generate data and further research on suicide and its management across cultures, thereby contextualizing suicide prevention policy initiatives within specific cultural realities. In LAMICs, suicide research lacks focus [56] and needs to address reliability concerns due to low base rates and small sample sizes. Thus, experts recommend the establishment of national and international networks to enable large-scale evaluation and trials, utilization of novel technologies and social media in the study of suicide risk and behavior, and the development of new theories of suicidal behaviour, including developments in brain imaging and epigenetics, and identification of biomarkers and endophenotypes [2, 56].

6   Caring for Suicidal Persons at Risk of Self-immolation

Since almost all people who self-immolate live in LAMICs, interventions can be challenging due to limited access to care and scarcity of clinicians. If medications and mental health providers are unavailable, psychosocial interventions delegated to community workers should include minimal basic training when task-shifting.

Interventions at the national level need to incorporate the following:

- Promoting responsible media reporting to mitigate the contagion effect
- Legislation to protect human rights
- Decriminalization of suicide
- Enacting a national suicide prevention strategy into law

At the community level, religious and community leaders will benefit from being tasked with identifying and protecting individuals at risk. When intimate partner violence is rampant, programs need to be designed to sensitize men to avoid violence and encourage strengthening of social ties among women who need support and protection.

When people feel expendable, suicide may follow, and with self-immolations the glorification of the act is problematic. Perceptions of self-sacrifice suicides as altruistic or deserving of martyrdom provides a social endorsement that could increase suicide risk. Clinicians should influence politicians and activists to understand that nonviolent forms of protest that spare human life may also be effective to communicate dissent.

The most important precipitating and enabling factors contributing to self-immolation suicides are intimate partner violence and other forms of violence in the household. Working with families, non-governmental organizations and community leaders to mitigate the epidemic of domestic is of essence to prevent self-immolations. Given the intergenerational transmission of suicide, probably mediated by epigenetic changes during vulnerable periods of development and retraumatization later in life, attention to identifying family units with history of self-immolation is perhaps the best way to signal risk and effectively allocate resources. When entire regions are beleaguered by self-immolations, such as the Herat province in Afghanistan, most of Tunisia, parts of South Africa, and the Tibetan plateau, group interventions may be the only way to preserve resources and effect change. It is our experience that religious leaders can be easily trained by mental health clinicians to provide effective supportive group psychotherapy. Collaborative models of care and task-shifting efforts are indispensable in order to properly outsource suicide prevention interventions in LAMICS with high prevalence of self-immolation.

7 Conclusion

The care of the suicidal person draws its urgency from the universal value of human life and its preservation. Suicide, as a threat to human life, elicits collective preventive action from societies, communities, loved ones, and carers. Notwithstanding the widespread notion of the undesirability of suicide, its phenomenology and its care differ across cultures.

Suicide rates vary from global estimates when stratified according to country economic level, sex, age, religion, and geography. The figures boggle the mind further when subjected to cross-sectional analysis, reinforcing the need to contextualize the study of suicide within diverse biological, social, and cultural settings.

The conceptual framework for the care of the suicidal person appears standard enough. It views the suicidal person as part of a relationship, within a community that is part of society-at large. Correspondingly, the care interventions follow a systemic, multi-level approach, from universal to selective to indicated. These interventions shift focus from prevention and management of protective and risk factors in health systems to early detection in at-risk communities to pharmacological, psychological, and social interventions in vulnerable individuals. However, given the complexity of the suicide experience, the relevance of this organized approach hinges on greater comprehension of culture, the interactive multi-level systems and structures shaping human life.

Similarly, the list of suicide risk factors and protective factors consisting of personal attributes and environmental factors appears inclusive and holistic, reflecting the systemic approach to suicide management. But once again, since different cultures interpret risk and protective factors differently, the nuanced suicide risk assessor is cautioned to be sensitive to cultural diversity. The psychopharmacotherapy and psychosocial interventions for the suicidal person requires the same awareness of cultural variations. Studies on genotyping studies and drug interactions with diet, culture, and environment challenge standardized CPGs for suicidal persons as more evidence demonstrates that psychopharmacology across cultures may vary. Psychosocial care for the suicidal person changes rationale as one considers unique social contexts that drive suicide. National level and community-based suicide care programs succeed when they blend holistic, inclusive, standardized perspectives with culturally-informed community-specific values.

References

1. Brodsky BS, Spruch-Feiner A, Stanley B. The zero suicide model: applying evidence-based suicide prevention practices to clinical care. Front Psych. 2018;9:33.
2. World Health Organization. Preventing suicide: a global imperative. Geneva: World Health Organization; 2014.
3. Hjelmeland H. Cultural aspects of suicide. In: Bhugra D, Bhui K, editors. Textbook of cultural psychiatry. Cambridge: Cambridge University Press; 2018. p. 482–92.
4. Bachmann S. Epidemiology of suicide and the psychiatric perspective. Int J Environ Res Public Health. 2018;15(7):1425.
5. Jacobs DG, Baldessarini RJ, Conwell Y, Fawcett JA, Horton L, Meltzer H, et al. Practice guideline for the assessment and treatment of patients with suicidal behaviors. In: APA practice guidelines for the treatment of psychiatric disorders: comprehensive guidelines and guideline watches; 2010.
6. U.S. Department of Health and Human Services (HHS) Office of the Surgeon General and National Action Alliance for Suicide Prevention. National strategy for suicide prevention: goals and objectives for action. Washington, DC: HHS; 2012.
7. Carter G, Page A, Large M, Hetrick S, Milner AJ, Bendit N, et al. Royal Australian and New Zealand College of Psychiatrists clinical practice guideline for the management of deliberate self-harm. Austral N Z J Psychiatry. 2016;50(10):939–1000.
8. Wexler L, Mceachern D, Difulvio G, Smith C, Graham LF, Dombrowski K. Creating a community of practice to prevent suicide through multiple channels: describing the theoretical foundations and structured learning of PC CARES. Int Q Community Health Educ. 2016;36(2):115–22.
9. Ruiz P. Global epidemiology of suicide. In: Koslow SH, Ruiz P, Nemeroff CB, editors. A concise guide to understanding suicide: epidemiology, pathophysiology, and prevention. Cambridge: Cambridge University Press; 2014. p. 13–6.
10. Patel V, Ramasundarahettige C, Vijayakumar L, Thakur J, Gajalakshmi V, Gururaj G, et al. Suicide mortality in India: a nationally representative survey. Lancet. 2012;379(9834):2343–51.
11. Mars B, Burrows S, Hjelmeland H, Gunnell D. Suicidal behaviour across the African continent: a review of the literature. BMC Public Health. 2014;14(1):606.
12. Redaniel MT, Lebanan-Dalida MA, Gunnell D. Suicide in the Philippines: time trend analysis (1974–2005) and literature review. BMC Public Health. 2011;11(1):536.
13. Lotrakul M. Suicide in Thailand during the period 1998–2003. Psychiatry Clin Neurosci. 2006;60(1):90–5.
14. Ministry of Health Malaysia. National suicide registry Malaysia (NSRM) annual report 2009. Kuala Lumpur: National Suicide Registry Malaysia; 2011.
15. Ajdacic-Gross V. Methods of suicide: international suicide patters derived from the WHO mortality database. Bull World Health Organ. 2008;86(9):726–32.
16. World Health Organization. Mental health action plan 2013–2020. Geneva: World Health Organzation; 2013.
17. Iyengar U, Snowden N, Asarnow JR, Moran P, Tranah T, Ougrin D. A further look at therapeutic interventions for suicide attempts and self-harm in adolescents: an updated systematic review of randomized controlled trials. Front Psych. 2018;9:583.
18. National Action Alliance for Suicide Prevention: Transforming Health Systems Initiative Work Group. Recommended standard care for people with suicide risk: Making health care suicide safe. Washington, DC: Education Development Center, Inc.; 2018.

19. Barnes DH, Lawson WB, Ball K. Ethnicity: how much of our understanding of suicide is applicable across ethnic cultures? In: Koslow SH, Ruiz P, Nemeroff CB, editors. A concise guide to understanding suicide: epidemiology, pathophysiology, and prevention. Cambridge: Cambridge University Press; 2014. p. 62–5.

20. Centers for Disease Control and Prevention. Suicide risk and protective factors. Centers for Disease Control and Prevention. 2019 [cited 2020 Apr 9]. https://www.cdc.gov/violenceprevention/suicide/riskprotectivefactors.html

21. Glenn CR, Cha CB, Kleiman EM, Nock MK. Understanding suicide risk within the research domain criteria (RDoC) framework: insights, challenges, and future research considerations. Clin Psychol Sci. 2017;5(3):568–92.

22. Runeson B, Odeberg J, Pettersson A, Edbom T, Adamsson IJ, Waern M. Instruments for the assessment of suicide risk: a systematic review evaluating the certainty of the evidence. PLoS One. 2017;12(7):e0180292.

23. Zaleski ME, Johnson ML, Valdez AM, Bradford JY, Reeve NE, Horigan A, et al. Clinical practice guideline: suicide risk assessment. J Emerg Nurs. 2018;4(5):505.e1–505.e33.

24. Chu J, Floyd R, Diep H, Pardo S, Goldblum P, Bongar B. A tool for the culturally competent assessment of suicide: The Cultural Assessment of Risk for Suicide (CARS) Measure. Psychol Assess. 2013;25(2):424–34.

25. Kreuze E, Lamis DA. A review of psychometrically tested instruments assessing suicide risk in adults. OMEGA—J Death Dying. 2017;77(1):36–90.

26. Griffiths JJ, Zarate CA, Rasimas J. Existing and novel biological therapeutics in suicide prevention. Am J Prev Med. 2014;47(3):S195–203.

27. Lewitzka U, Severus E, Bauer R, Ritter P, Müller-Oerlinghausen B, Bauer M. The suicide prevention effect of lithium: more than 20 years of evidence—a narrative review. Int J Bipolar Disorders. 2015;3(1):1–6.

28. DiazGranados N, Ibrahim LA, Brutsche NE, Ameli R, Henter ID, Luckenbaugh DA, et al. Rapid resolution of suicidal ideation after a single infusion of an NMDA antagonist in patients with treatment-resistant major depressive disorder. J Clin Psychiatry. 2010;71(12):1605–11.

29. Strong CE, Kabbaj M. On the safety of repeated ketamine infusions for the treatment of depression: effects of sex and developmental periods. Neurobiol Stress. 2018;9:166–75.

30. Ng CH, Bousman CA. Cross-cultural psychopharmacotherapy. In: Bhugra D, Bhui K, editors. Textbook of cultural psychiatry. Cambridge: Cambridge University Press; 2018. p. 432–41.

31. Taylor D, Werneke U. Ethnopharmacology. Nord J Psychiatry. 2018;72(1):30–2.

32. Poolsup N, Li Wan Po A, Knight TL. Pharmacogenetics and psychopharmacotherapy. J Clin Pharm Therapeut. 2000;25(3):197–220. https://doi.org/10.1046/j.1365-2710.2000.00281.x.

33. Bradford LD. CYP2D6 allele frequency in European Caucasians, Asians, Africans and their descendants. Pharmacogenomics. 2002;3(2):229–43.

34. Teh LK, Bertilsson L. Pharmacogenomics of CYP2D6: molecular genetics, interethnic differences and clinical importance. Drug Metab Pharmacokinet. 2012;27(1):55–67.

35. Ng CH, Ng CH, Schweitzer I, Norman T, Easteal S. The emerging role of pharmacogenetics: implications for clinical psychiatry. Austral N Z J Psychiatry. 2004;38(7):483–9.

36. Fricke-Galindo I, Céspedes-Garro C, Rodrigues-Soares F, Naranjo MEG, Delgado Á, Andrés FD, et al. Interethnic variation of CYP2C19 alleles, 'predicted' phenotypes and 'measured' metabolic phenotypes across world populations. Pharmacogenomics J. 2015;16(2):113–23.

37. Lin HJ, Han C-Y, Lin BK, Hardy S. Slow acetylator mutations in the human polymorphic n-acetyltransferase gene in 786 Asians, Blacks, Hispanics, and Whites: application to metabolic epidemiology. Am J Hum Genet. 1993;52:827–34.

38. Bousman CA, Sarris J, Won E-S, Chang H-S, Singh A, Lee H-Y, et al. Escitalopram efficacy in depression. J Clin Psychopharmacol. 2014;34(5):645–8.

39. Goldman N, Glei DA, Lin Y-H, Weinstein M. The serotonin transporter polymorphism (5-HTTLPR): allelic variation and links with depressive symptoms. Depress Anxiety. 2010;27(3):260–9.

40. Perera V, Gross AS, Mclachlan AJ. Influence of environmental and genetic factors on CYP1A2 activity in individuals of South Asian and European ancestry. Clin Pharmacol Therapeut. 2012;92:511–9.
41. Stewart S, Simmons A, Habibpour E. Treatment of culturally diverse children and adolescents with depression. J Child Adolesc Psychopharmacol. 2012;22(1):72–9.
42. National Collaborating Centre for Mental Health. Self-harm: the short-term physical and psychological management and secondary prevention of self-harm in primary and secondary care. Leicester: The British Psychological Society; 2004.
43. Schechter R, Herbstman G. Psychotherapy with suicidal patients: the integrative psychodynamic approach of the Boston suicide study group. Medicina. 2019;55(6):303.
44. Gamarra JM, Luciano MT, Gradus JL, Stirman SW. Assessing variability and implementation fidelity of suicide prevention safety planning in a regional VA healthcare system. Crisis. 2015;36(6):433–9.
45. Fang Y, Zeng B, Chen P, Mai Y, Teng S, Zhang M, et al. Mindfulness and suicide risk in undergraduates: exploring the mediating effect of alexithymia. Front Psychol. 2019;10:2106.
46. Prada P, Perroud N, Rüfenacht E, Nicastro R. Strategies to deal with suicide and non-suicidal self-injury in borderline personality disorder, the case of DBT. Front Psychol. 2018;9:2595.
47. Witt K, Spittal MJ, Carter G, Pirkis J, Hetrick S, Currier D, et al. Effectiveness of online and mobile telephone applications ('apps') for the self-management of suicidal ideation and self-harm: a systematic review and meta-analysis. BMC Psychiatry. 2017;17(1):297.
48. King CA, Arango A, Foster CE. Emerging trends in adolescent suicide prevention research. Curr Opin Psychol. 2018;22:89–94.
49. Beck JS. Cognitive behavior therapy basics and beyond. 2nd ed. New York: The Guilford Press; 2011.
50. Heisel MJ, Talbot NL, King DA, Tu XM, Duberstein PR. Adapting interpersonal psychotherapy for older adults at risk for suicide. Am J Geriatr Psychiatry. 2015;23(1):87–98.
51. Hawton K, Witt KG, Salisbury TLT, Arensman E, Gunnell D, Hazell P, et al. Psychosocial interventions following self-harm in adults: a systematic review and meta-analysis. Lancet Psychiatry. 2016;3(8):740–50.
52. Mewton L, Andrews G. Cognitive behavioral therapy for suicidal behaviors: improving patient outcomes. Psychol Res Behav Manag. 2016;9:21–9.
53. Decou CR, Comtois KA, Landes SJ. Dialectical behavior therapy is effective for the treatment of suicidal behavior: a meta-analysis. Behav Ther. 2019;50(1):60–72.
54. Wong J, Bahji A, Khalid-Khan S. Psychotherapies for adolescents with subclinical and borderline personality disorder: a systematic review and meta-analysis. Can J Psychiatry. 2019;65(1):5–15.
55. Ewing ESK, Diamond G, Levy S. Attachment-based family therapy for depressed and suicidal adolescents: theory, clinical model and empirical support. Attachment Human Develop. 2015;17(2):136–56.
56. O'Connor RC, Portzky G. Looking to the future: a synthesis of new developments and challenges in suicide research and prevention. Front Psychol. 2018;9:2139.
57. Tarrier N, Taylor K, Gooding P. Cognitive-behavioral interventions to reduce suicide behavior. Behav Modif. 2008;32(1):77–108.
58. Comtois KA, Linehan MM. Psychosocial treatments of suicidal behaviors: a practice-friendly review. J Clin Psychol. 2005;62(2):161–70.
59. Tantam D, Sayar K. Psychotherapy across cultures. In: Bhugra D, Bhui K, editors. Textbook of cultural psychiatry. Cambridge: Cambridge University Press; 2018. p. 442–57.
60. Marecek J, Senadheera C. 'I drank it to put an end to me': narrating girls' suicide and self-harm in Sri Lanka. Contribut Indian Sociol. 2012;46(1–2):53–82.
61. Hjelmeland H, Dieserud G, Dyregrov K, Knizek BL, Leenaars AA. Psychological autopsy studies as diagnostic tools: are they methodologically flawed? Death Stud. 2012;36(7):605–26.
62. Staples J, Widger T. Situating suicide as an anthropological problem: ethnographic approaches to understanding self-harm and self-inflicted death. Cult Med Psychiatry. 2012;36(2):183–203.

63. Kral MJ. Postcolonial suicide among inuit in Arctic Canada. Cult Med Psychiatry. 2012;36(2):306–25.
64. Mehl-Madrona L. Indigenous knowledge approach to successful psychotherapies with aboriginal suicide attempters. Can J Psychiatry. 2016;61(11):696–9.
65. Lewitzka U, Sauer C, Bauer M, Felber W. Are national suicide prevention programs effective? A comparison of 4 verum and 4 control countries over 30 years. BMC Psychiatry. 2019;19(1):158.
66. Malakouti SK, Nojomi M, Ahmadkhaniha HR, Hosseini M, Fallah MY, Khoshalani MM. Integration of suicide prevention program into primary health care network: a field clinical trial in Iran. Med J Islam Repub Iran. 2015;29:208.
67. Schaffer A, Sinyor M, Kurdyak P, Vigod S, Sareen J, Reis C, et al. Population-based analysis of health care contacts among suicide decedents: identifying opportunities for more targeted suicide prevention strategies. World Psychiatry. 2016;15(2):135–45.
68. Hegerl U, Wittenburg L, Arensman E, Audenhove CV, Coyne JC, Mcdaid D, et al. Optimizing Suicide Prevention Programs and Their Implementation in Europe (OSPI Europe): an evidence-based multi-level approach. BMC Public Health. 2009;9(1):51–9.
69. Fleischmann A, Arensman E, Berman A, Carli V, De Leo D, Hadlaczky G. Overview evidence on interventions for population suicide with an eye to identifying best-supported strategies for LMICs. Global Mental Health. 2016;3:e5. https://doi.org/10.1017/gmh.2015.27.

The Role of Mental Health Professionals in Burn Centers and Units

Feranindhya Agiananda and Irmia Kusumadewi

1 Introduction

Psychiatric disorders are more common in persons with burn injuries, adding to the burden of disease in burn centers. Even in the absence of underlying psychiatric illness it may still be advantageous for patients with burn injuries to have a comprehensive psychiatric examination during hospitalization, and multiple studies demonstrate that receiving psychological support in medical and surgical intensive care specialized burn units decreases length of stay and positively impacts morbidity. Expert psychiatrists, either with added qualifications in consultation and liaison psychiatry or with extensive experience in the psychiatric care of the critically ill, have the necessary proficiency to enhance the care for patients with burn wounds and offer invaluable help as members of multidisciplinary teams in burn centers [1, 2].

Depressive disorders, anxiety disorders, substance use disorders and post-traumatic stress disorder (PTSD) are the most common mental disorders observed in patients with burns. Collaborative care among medical specialists is essential in specialized units [3]. Certain demographic characteristics, degree of burns, and pre-existing psychiatric disorders are important predictors of developing mental disorders after burn injuries. Approximately 25–50% of all burn patients experience a mental health disorder after a burn injury [4].

Psychiatric disorders that complicate the recovery from burn injuries include depressive disorders, acute stress disorder (ASD), PTSD, schizophrenia, anxiety disorders, bipolar disorder, and substance use disorders [3, 5–7]. Pre-injury factors,

F. Agiananda (✉) · I. Kusumadewi
Consultation Liaison Psychiatry Division, Department of Psychiatry, Faculty of Medicine, Universitas Indonesia, Jakarta, Indonesia

Dr. Cipto Mangunkusumo National General Hospital, Jakarta, Indonesia
e-mail: feranindhya@gmail.com; irmiakusumadewi@yahoo.com

© The Author(s), under exclusive license to Springer Nature Switzerland AG 2021
C. A. Alfonso et al. (eds.), *Suicide by Self-Immolation*,
https://doi.org/10.1007/978-3-030-62613-6_16

important in predicting higher risk for complications (morbidity and mortality), include pre-morbid psychiatric disorders, maladaptive personality characteristics, impulsivity, a suicide history, peri-traumatic factors and post-burn factors. The prevalence of premorbid psychiatric morbidity in patients admitted to specialized burn units is in the range of 28% and 75% [3, 7].

There are many distressing factors that can contribute to psychiatric disorders in patients with burns. Disfigurement caused by the burn itself, pain arising from treatments such as multiple protective dressing changes, combined with physical isolation to prevent infection can contribute to the psychological sequelae of burn injuries. These traumatic experiences are complex and require problem-focused coping mechanisms. Failure of adaptation could lead to the development of acute, recurrent or chronic mental disorders [3, 8, 9].

Furthermore, there is a paucity of studies that systematically investigate the relationship between type and extent of burn injury and mental disorders following burns. The relationship therefore remains complex and unclear. Similarly, few clinical observational reports describe the care of patients who self-immolate after surviving this highly lethal suicide method. This chapter will elaborate role of mental health professionals in treating patients with burn injuries, as well as reviewing the comprehensive medical management of psychopathology in patients with burns.

2   Psychiatric Disorders and Burn Injuries

Cytokine-induced activation of the hypothalamic-pituitary-adrenal (HPA) axis correlates with depressive disorders and PTSD in patients who experience physical trauma including burn injury. Disfiguring scars, pain, pruritus, muscle dystrophy and atrophy, contractures, changes in heat sensitivity and other sensory deficits are common results from burn trauma and injuries [10, 11]. It is not surprising that persons with burns, even if injuries are minor and recovery uncomplicated, are at risk of developing depressive disorders, anxiety disorders, delirium and PTSD. Psychological distress after burns is modulated in part by the patient's personality traits, coping strategies and perception of body image following injury. A high tendency towards neuroticism and low tendency to extraversion are predisposing factors for burn injuries. These personality traits correlate with experiencing more traumatic events in general, but it is unclear if the link with burn injuries is a causative association [10, 12, 13]. Common symptoms during the acute phase of burn injury recovery include sleep disturbance, behavioural disinhibition, delirium, intrusive recollections, depression, and anxiety. These may be caused by a combination of the burn experience itself, the treatment given, or pre-existing conditions [14]. Although mental disorders after burn injuries generally decline over time, from 45% during the acute phase of recovery to 33% at 6 months post-injury, psychiatric interventions during the acute phase may significantly reduce morbidity. [5] The prevalence of some psychiatric disorders such as PTSD and major depression steadily increase over time post-injury, alerting clinicians of the need for long-term psychosocial and psychopharmacological interventions.

2.1 Depressive Disorders

Depressed patients experience symptoms such as low mood, loss of interest or pleasure in activities (anhedonia), hopelessness, and general distress. Other variable symptoms include changes in appetite or sleep (insomnia or hypersomnia), psychomotor retardation or agitation, impaired concentration, feelings of worthlessness, guilt or suicidal behaviour. For a diagnosis of major depression (with a higher morbidity and mortality) symptoms must be consistently present for at least 2 weeks and cause clinically significant impairment in daily functioning [15–17].

Rates of depression in burn centers vary considerably between studies, ranging from 6% to 42% post injury. Depressive symptoms tend to decline in the short-term period after a traumatic event. While 78% and 72% of injury survivors experience symptoms depression and anxiety in the first week post-trauma, by the sixth week the incidence declines to 63% and 59%, respectively [15, 18].

In the long-term, however, the prevalence of major depression in patients with burns increases from about 4% at the time of discharge from burn units to between 10% and 23% at 1 year after injury. In the second year following injury, up to 42% of patients with burns have symptoms of moderate to severe depression. This alarming trend indicates the need for continuous and long-term psychiatric follow of patients with burn injuries [16, 19].

Somatic symptoms, key elements in the diagnosis of major depression, may occur in patients who sustained burn injuries with or without other depressive symptoms. Many patients in burn units will have difficulty sleeping, daytime fatigue, and appetite changes as an effect of their injury or side effect of medications such as opioid analgesics. Under-recognition of depression may also occur in those presenting with primarily somatic symptoms. The overlap of subjective and observable symptoms of depression with symptoms caused by other medical conditions may explain why psychiatric disorders are so frequently underdiagnosed in primary care settings and intensive care specialized medical-surgical units.

2.2 Acute Stress Disorder and Posttraumatic Stress Disorder

The difference between a diagnosis of acute stress disorder (ASD) and posttraumatic stress disorder (PTSD) as per *Diagnostic and Statistical Manual of Nervous and Mental Disorders* (DSM-V) criteria is that duration of symptoms in ASD is up to 1 month and in PTSD symptoms last longer than 1 month after the traumatic event. Diagnostic criteria include exposure to a traumatic event either by learning of, witnessing or directly experiencing trauma, in combination with associated symptoms of intrusive recollections, negative mood, dissociation, avoidance, and arousal. [15, 17] ASD is a common psychiatric disorder in patients with burn injuries, with a prevalence as high as 19% [20, 21].

PTSD core features are the same as the ASD diagnostic criteria. People with PTSD develop irritability, concentration problems, sleep disturbance and negative alterations in cognitions and mood. Individuals with PTSD have persistent negative beliefs and expectations, a sense of foreshortened future, persistent distorted blame of self or others, dissociative symptoms, feelings of detachment and a constricted affective range [17, 22].

In persons who sustain non-burn injuries, the prevalence of PTSD remains stable at approximately 30% 1 month to 1-year post-injury. In persons who sustain burn injuries, the prevalence of PTSD increases from 26% 1 month after injury to 45% by the 12th month after burn injury [7, 18, 22]. Most patients recovering from a traumatic injury develop post-traumatic stress symptoms that are subsyndromal, which include shock, anxiety, and agitation. These symptoms are similar to those experienced by patients with PTSD and depression on the their first to second day post-trauma [23, 24].

PTSD, like depressive disorders, is an incapacitating condition associated with high morbidity and mortality. ASD and PTSD are frequently unrecognized and underdiagnosed, a clinical oversight that could dangerously complicate the recovery process of patients who sustain burns injuries [18, 25]. The authors and editors postulate that PTSD that relates to early childhood trauma and adverse life events, with subsequent adult retraumatization, poses a particular clinical challenge to psychiatrists and health care professionals caring for critically ill patients, as these patients with a lifelong history of traumatic experiences may become non-adherent, have difficulty establishing trusting relationships, and resist collaborative care. The intergenerational transmission of trauma is discussed in Chap. 12.

2.3 Anxiety Disorders

Anxiety can be both adaptive and maladaptive. Adaptive anxiety signals the brain to increase levels of alertness, focus, and attention, helping to secure oneself against dangerous or challenging situations. Excessive anxiety causes distress and incapacity. Anxiety symptoms arise as a result of one's response to the perception of imminent or chronic danger and usually manifest with a variety of somatic and subjective symptoms. Somatic symptoms include muscle tension, breathing difficulty, hyperventilation, increased rate of peristalsis, diarrhea, shivering of upper and lower extremities, excessive sweating, rhinorrhoea, flushing of the skin, a sensation of choking, and dry mouth. Subjective symptoms include agitation, fear, distress, fear of losing one's mind, fear of death, and a sense of dread or impending doom [26].

Anxiety disorders are common in persons with burn injuries. These include panic disorder, agoraphobia, social anxiety disorder, phobias and generalised anxiety disorder. All may develop after burn injuries, but generalized anxiety disorder has the highest prevalence in this population. One year after the burn injury, the prevalence of general anxiety disorder in persons with burns can be close to 35%. Prevalence rates increase over time, from 2.2% at 2 weeks after injury to 19% at 3 months after injury and to approximately one in three persons at 12 months after injury [3, 18].

Pain experienced by patients with burn injuries coexists with anxiety. Nociceptive and neuropathic pain caused by burns can be exacerbated by treatments and procedures such as frequent dressing changes, escharotomies, intravenous line placement, and physical and occupational therapy. Burn injuries require expert pain control and attention to treatment guidelines. When anxiety compounds burn pain, it triggers a physiological stress response that delays wound healing. Moreover, anticipatory anxiety during burn procedures increases the perception of pain and overall levels of distress [9, 14]. All physicians working in burn centers should be familiar with the updated WHO guidelines for pain management (https://www.who.int/news-room/detail/27-08-2019-who-revision-of-pain-management-guidelines).

The undertreatment of pain increases risk of developing depressive and anxiety disorders. Other factors associated with the development of anxiety disorders in patients who sustained burn injuries include fear of loss of love and approval, fear of loss of body parts, a threat to the narcissistic integrity of the self, fear of loss of loved ones, separation and abandonment, and fear of loss of function and generativity [9, 14].

2.4   Substance Use Disorders

Patients in burn centers commonly have pre-existing substance use disorders and burns often occur in states of inebriation, intoxication or drug withdrawal. The reported prevalence of substance use disorders (alcohol and illicit substances) in persons who are admitted to burn centers is up to 15% [2, 27]. Tobacco use disorder also increases the risk of burns. People who smoke more than 10 cigarettes a day have a risk of burns six times higher than non-smokers [28].

The incidence of alcohol-related burns in patients with history of alcohol dependence is 54%. Up to 33% of patients with burn injuries are intoxicated with alcohol at the time of burns. Alcohol dependence occurs in 11.6% of patients recovering from burn injuries and 8% of all patients develop alcohol dependence *de novo* after burn injuries. There is a greater risk of infection, sepsis and multi-system organ failure in patients who had alcohol intoxication at the time of burn injuries.

Individuals with substance use disorders that develop or worsen after burn injuries benefit from multidisciplinary mental health interventionists that include addiction specialists. Tailored treatments that coordinate addiction recovery and rehabilitation services help optimize the overall health outcomes and survival of patients in inpatient burn centers and outpatient aftercare programs. The self-medication hypothesis postulates that addiction results from a failed attempt at self-medicating with intoxicants in order to escape distressing affective states. Maladaptive coping mechanisms and avoidant behaviours that characterize substance use disorders are related to poor health outcomes in patients recovering from burn injuries [2, 29].

2.5 Dementia and Delirium

Patients in burn centers often have cognitive deficits that present as objective findings in mental status examinations in addition to subjective complaints of problems with memory, attention and concentration. Cognitive deficits compound the incapacity caused by sensory and motor deficits, often presenting as poor registration and recall, dyscalculia, disorientation, constructional apraxia, word finding difficulty, speech and language disturbance and problems with executive functioning. Delayed onset post-burn amnesia is a reported complication in patients with burn injury. Possible causes include prolonged hypoxia and dissociative states [3, 30].

Disorientation, confusion, delirium, and sleep disorders are commonly observed during the acute treatment of burn injuries [31]. About 20% patients in burn centers potentially reversible acute confusional states- delirium [3]. The aetiology of delirium is multifactorial and could include hypoglycaemia, sepsis and infectious causes, metabolic abnormalities such as hypercalcemia and hyponatremia, hepatic encephalopathy, uraemia and hypoxia. Delirium in patients in burn units, with a history of substance use disorders, could be caused by intoxication of drug withdrawal states. Delirium is also more common in persons with extensive burns over larger body surface areas [28, 32].

3 Role of Mental Health Professionals

Mental health interventions for patients with burn injuries need to account for social, economic and cultural gaps in order to provide health treatment that is patient-centred and culturally informed. Barriers to care in underserved communities include patients' lack of knowledge about mental health services and understanding of mental disorders, and barriers within the medical system such as lack of mental health training, tense physician-patient relationships, and cultural stereotypes about mental illness among colleagues in medicine and surgery specialized services. Culturally endorsed attitudes that promote somatization and aversion to verbally express feelings, low education and living in poverty also result in difficulty accessing adequate care. Lack of access to mental health professionals during hospitalizations in burn centers is most problematic [33].

Mental health professionals in burn care units could enhance therapeutic medical-surgical efforts from admission until discharge and in the aftercare of patients who sustained burn injuries. Table 1 summarizes the stages of mental health care for patients in burn centers.

Table 1 Stages of recovery and mental health recommendations for patients in Burn Care Units [34]

Stage	Course, symptoms, diagnoses	Treatments
I—Admission and critical care	– Length of this stage varies between individuals, depends on the severity of burn injury – Patient's dependent and passive behaviour – Burn pain, grief, and anxiety – Acute stress disorder, delirium	– Antianxiety medication – Analgesic medication – Psychological support (reassurance, normalization, relaxation techniques) – Spiritual guidance and religious services – Medication targeting acute stress disorder symptoms
II—In-hospital recuperation	– This stage ends upon the patient's discharge from the burn unit – Burn pain, grief, and anxiety – Acute stress disorder, delirium – Major depression, PTSD	– Targeted administration of analgesics – Physiotherapy – Psychotherapy (cognitive-behavioural, supportive, interpersonal, psychodynamic and family therapy) – Spiritual guidance and religious services – Pharmacological treatment of anxiety and depression
III—Rehabilitation and reintegration	– It takes several years – Adjustment disorders – Post-traumatic stress disorder – Anxiety disorders – Depressive disorders – Substance use disorders – Heightened suicide risk	– Re-entry and follow up programs – Medication targeting PTSD – Psychotherapy (cognitive-behavioural, supportive, interpersonal, psychodynamic and family therapy) – Spiritual guidance and religious services – Anxiolytics tapered off over time – Anti-depressant medication – Medications to curb drug cravings – Suicide prevention interventions

3.1 Critical Care

The stage of acute and critical care focuses on life saving, supportive medical and surgical care while the patient is sedated and psychologically in a dependent, vulnerable and passive state, usually experiencing the fluctuations in level of consciousness that characterize delirium. Essential treatments include vigorous analgesia, sedation and respiratory support and infection prevention treatments. Mental health professionals provide support, encourage palliative interventions and attend to the needs of family members. If patients are awake and responsive repetitive reassurance and relaxation techniques are helpful to lower anxiety and maximize analgesia, as patients need to endure excruciatingly painful procedures such as dressing changes, debridement, and skin grafts. It is also important to serve as patient advocates and liaison agents, providing medical information with clarity and facilitating communication with other healthcare workers. About 50% of family members of patients in burn centers develop acute stress disorder, anxiety and depressive symptoms. Therapeutic interventions with family members are integral to the treatment plan during this stage. Assessment of pre-injury medical history including psychological health, coping skills, and level of family or social support takes place during this stage of treatment [34–37].

3.2 In-Hospital Recuperation

The second stage is associated with an increment in patients' activity levels. This stage begins with identification of patients at risk to prioritize those who would benefit from mental health interventions. Those with identified pre-injury mental disorders and suicide history are at risk and should be offered treatment. During this stage patient's experience distress caused by disfigurement and physical limitations, which lead to psychopathological symptoms that interfere with recovery. Painful physiotherapy feels like torture but is essential to prevent further physical limitations due to contractures. During this stage, psychotropic medications are judiciously prescribed to alleviate symptoms and mental health interventions are supportive and focus on maximizing cooperation, alleviating distress and improving adherence to medical-surgical care [34, 35].

3.3 Rehabilitation and Reintegration

The rehabilitation phase is the last stage of mental health treatment and occurs largely after hospital discharge. It is a long-term treatment process that consists on optimizing physical and mental adjustment to return adaptively to the previous pre-hospitalization environment. Unfortunately, 50% of persons with severe burn injuries experience impairment in many aspects of their life including self-worth, employment, and social status due to decreased body functioning capacity. This results in reduced income, less independence, poor self-esteem, and social withdrawal. Suicidal persons are at heightened risk after discharge from burn centers. Dissatisfaction with body-image lowers self-esteem and leads to social withdrawal and avoidance, which could further compound depressive disorders and negatively affect sexual health and interpersonal relationships. Mental health professionals are trained to address all facets of the psychological care of persons with burn injuries and are most helpful during this phase of treatment [4, 34, 35].

4   Psychopharmacological Considerations

Multiple complications and comorbidities in patients with burn injuries make psychopharmacological interventions challenging. Multimorbidities that impact medication management with psychotropics include electrolyte imbalances, renal insufficiency or failure, acute respiratory distress syndrome (ARDS), central nervous system dysfunction, gastrointestinal disorders and hepatic failure. The most common condition found following burn injury is acute kidney injury. The Risk, Injury, Failure, Loss, End-Stage Renal Disease (RIFLE) or Acute Kidney Injury Network (AKIN) criteria are helpful tools to identify grade kidney dysfunction from risk, injury, to failure [38–40].

Recent studies show that patients with total body surface area burns greater than 30% have an increased risk of developing delirium during treatment. The risk factors for delirium vary and include severity of illness, pre-existing psychological problems, and receiving medications. Use of benzodiazepines for managing neuropathic burn pain or anxiety symptoms worsens or triggers delirium and should be used with extreme caution in burn centers [32].

When psychopharmacological treatment is needed, psychiatrists need to carefully consider the totality of the patient's medical condition. Antidepressant, antipsychotic and antianxiety therapy coupled with psychotherapy are considered safe for patients with acute kidney injury. Adjusted dosages of these medications for patients with renal dysfunction and concomitant delirium, depressive, anxiety, and psychotic symptoms are listed in Table 2 [38].

Another condition associated with burn injuries is hypovolemic shock. It commonly occurs in patients with burns greater than 20% of total body surface area. Intravascular volume is greatly reduced after burns due to increased capillary permeability, which leads to shock. The main treatment for hypovolemic shock is fluid resuscitation regardless of solution type. If untreated, hypovolemic shock worsens acute kidney injury and may lead to death. Attention to AKI merits careful dosing of psychotropic medications [41].

Liver dysfunction is common in patients who sustain burn injuries. It results from hepatic cell apoptosis. Hypoperfusion in the range of 60% for 4 h could result in cell apoptosis. It is unclear if psychopharmacological interventions need to be adjusted for this reason, but judicious practices dictate dose reductions for patients with liver dysfunction signalled by elevated liver function tests [42].

5   The Suicidal Patient in the Burn Unit

Suicide by self-immolation is almost always lethal but those who survive require aggressive interventions that should begin while admitted in burn centers and continue upon discharge during the rehabilitation and recovery phase of treatment. Countertransference reactions elicited by self-immolators include avoidance, denial, fear, terror, dissociation, and rage. Empathic misalignment between clinician and patient, triggered by these negative affective states, leads to dismissing the serious risk of suicide that persists when ambivalently suicidal self-immolators face disfigurement, stigma, discrimination and alienation from their family members and community that complicate pre-existing psychiatric disorders.

Table 2 Psychotropics used in burn units adjusted for renal dysfunction [38]

Medications	Daily dosage range for patients with burns (mg)	Daily dosage range for patients with burns and renal dysfunction (mg)
Antidepressants—selective serotonin reuptake inhibitors (SSRIs)		
Citalopram	20–60	10–40
Escitalopram	10–20	5–10
Fluoxetine	20–60	10–40
Fluvoxamine	50–300	50–200
Sertraline	50–150	25–100
Paroxetine	20–60	10–30
Antidepressant drugs—tricyclic antidepressants		
Amitriptyline	25–150	10–75
Imipramine	25–150	25–75
Doxepin	25–75	10–75
Nortriptyline	25–75	25–75
Trazodone	150–400	50–300
Antidepressants—newer antidepressants		
Venlafaxine	37.5–225	37.5–150
Mirtazapine	15–45	7.5–30
Duloxetine	20–80	20–60
Antipsychotics		
Haloperidol	0.5–15	0.5–15
Clozapine	25–400	Titrate dose as needed
Olanzapine	5–20	5–20
Quetiapine	150–600	150–600
Risperidone	1–4	0.5–2
Ziprasidone	20–80	20–60
Antianxiety medication		
Alprazolam	0.25–4	0.25–2
Clonazepam	0.5–2.0	0.5–1.5
Lorazepam	0.5–4	0.5–4
Diazepam	5–40	5–25
Buspirone	5–20	5–20
Zolpidem	5–10	5–10
Zaleplon	5–10 HS	5–10

The affective state of hopelessness is highly contagious, and clinicians need to navigate their own emotions carefully not to become apathetic or withdrawn. Maximizing life's potentials is a theme that provides therapeutic comfort to suicidal patients. Extending the person's supportive network may provide necessary temporary relief to anchor the suicidal patient while he or she searches for a meaningful existence. All psychotherapies are suicide protective, and more important than clinical expertise is continuity of effort, consistency, and validation of distress in nonjudgmental ways. Spiritual counselling and incorporating clergy as an integral part of the treatment team may facilitate suicide prevention, especially when clinical services face high demand.

6 Conclusion

Most persons who sustain burn injuries have a high prevalence of pre-existing mental disorders compounded by a higher prevalence of post-injury ASD, PTSD, depressive disorders, anxiety disorders, delirium and substance use disorders. Burn care unit patients are inappropriately deprived of appropriate psychiatric care due to socio-economic-cultural barriers that limit access to comprehensive care. Persons who recover from burn injuries benefit from psychiatric interventions during the rehabilitation stage when mental disorders like PTSD, generalized anxiety disorders and major depression increase in prevalence after discharge, and suicide risk intensifies. Liaison psychiatrists are uniquely trained to orchestrate the complex mental health needs of persons who sustain burn injuries.

References

1. Moore M, Fagan S, Nejad S, Bilodeau M, Goverman L, Ibrahim AE, Beresneva O, Sarhane KA, Goverman J. The role of a dedicated staff psychiatrist in modern burn centers. Ann Burns Fire Disasters. 2013;26(4):213.
2. Low JA, Meyer IIIWJ, Willebrand M, Thomas CR. Psychiatric disorders associated with burn injury. Total Burn Care. 2018;1:700–8.
3. Van Loey NE, Van Son MJ. Psychopathology and psychological problems in patients with burn scars. Am J Clin Dermatol. 2003;4(4):245–72.
4. Mahendraraj K, Durgan DM, Chamberlain RS. Acute mental disorders and short and long term morbidity in patients with third degree flame burn: a population-based outcome study of 96,451 patients from the Nationwide Inpatient Sample (NIS) database (2001–2011). Burns. 2016;42(8):1766–73.
5. Palmu R, Suominen K, Vuola J, Isometsä E. Mental disorders after burn injury: a prospective study. Burns. 2011;37(4):601–9.
6. Falder S, Browne A, Edgar D, Staples E, Fong J, Rea S, Wood F. Core outcomes for adult burn survivors: a clinical overview. Burns. 2009;35(5):618–41.
7. Dyster-Aas J, Willebrand M, Wikehult B, Gerdin B, Ekselius L. Major depression and post-traumatic stress disorder symptoms following severe burn injury in relation to lifetime psychiatric morbidity. J Trauma Acute Care Surg. 2008;64(5):1349–56.
8. Menzies V. Depression and burn wounds. Arch Psychiatr Nurs. 2000;14(4):199–206.
9. Byers JF, Bridges S, Kijek J, LaBorde P. Burn patients' pain and anxiety experiences. J Burn Care Rehabil. 2001;22(2):144–9.
10. Palmu R. Mental disorders among burn patients. Raimo Palmu and National Institute for Health and Welfare: Helsinki; 2010.
11. Capuron L, Raison CL, Musselman DL, Lawson DH, Nemeroff CB, Miller AH. Association of exaggerated HPA axis response to the initial injection of interferon-alpha with development of depression during interferon-alpha therapy. Am J Psychiatr. 2003;160(7):1342–5.
12. Kildal M, Willebrand M, Andersson G, Gerdin B, Ekselius L. Personality characteristics and perceived health problems after burn injury. J Burn Care Rehabil. 2004;25(3):228–35.
13. Willebrand M, Andersson G, Kildal M, Ekselius L. Exploration of coping patterns in burned adults: cluster analysis of the coping with burns questionnaire (CBQ). Burns. 2002;28(6):549–54.
14. Lončar Z, Braš M, Mičković V. The relationships between burn pain, anxiety and depression. Collegium Antropologicum. 2006;30(2):319–25.

15. Wang CH, Tsay SL, Elaine Bond A. Post-traumatic stress disorder, depression, anxiety and quality of life in patients with traffic-related injuries. J Adv Nurs. 2005;52(1):22–30.
16. Wiechman S, Kalpakjian CZ, Johnson KL. Measuring depression in adults with burn injury: a systematic review. J Burn Care Res. 2016;37(5):e415–26.
17. American Psychiatric Association. American Psychiatric Association: Diagnostic and Statistical Manual of Mental Disorders. Arlington: American Psychiatric Association; 2013.
18. O'Donnell ML, Bryant RA, Creamer M, Carty J. Mental health following traumatic injury: toward a health system model of early psychological intervention. Clin Psychol Rev. 2008;28(3):387–406.
19. Wiechman SA, Ptacek JT, Patterson DR, Gibran NS, Engrav LE, Heimbach DM. Rates, trends, and severity of depression after burn injuries. J Burn Care Rehabil. 2001;22(6):417–24.
20. McKibben JB, Bresnick MG, Wiechman Askay SA, Fauerbach JA. Acute stress disorder and posttraumatic stress disorder: a prospective study of prevalence, course, and predictors in a sample with major burn injuries. J Burn Care Res. 2008;29(1):22–35.
21. Giannoni-Pastor A, Eiroa-Orosa FJ, Fidel Kinori SG, Arguello JM, Casas M. Prevalence and predictors of posttraumatic stress symptomatology among burn survivors: a systematic review and meta-analysis. J Burn Care Res. 2016;37(1):e79–89.
22. Sareen J. Posttraumatic stress disorder in adults: impact, comorbidity, risk factors, and treatment. Can J Psychiatry. 2014;59(9):460–7.
23. Van Loey NE, Maas CJ, Faber AW, Taal LA. Predictors of chronic posttraumatic stress symptoms following burn injury: results of a longitudinal study. J Traumatic Stress. 2003;16(4):361–9.
24. Shalev AY. Acute stress reactions in adults. Biol Psychiatry. 2002;51(7):532–43.
25. Schell TL, Marshall GN, Jaycox LH. All symptoms are not created equal: the prominent role of hyperarousal in the natural course of posttraumatic psychological distress. J Abnorm Psychol. 2004;113(2):189.
26. Deniz S, Arslan S. Pain and anxiety in burn patients. Int J Caring Sci. 2017;10(3):1723.
27. Salehi SH, As'adi K, Musavi J, Ahrari F, Nemazi P, Kamranfar B, Gaseminegad K, Faramarzi S, Shoar S. Assessment of substances abuse in burn patients by using drug abuse screening test. Acta Med Iran. 2012;50:257–64.
28. Blank K, Perry S. Relationship of psychological processes during delirium to outcome. Am J Psychiatry. 1984;141(7):843–7.
29. Sveen J, Öster C. Alcohol consumption after severe burn: a prospective study. Psychosomatics. 2015;56(4):390–6.
30. Duff K, McCaffrey RJ. Electrical injury and lightning injury: a review of their mechanisms and neuropsychological, psychiatric, and neurological sequelae. Neuropsychol Rev. 2001;11(2):101–16.
31. Patterson DR, Everett JJ, Bombardier CH, Questad KA, Lee VK, Marvin JA. Psychological effects of severe burn injuries. Psychol Bull. 1993;113(2):362.
32. Agarwal V, O'Neill PJ, Cotton BA, Pun BT, Haney S, Thompson J, Kassebaum N, Shintani A, Guy J, Ely EW, Pandharipande P. Prevalence and risk factors for development of delirium in burn intensive care unit patients. J Burn Care Res. 2010;31(5):706–15.
33. Ren Z, Zhang P, Wang H, Wang H. Qualitative research investigating the mental health care service gap in Chinese burn injury patients. BMC Health Serv Res. 2018;18(1):902.
34. Blakeney P, Rosenberg L, Rosenberg M, Faber A. Psychosocial care of persons with severe burns. Burns. 2008;34(4):433–40.
35. Bryant R, Touyz S. The role of the clinical psychologist on a burn unit in a general teaching hospital. J Clin Psychol Med Settings. 1996;3(1):41–55.
36. Johnson R, Taggart S, Gullick J. Emerging from the trauma bubble: redefining 'normal' after burn injury. Burns. 2016;42:1223–32.
37. McLean L, Chen R, Kwiet J, Vandervord J, Kornhaber R. A clinical update on posttraumatic stress disorder in burn injury survivors. Australas Psychiatry. 2017;25(4):348–50.
38. De Sousa A. Psychiatric issues in renal failure and dialysis. Indian J Nephrol. 2008;18(2):47–50.

39. Clark A, Neyra J, Madni T, Imran J, Phelan H, Arnoldo B, Wolf S. Acute kidney injury after burn. Burns. 2017;43:898–908.
40. Nielson C, Duethman N, Howard J, Moncure M, Wood J. Burns. J Burn Care Res. 2017;38(1):e469–81.
41. Pham T, Cancio L, Gibran N. American Burn Association Practice Guidelines Burn Shock Resuscitation. J Burn Care Res. 2008;29(1):257–66.
42. Jeschke MG, Herndon D. The hepatic response to severe injury. In: Vincent JL, editor. Intensive care medicine, vol. 2007. New York: Springer; 2007. p. 651–65.

Media, Suicide and Contagion: Safe Reporting as Suicide Prevention

Yin Ping Ng, Ravivarma Rao Panirselvam, and Lai Fong Chan

Reporters get numbed after a long time, we no longer experience the nausea, appetite loss or insomnia as when we first started. It's just that I don't want to be emotionally insensitive. I deeply feel the grief of the family members in the tragedy. There was no need to expose the private affairs of others, I did not want to let the family members of the deceased feel pain.

(translated excerpt from Sin Chew Daily, "Interviewing Suicide Cases" by senior reporter, Ooi Lye Lau)

Y. P. Ng (✉)
Pantai Hospital Penang, Penang, Malaysia

Suicide Prevention Research Malaysia (SUPREMA), National University (UKM), Kuala Lumpur, Malaysia
e-mail: dr.ngyinping@pantaipg.com.my, pingingfeline@gmail.com

R. R. Panirselvam
Suicide Prevention Research Malaysia (SUPREMA), National University (UKM), Kuala Lumpur, Malaysia

Department of Psychiatry & Mental Health, Hospital Miri, Miri, Sarawak, Malaysia
e-mail: ravivarmarao@gmail.com

L. F. Chan
Suicide Prevention Research Malaysia (SUPREMA), National University (UKM), Kuala Lumpur, Malaysia

Department of Psychiatry, Faculty of Medicine, National University of Malaysia, Kuala Lumpur, Malaysia

Malaysian National Representative of the International Association of Suicide Prevention (IASP), WA, USA
e-mail: laifchan@ppukm.ukm.edu.my

1 Introduction

Media reporting of suicide is evolving in quality across the globe. Commonly observed problematic characteristics of suicide news reports include: sensationalism [1] and explicit reporting of suicide methods, sometimes prominently in headlines [2–4]; over-representing depictions of violent methods [3, 5]; displaying graphic materials such as victims' photos, suicide notes and locations including public places; and detailed characterisation of the decedent and attribution to a single cause [5–7].

Selective and stereotypical reporting still occurs. In Hong Kong, for example, suicide news have a tendency to focus on student suicides or institutions with multiple fatalities [8]. In South India, Armstrong's 2018 review of Tamil Nadu papers demonstrated a trend of repetitively reporting the same news (68.6%) as well as frequent inaccuracies in terms of risk factors (>54%) inconsistent with psychological autopsy findings [3]. There are no studies specifically examining media reporting of self-immolation suicides to determine if safer reporting guidelines could reduce the prevalence of these suicides. We, as others, believe that suicide contagion is of relevance in self-immolations, especially when these are culturally, politically and socially motivated. The authors of this chapter, therefore, will take a general approach reviewing existing studies that could inform *safe reporting of all suicides*, which is an important aspect of suicide prevention.

2 Impact

Media reporting of suicides can exert considerable impact on individuals, especially in those with a higher vulnerability to suicide [6, 9–11]. Subgroups with an increased vulnerability include people suffering from mental disorders, young people, those with a history of suicidal behaviour and the suicide-bereaved [12]. Depending on the quality of reporting, suicide coverage of suicides can result in negative (harmful) effects or positive (preventive) effects. Other terms used are *Werther* effects to represent harmful effects; and *Papageno* effects for preventive effects.

2.1 Werther *Effect*

Phillips first described the *Werther* effect phenomenon, where exposure to a media suicide reporting leads to the occurrence of other suicides; in reference to Goethe's 1774 novella [13]. In Goethe's book, Werther ended his life following unrequited love from his beloved and the suicide was described in a detailed and romanticised manner. Several suicides took place following the book's publication in a manner similar to Werther's death [13]. This imitative or contagion effect is thought to be mediated by social learning where a vulnerable person identifies with the decedent and proceeds to act in the same way [13]. Others postulate that individuals with ambivalent ideas about suicide may be influenced by media messages to end their lives by suicide [9, 14, 15].

In this chapter we will refer to suicide contagion as imitative suicidal behaviour resulting from exposure to media content relating to suicide [13, 16, 17]. Suicide contagion is well documented [1, 2, 16] and is particularly significant in teenagers [18]. There is a strong association between increased suicide rates and media suicide reporting that covers prominent persons, is repetitive and sensationalistic, provides explicit details (e.g. methods or graphic images) or inaccurate information, involves novel methods, and frames suicide positively or idolizes the decedent [6, 10, 19–21]. A recent meta-analysis showed that reporting of celebrity suicides correlates with an increase of 8–18% of suicides in the ensuing 1–2 months, and suicide method information is linked to a 18–44% rise in suicide risk by the same method [10]. Such contagion effects tend to persist long term [22]. The association is greater especially among persons with similar characteristics who may identify with the decedent [1, 6, 19]. For example, in a sample of 438 depressed patients, 38.8% were influenced in their subsequent suicidal behaviour by a sensationalistic and explicitly written celebrity suicide media report; and 24 attempted suicide [19].

Internet use further compounds the contagion effect, facilitating easy on-demand access and dissemination of online information about suicides, concealment of user identity, and interactive, real time responses to published online posts [23, 24]. Ueda and colleagues found increased suicide rates following a celebrity suicide death that generated an immense number of tweets; while no increase was noted when another suicide death (which had considerable reportage in traditional media) generated little interest on Twitter [25]. Unlike print media, new media content is not constrained by space and is permanently available in cyberspace. Social media platforms also allow content curation (via click-baits) to attract attention, repetitive viewing [26] and sharing of graphics and videos not usually available on print media [24].

2.2   Trauma Effects

Exposure to suicide stories or reports can be emotionally disturbing especially to people with lived experience (PLE) [19], even to the point of triggering suicidal behaviour [19, 27], and may worsen the distress of grieving in the suicide-bereaved [28, 29]. Qualitative studies show that media reports can exacerbate the distress of the suicide-bereaved [28, 30, 31], particularly when published in an insensitive or inaccurate manner [28]. By identifying with the suicide-bereaved when reading suicide reports, some describe a massive intrusion into their grieving process [28] while others experience re-traumatisation and increased grief symptoms [30].

Mental health professionals are equally as likely to be affected by media suicide reporting, especially when it involves one of their own patients [32]. A mental health professional's occupation involves forming strong therapeutic relationships, sharing of personal information and carrying patients through crises. From the author's own experience (Ng) and personal communication with local Malaysian psychiatrists, mental health professionals can be affected by suicide news reports, especially those involving explicit descriptions of their patients. Such reports can trigger distressing memories of previous patient suicides, complicate grief and affect the therapist personally and professionally.

Media practitioners are not spared when it comes to suicide reporting-related trauma [33]. Some report distress upon being exposed and in close proximity to the subject of suicide [33], particularly when caught unprepared in terms of emotional intelligence and knowledge to support a recently suicide-bereaved person [34]. At least two Malaysian vernacular newspaper journalists describe similar experiences [35, 36]. For some, suicide remains a disturbing topic long after the completed journalistic reporting [33].

2.3 Propagating Stigma and Myths

Apart from contagion and trauma effects, reporting of suicides may propagate myths [37] or inaccurate information about suicide (monocausal attribution, selective reporting, apportioning blame, misreporting suicide risk factors) [5, 8, 38], which in turn worsens the stigma surrounding suicides.

2.4 Papageno Effect

Suicide reporting can confer protective effects [9]. Niederkrotenthaler (2010) reported a protective phenomenon linked to news reports focused on individuals who successfully overcame their suicide crises [21]. He named it the Papageno effect, based on Mozart's character from the opera The Magic Flute who overcame his suicidal crisis after three boys reminded him of other ways to resolve his problems. Niederkrotenthaler posited that stories of hope and recovery that encourage coping facilitate the Papageno effect and may prevent suicide [39]. There is international evidence for the Papageno effect of suicide reporting resulting in gains in knowledge about determinants of suicide, suicidal behaviour reductions or improved help-seeking behaviour [9, 40]. It is worth noting, however, that we need additional high-quality studies to better understand how positive media portrayals affect vulnerable individuals [9].

Other beneficial effects of suicide reporting include improving mental health literacy, correcting myths, disseminating help-seeking information and providing a platform for discussion of an otherwise stigmatised issue [39, 41]. Internet and social media platforms may facilitate access to otherwise hard-to-engage individuals, and be used as a modality for suicide prevention [42]. In addition, reporting of suicides may serve as a platform for the bereaved to share their views, process grief and advocate for suicide prevention [28, 30].

3 Reasons for Harmful Reporting

3.1 Commercial Competitiveness

It is undeniable that economic pressures influence news publications. With increasing competition for consumer attention and advertising, media production is now largely audience-oriented and commercial, focusing on events with broad audience appeal, i.e. newsworthy events [43, 44]. In essence, news is for sale [43]. Values that make an event newsworthy include timeliness, proximity to target consumer, appeal to human interest, currency (trending issues), prominence, significance, unusualness and conflict element content [45]. To capitalise on sales and remain competitive and cost-effective, media companies often focus on producing exclusive and sensationalistic news, with reporters working under intense time pressure and editors making quick decisions on sensitive issues [43, 46, 47]. The stories are often simplified and personified to make them comprehensible and relatable to a broad segment of the general public, resulting in "a version of reality that is less complex than it may actually be" [43, 48].

Suicide stories that are deemed newsworthy commonly involve public figures, vulnerable populations, public locations, violent or unusual methods or important social issues that impact the community [5, 33, 49]. Since space availability relates to cost, which is often limited, the resultant focus will likely be on the death event itself rather than the factors which led to the suicide [46]. In a qualitative study [48], some journalists had to accept their organization's commercial practices to safeguard their jobs even if these were in conflict with their own values and professional judgment. They reported that media organisations employ inexperienced graduates with little understanding of journalism ethics as frontline reporters with less pay, resulting in a high turnover further compromising the quality of reporting [48].

3.2 Lack of Awareness and Knowledge

Some studies describe that media practitioners are skeptical of the potentially harmful or contributory nature of media reporting to imitative suicides [33, 46, 48]. Some media outlets view it as their right to report suicide stories as a way to empower society by providing information to support the public's right to know [33]. Journalists may feel that excluding suicide news may be more damaging [33, 46], believing that reporting disturbing and graphic details of suicides may serve to deter people from the notion of suicide being a 'solution to their problems', and that 'sanitized' reports may actually encourage suicidal behaviour [46].

It is possible that reporters who do not have lived experience or prior engagement with the suicide-bereaved, might find it difficult to appreciate how their reporting may impact the bereaved. Luce (2018) shared how losing a dear friend to suicide brought about awareness of the negative impact of sensationalistic reporting on the suicide bereaved. She later reflected in hindsight that the suicide stories she wrote prior to the loss were "unfortunately stigmatising, sensationalistic and did not take into account how the bereaved might feel" and the reports did not provide support helplines [34].

In some cases, media practitioners' misconceptions about suicide may also contribute to inappropriate reporting. For example, a study participant covered a story involving a student who attended an orientation camp prior to her suicide. Based on the reporter's own beliefs, speculations were made that linked the suicide to the orientation camp. Although eventually no causal connections were found, the editor made the decision to mention 'orientation camp' in the publication headline [48].

Interestingly, although some journalists may see detailed reporting as helpful, this view is not necessarily supported by the public. For example, a national survey conducted by the American Society of Newspaper Editors found that while 75% of the public preferred to respect a family's wishes to not publish a story on a child's fatal accident, 70% of the editors opined otherwise and would run the story [50].

Media practitioners who are aware of the potential harm of suicide reporting are often faced with the dilemma of what to report and what to exclude. It is not easy to strike a balance between what is deemed public versus private; or safe versus harmful [47].

3.3   Lack of Training

Related to poor awareness or knowledge is lack of training in journalism schools on safe suicide reporting [46, 50]. Most media organisations have some form of general media ethics guidelines, however, none specifically address how to report issues related to mental health or suicide [46, 50]. Similarly, the topic of suicide is also not covered in the syllabus of most journalism programs [50]. Media professionals would appreciate guidance to be able to understand grief and provide support when interviewing the bereaved [30]. Luce describes her first experience reporting a suicide story—she had planned her approach, i.e. to do background work, find sources, get quotes, "write it and move on", only to be "taken aback by the depth of grief", "caught completely unprepared" and certainly lacking "the knowledge and emotional intelligence necessary to support a source who was suffering enormously" [34].

3.4   Absence of Reporting Quality Monitoring

Absence of monitoring of suicide reporting quality is problematic in some countries, notably in those that do not have a national suicide prevention strategy [7]. Even more challenging is keeping track of suicide news stories and interactive comments published in social media whose content creators and end users are not necessarily familiar with or bound by professional journalism ethics [48, 51]. There is also the issue of the increasing amorphous nature of what constitutes truthful and fake news on the internet. Fact checking is becoming increasingly difficult and misleading information often becomes viral [52].

4   Safe Suicide-Reporting in the Media: Concepts and Components

Safe reporting as it relates to suicide prevention encompasses elements of the *Papageno* effect and takes into consideration the *Werther* effect. The World Health Organization (WHO) recognizes the significance of safe reporting and includes interaction with the media towards responsible reporting as one of the core interventions within *LIVE LIFE*, a framework outlining their organization's strategic approach to suicide [53].

Cheng and colleagues' [40] study of students in Hong Kong is an elegant case example of what constitutes safe reporting and how real-world interaction with the media may moderate suicide reporting to have a significant impact on suicide prevention. This phenomenon, illustrated in Fig. 1, demonstrates that narrowing the gap between descriptive-reporting and preventive-reporting correlates with lower rates of student suicides. The authors' operational definition of preventive reporting intensity includes the quality (type of information) and quantity (word count) of sentences in news reports such as suicide prevention information and research from both expert opinion and local community resources, as well as stories of how people in suicidal crises overcame their difficulties. Descriptive reporting is broadly defined as sensationalistic and prominent reporting of student suicides that includes many details such as suicide methods and personal information about the deceased without careful consideration of suicide risk factors [8]. Cheng and colleagues concluded the following:

- Safe reporting of suicide results in a reduction of student suicides when it includes preventive reporting and avoids descriptive reporting practices.
- Media engagement is an effective strategy that influences a change in media practices towards safer reporting of student suicides [8, 40].

Level of safety in suicide news reporting also relates to how the media frames the story. Findings from content analysis studies based on established media guidelines are helpful in characterising the components of safe reporting of suicide news.

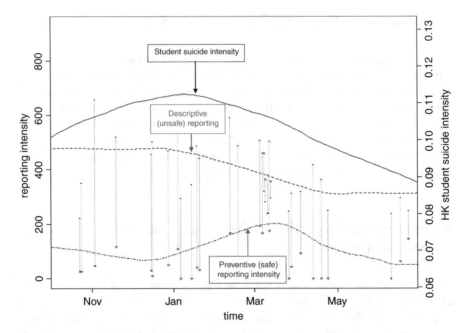

Fig. 1 Correlation between intensity of student suicide with level of safe reporting (modified with permission from Cheng and colleagues [40])

Table 1 provides a summary of findings from relevant studies that assess the quality/ framing of suicide news reporting [3, 4] establishing an association between media content and suicide rates, identifying protective and harmful indicators [8, 21, 40].

Politicians, policymakers, health and medical experts, journalists, editors, and lay people are the prime agents in news agenda-setting and dissemination. Contextual factors such as the narrative structure and sub-textual features within a news report featuring suicide affect the process of how meaning is interpreted by the readership or audience [55]. Therefore, before concluding whether a particular news report about suicide is safe or not, one needs to consider the diversity of sub-populations within the general public. Varying degrees of vulnerability to suicidal behaviour could be dependent on the individual's level of exposure to suicide or PLE. Thus, a more pragmatic view of safe reporting should take into account a dimensional approach rather than a rigid categorization of risks.

5   Intervention

5.1   Media Guidelines

Media guidelines for suicide reporting aim to promote responsible coverage of suicide news. Guidelines are helpful to raise awareness, provide recommendations and serve as a reference source for reporting suicide-related news. Most guidelines

Table 1 Protective and harmful indicators in media suicide reporting[a]

	Indicators	
	Suicide-preventive: protective [21, 40]	Suicide-descriptive: harmful [21, 40]
Suicidal act [3]		Detailed account of suicide method Step-by-step description of suicide Description of novel type of suicide method [54] Named public site location of suicide Event reported as a suicide pact Event reported as a mass suicide
Prominence [3]		Front coverage or in the first three pages Headlines include the term "suicide" Headlines include the suicide method Headlines referring to life event(s)
Identity of suicidal person/ deceased [3, 21]		Coverage includes photograph Coverage includes detailed personal characteristics Sensationalised and glorified coverage of celebrity/high-profile suicides [54]
Epidemiology and (/or) expert opinion [3, 21]	Suicide statistics presented in context that highlights suicide prevention research findings	Suicide research statistics framed as an epidemic, attributed to increasing societal problems or presented in a sensationalist tone
Style [21]		Use of lengthy articles Repetitive reporting of the same suicide story
Raising awareness of prevention services [3, 21, 40, 54]	Reporting includes description of suicide prevention programme and strategies Reporting includes information detailing how to seek help, including contacts for help resources Reporting includes accounts of adaptive coping, including lived experience stories of suicidal individuals who adapted positively when faced with adverse circumstances Reporting includes accurate information on how suicide is preventable and dispel myths such as "suicide is not preventable", "there are no warning signs", etc.	
Causes of suicidal behaviour [3, 8, 21]	Recognises link with poor mental health Recognises link with harmful use of substances	Monocausal explanation for suicidal behaviour such as a single negative life event Causes cited from suicide note

(continued)

Table 1 (continued)

	Indicators	
	Suicide-preventive: protective [21, 40]	Suicide-descriptive: harmful [21, 40]
Consideration for bereaved persons [3, 21, 54]	Respecting grief and privacy Delaying interviews for the bereaved Support services made available	Reporting may re-traumatise the bereaved Reporting may be an invasion of privacy
Criminalisation [4]		Framing suicide as a criminal offence that will be met with police action

ªCompiled and adapted from [3, 4, 8, 21, 40, 54]

Table 2 Media suicide reporting summary of recommendations [12, 54, 56–58]

Dos	Don'ts
Do provide helpful information related to suicide and its prevention	Don't describe method explicitly or provide any details relating to the method/location
Do highlight stories which promote positive coping, hope and help-seeking	Don't use a simplistic or monocausal explanation for suicide
Do provide accurate information on how and where to get help such as helplines	Don't frame suicide in a normalised or glamourized manner, or present it as a solution to problems
Do use caution when reporting celebrity suicides	Don't publish photographs/graphic images or use video links
Do consider impact on readers especially people at-risk or the bereaved	Don't report or place news prominently or repeatedly
Do exercise care when interviewing the bereaved	
Do recognise that media professionals can be affected by reporting suicides	
Do choose appropriate language	

share similar content in terms of recommendations of what is considered helpful (dos) and harmful (don'ts) practices (see Table 2). Guidelines are frequently updated to incorporate emerging evidence on how to report on social media and advocate greater awareness on the effect of suicide reporting on media professionals. Cultural differences and the strength of the imitative effect in a particular society or region need to be considered during development, dissemination and implementation of guidelines.

There is evidence showing the effectiveness of media guidelines for improving reporting style and reducing suicide contagion and suicide rates, for example in countries like Australia and Austria [59]. The extent of media involvement in the development, promotion and dissemination of guidelines appears to be crucial in influencing utilisation and effectiveness of the guidelines [56]. Australia's Mindframe guidelines, developed with significant media input and collaboration, were well-received by the media [54]. In China and New Zealand, however, media guidelines were developed without media collaboration, resulting in little media buy-in and in turn, minimal improvement on the quality of reporting [59, 60].

5.2 Engagement with the Media and Other Relevant Stakeholders

Findings from qualitative studies suggest that in order to engage media buy-in, any proposed guideline or change in media practice has to take into consideration the freedom of the press and the interests of media organisations [33, 46, 49]. The guidelines themselves should not appear to dictate what or how journalists should write, but rather serve as guidance for them to write in a way that promotes suicide prevention, while remaining appropriate to the local cultural context [57].

Strategies to promote media engagement include:

- Inviting media representatives (including social media organisations) and other relevant stakeholders for input during guideline development and discussions related to safe reporting [7, 57].
- Partnering with media organisations for the dissemination and promotion of guidelines [7].
- Facilitating ongoing journalistic education by providing:
  - Regular, interactive and targeted 'refresher' media training on guideline use, especially in organizations where reporter turnover is high [7, 48].
  - Ready resources on suicide and suicide prevention [48].
- Organising sharing sessions between suicide survivors and journalists to facilitate insight into how suicide reports might impact survivors. Interventions incorporating contact-based advocacy by PLEs are effective in promoting attitudinal change [61]. This empathic engagement may help strengthen media accountability towards the community in their reporting of suicide stories [31, 33, 34, 48].
- Providing incentives such as media awards [7].
- Starting education on safe suicide reporting early in journalism schools by incorporating the topic in the school syllabus [57].
- Enlisting assistance from mental health professionals who may be contacted to comment on suicide-related issues in the press and provide media training with emphasis on safe reporting [57].

It is helpful to emphasize that inspiring stories emphasizing adaptive coping and overcoming adversity can be as newsworthy and attract readership [62] without necessarily relying on sensationalism. Media organizations should be encouraged to publish more *Papageno*-like news that can help save lives [9]. It is important to specifically engage middle level management media personnel such as copyeditors and chief reporters who could positively influence changes in suicide reporting styles [46, 48]. Appealing to the media organizations' sense of social responsibility in promoting suicide prevention could improve engagement [48]. In an encouraging recent development, some social media platforms developed avenues for end-users to report suicidal content that will then be flagged and activate support messages [63].

It is also important to engage other relevant stakeholders to promote safe reporting [7, 57]. Strategies to improve mental health literacy on suicide prevention and safe reporting should involve:

- Policymakers, advocating for and working on sustainable national suicide prevention strategies (incorporating safe reporting).
- First responders, police, and coroner officials, exercising care in releasing sensitive information to the media as not all details are helpful to the public.
- NGOs, providing advocacy, expertise and resources.
- PLEs, providing feedback on media reporting, sharing experiences of mastery over crisis.
- Mental healthcare professionals, providing expertise on suicide prevention and mental health issues.

5.3 Monitoring

It is essential for have some level of regular monitoring or surveillance of quality of reporting in order to establish a baseline quality of suicide reporting, evaluate the effectiveness of interventions conducted to improve suicide reporting, and ensure that safe reporting is sustained over the long term [7, 59].

Countries such as Australia and Taiwan carry out national level media surveillance, which are helpful in informing intervention strategies to improve guideline adherence and reporting quality [64, 65]. These media surveillance programs are organised at a national level, utilise a standard set of evidence-based criteria (based on media guidelines), and provide funding and training to ensure that the monitoring can be maintained to facilitate evaluation of long-term outcomes [64, 65].

5.4 Legislation

There are mixed views about legislative restrictions implemented in some countries to deter harmful reporting of suicides. In New Zealand, the Coroners Act of 2006 forbade any reports relating to suicide particulars without the coroner's permission [66]. The media protested that the ban was against current international practice, restricted freedom of the press, and discouraged public suicide discourse [66]. The restrictions have since been revised to allow mention of suicides, but without mentioning of methods or related details [67]. Meanwhile, Australia banned pro-suicide websites. Although concerns were raised that the law interfered with the autonomy of those who wished to die and did not deter people from sourcing offshore websites, its proponents argued the ban raised awareness on cyber-suicide, limited access to domestic pro-suicide websites and acted as a deterrent to suicide [68].

6 Conclusion

Harmful reporting of suicides is relatively well-established as a risk factor for suicide, with increasing evidence of safe reporting potentially being suicide-preventive. Media guidelines offer a roadmap for safe reporting practices. To implement such guidelines in a sustainable and feasible way requires mutual understanding and multi-lateral collaboration from all stakeholders. Other related areas with public health and suicide prevention implications include the expanding scope of safe reporting beyond suicide news, to encompass safe messaging of fictional suicide-related media content, for example in film, television programs, music, and other expressions of popular culture. Lastly, there is a need for research studies to examine how media reporting practices may influence imitative suicides in regions of the world with a high prevalence of self-immolations, such as Tibetan diaspora, Arab League countries, Western and South Asia and Southern Africa.

References

1. Niederkrotenthaler T, Fu K-w, Yip PS, Fong DY, Stack S, Cheng Q, et al. Changes in suicide rates following media reports on celebrity suicide: a meta-analysis. J Epidemiol Community Health. 2012;66(11):1037–42.
2. Cheng Q, Chen F, Yip PS. Media effects on suicide methods: a case study on Hong Kong 1998–2005. PLoS One. 2017;12(4):e0175580.
3. Armstrong G, Vijayakumar L, Niederkrotenthaler T, Jayaseelan M, Kannan R, Pirkis J, et al. Assessing the quality of media reporting of suicide news in India against World Health Organization guidelines: a content analysis study of nine major newspapers in Tamil Nadu. Austral N Z J Psychiatry. 2018;52(9):856–63.
4. Victor J, Koon JHG, Govindaraju GM, Ling TP, Rajaratnam UD, Fong YL. Media reporting of suicide: a comparative framing analysis of Malaysian newspapers. 2019.
5. Machlin A, Pirkis J, Spittal MJ. Which suicides are reported in the media—and what makes them "newsworthy"? Crisis. 2013;34(5):305–13.
6. Sisask M, Värnik A. Media roles in suicide prevention: a systematic review. Int J Environ Res Public Health. 2012;9(1):123–38.
7. Beautrais A, Hendin H, Yip P, Takahashi Y, Chia BH, Schmidtke A, et al. Improving portrayal of suicide in the media in Asia. In: Hendin H, Phillips MR, Vijayakumar L, Pirkis J, Wang H, Yip P, Wasserman D, Bertolote J, Fleischmann A, editors. Suicide and Suicide Prevention in Asia. Geneva: World Health Organization; 2008. p. 39–50.
8. Cheng Q, Yip PS. Suicide news reporting accuracy and stereotyping in Hong Kong. J Affect Disord. 2012;141(2–3):270–5.

9. Niederkrotenthaler T, Till B. Suicide and the media: from Werther to Papageno effects—a selective literature review. Suicidologi. 2019;24(2).

10. Niederkrotenthaler T, Braun M, Pirkis J, Till B, Stack S, Sinyor M, et al. Association between suicide reporting in the media and suicide: systematic review and meta-analysis. BMJ. 2020;368:m575.

11. Pirkis J, Blood W. Suicide and the news and information media. Suicide. 2018.

12. World Health Organisation. Preventing suicide: a resource for media professionals. Geneva: World Health Organization; 2017.

13. Phillips DP. The influence of suggestion on suicide: substantive and theoretical implications of the Werther effect. Am Sociol Rev. 1974;39(3):340–54.

14. Ringel E. The presuicidal syndrome. Suicide Life Threat Behav. 1976;6(3):131–49.

15. Shneidman ES. Suicide as psychache: a clinical approach to self-destructive behavior. Northvale, NJ: Jason Aronson; 1993.

16. Ortiz P, Khin Khin E. Traditional and new media's influence on suicidal behavior and contagion. Behav Sci Law. 2018;36(2):245–56.

17. Stack S. Suicide in the media: a quantitative review of studies based on nonfictional stories. Suicide Life Threat Behav. 2005;35(2):121–33.

18. Phillips DP, Carstensen LL. The effect of suicide stories on various demographic groups, 1968–1985. Suicide Life Threat Behav. 1988;18(1):100–14.

19. Cheng AT, Hawton K, Chen TH, Yen AM, Chang J-C, Chong M-Y, et al. The influence of media reporting of a celebrity suicide on suicidal behavior in patients with a history of depressive disorder. J Affect Disord. 2007;103(1–3):69–75.

20. Tsai C-W, Gunnell D, Chou Y-H, Kuo C-J, Lee M-B, Chen Y-Y. Why do people choose charcoal burning as a method of suicide? An interview based study of survivors in Taiwan. J Affect Disord. 2011;131(1–3):402–7.

21. Niederkrotenthaler T, Voracek M, Herberth A, Till B, Strauss M, Etzersdorfer E, et al. Role of media reports in completed and prevented suicide: Werther v. Papageno effects. Br J Psychiatry. 2010;197(3):234–43.

22. Hegerl U, Koburger N, Rummel-Kluge C, Gravert C, Walden M, Mergl R. One followed by many?—Long-term effects of a celebrity suicide on the number of suicidal acts on the German railway net. J Affect Disord. 2013;146(1):39–44.

23. Daine K, Hawton K, Singaravelu V, Stewart A, Simkin S, Montgomery P. The power of the web: a systematic review of studies of the influence of the internet on self-harm and suicide in young people. PLoS One. 2013;8(10):e77555.

24. Marchant A, Hawton K, Stewart A, Montgomery P, Singaravelu V, Lloyd K, et al. A systematic review of the relationship between internet use, self-harm and suicidal behaviour in young people: the good, the bad and the unknown. PLoS One. 2017;12(8):e0181722.

25. Ueda M, Mori K, Matsubayashi T, Sawada Y. Tweeting celebrity suicides: users' reaction to prominent suicide deaths on Twitter and subsequent increases in actual suicides. Soc Sci Med. 2017;189:158–66.

26. Blom JN, Hansen KR. Click bait: forward-reference as lure in online news headlines. J Pragmat. 2015;76:87–100.

27. Zimerman A, Caye A, Salum G, Passos I, Kieling C. Revisiting the Werther effect in the 21st century: bullying and suicidality among adolescents who watched 13 Reasons Why. J Am Acad Child Adolescent Psychiatry. 2018;57(8):610–3.e2.

28. Chapple A, Ziebland S, Simkin S, Hawton K. How people bereaved by suicide perceive newspaper reporting: qualitative study. Br J Psychiatry. 2013;203(3):228–32.

29. Jempson M, Cookson R, Williams T, Thorsen E, Khan A, Thevanayagam P. Sensitive coverage saves lives: improving media portrayal of suicidal behaviour. London: National Institute for Mental Health in England; 2007.

30. Skehan J, Maple M, Fisher J, Sharrock G. Suicide bereavement and the media: a qualitative study. Adv Ment Health. 2013;11(3):223–37.

31. Gregory P, Stevenson F, King M, Osborn D, Pitman A. The experiences of people bereaved by suicide regarding the press reporting of the death: qualitative study. BMC Public Health. 2020;20(1):1–14.
32. Séguin M, Bordeleau V, Drouin M-S, Castelli-Dransart DA, Giasson F. Professionals' reactions following a patient's suicide: review and future investigation. Arch Suicide Res. 2014;18(4):340–62.
33. Collings SC, Kemp CG. Death knocks, professional practice, and the public good: the media experience of suicide reporting in New Zealand. Soc Sci Med. 2010;71(2):244–8.
34. Luce A. Ethical reporting of sensitive topics. London: Routledge; 2019.
35. Lau OL. 采访自杀案. Sin Chew Daily. 2019.
36. Yang YY. 【記者室】我不想再報自殺新聞了 光明日报. Guang Ming Daily. 2018.
37. Till B, Wild TA, Arendt F, Scherr S, Niederkrotenthaler T. Associations of tabloid newspaper use with endorsement of suicide myths, suicide-related knowledge, and stigmatizing attitudes toward suicidal individuals. Crisis. 2018;39:1–10.
38. Pirkis J, Burgess P, Blood RW, Francis C. The newsworthiness of suicide. Suicide Life Threat Behav. 2007;37(3):278–83.
39. Niederkrotenthaler T, Reidenberg DJ, Till B, Gould MS. Increasing help-seeking and referrals for individuals at risk for suicide by decreasing stigma: the role of mass media. Am J Prev Med. 2014;47(3):S235–S43.
40. Cheng Q, Chen F, Lee ES, Yip PS. The role of media in preventing student suicides: a Hong Kong experience. J Affect Disord. 2018;227:643–8.
41. Arendt F, Scherr S, Niederkrotenthaler T, Krallmann S, Till B. Effects of awareness material on suicide-related knowledge and the intention to provide adequate help to suicidal individuals. Crisis. 2018;39(1):47.
42. Robinson J, Cox G, Bailey E, Hetrick S, Rodrigues M, Fisher S, et al. Social media and suicide prevention: a systematic review. Early Interv Psychiatry. 2016;10(2):103–21.
43. Allern S. Journalistic and commercial news values. Nordicom Rev. 2002;23(1–2):137–52.
44. Picard RG. Commercialism and newspaper quality. Newsp Res J. 2004;25(1):54–65.
45. Caple H, Bednarek M. Delving into the discourse: approaches to news values in journalism studies and beyond. Oxford: Reuters; 2013.
46. Crane C, Hawton K, Simkin S, Coulter P. Suicide and the media: pitfalls and prevention: report on a meeting organized by the Reuters Foundation Program at Green College and University of Oxford Centre for Suicide Research at Green College, Oxford, UK, November 18, 2003. Crisis. 2005;26(1):42–7.
47. O'Brien A. Reporting on mental health difficulties, mental illness and suicide: Journalists' accounts of the challenges. Journalism Stud. 2020;19:1447–65.
48. Cheng Q, Fu K-w, Caine E, Yip PS. Why do we report suicides and how can we facilitate suicide prevention efforts? Perspectives of Hong Kong media professionals. Crisis. 2014;35(2):74.
49. Tully J, Elsaka N. Suicide and the media: a study of the media response to suicide and the media: the reporting and portrayal of suicide in the media-a resource. Christchurch: School of Political Science and Communication, University of Canterbury; 2004.
50. Norris B, Jempson M, Bygrave L, Thorsen E. Reporting suicide worldwide: media responsibilities. The MediaWise Trust. 2006.
51. Luxton DD, June JD, Fairall JM. Social media and suicide: a public health perspective. Am J Public Health. 2012;102(S2):S195–200.
52. Pierri F, Piccardi C, Ceri S. Topology comparison of Twitter diffusion networks effectively reveals misleading information. Sci Rep. 2020;10(1):1–9.
53. World Health Organization. National suicide prevention strategies: progress, examples and indicators. Geneva: World Health Organization; 2018.
54. Hunter Institute of Mental Health Newcastle. Reporting suicide and mental illness: a mindframe resource for media professionals. Hunter Institute of Mental Health Newcastle, Newcastle; 2014.
55. Blood RW, Pirkis J. Suicide and the media: Part III. Theoretical issues. Crisis. 2001;22(4):163.

56. Pirkis J, Blood RW, Beautrais A, Burgess P, Skehan J. Media guidelines on the reporting of suicide. Crisis. 2006;27(2):82–7.
57. Sinyor M, Schaffer A, Heisel MJ, Picard A, Adamson G, Cheung CP, et al. Media guidelines for reporting on suicide: 2017 update of the Canadian Psychiatric Association Policy Paper. Can J Psychiatry. 2018;63(3):182–96.
58. The Hong Kong Jockey Club Centre for Suicide Research and Prevention. Recommendations on suicide reporting and online information dissemination for media professionals. Pokfulam, Hong Kong: The Hong Kong Jockey Club Centre for Suicide Research and Prevention; 2015. https://csrp.hku.hk/wp-content/uploads/2015/06/RecommendationsSuicideReport-en.pdf
59. India B, Wang X. Media guidelines for the responsible reporting of suicide. Crisis. 2012;33(4):190–8.
60. K-w F, Yip PSF. Changes in reporting of suicide news after the promotion of the WHO media recommendations. Suicide Life Threat Behav. 2008;38(5):631–6.
61. Corrigan PW, Morris SB, Michaels PJ, Rafacz JD, Rüsch N. Challenging the public stigma of mental illness: a meta-analysis of outcome studies. Psychiatr Serv. 2012;63(10):963–73.
62. Harcup T, O'neill D. What is news? News values revisited (again). Journal Stud. 2017;18(12):1470–88.
63. internetmatters.org. How to report suicidal content on social media www.internet-matters.org: internetmatters.org; 2020. https://www.internetmatters.org/resources/how-to-report-suicidal-content-on-social-media/.
64. Wu C-Y, Lee M-B, Liao S-C, Chan C-T, Chen C-Y. The trend of suicide reporting in the media: an effectiveness study of daily surveillance over nine years. bioRxiv. 2019:768945.
65. Pirkis J, Blood W, Dare A, Holland K. The Media Monitoring Project. Changes in reporting of suicide and mental illness in Australia: 2000/01–2006/07. 2008.
66. Hollings J. Reporting suicide in New Zealand: time to end censorship. Pac Journal Rev. 2013;19(2):136.
67. Ministry Of Justice. Making information about a suicide public. Ministry of Justice, New Zealand; 2020. https://coronialservices.justice.govt.nz/: updated 13/1/2020. https://coronialservices.justice.govt.nz/suicide/making-information-about-a-suicide-public/.
68. Pirkis J, Neal L, Dare A, Blood RW, Studdert D. Legal bans on pro-suicide web sites: an early retrospective from Australia. Suicide Life Threat Behav. 2009;39(2):190–3.

Suicide Prevention Strategies to Protect Young Women at Risk

Aruna Yadiyal and Prabha S. Chandra

1 Prevention of Suicide in Young Women: Is the Problem Unique Enough to Warrant a Separate Discussion?

Most epidemiological studies from diverse nations and cultures show distinct differences in suicidal behavior, across gender and life span, independent of methodological issues. The global age-standardized suicide rate for males (13.7 per 100,000) was higher by 1.8 times than that of females (7.5 per 100,000) in most countries [1, 2]. The prevalence of suicide attempts are two to three times higher than suicides and are clearly more in women everywhere. This gender paradox was found reversed in few countries like China, Bangladesh, Lesotho, Morocco, and Myanmar, according to recent most estimates by WHO. For young women aged 15–29 years, suicide was found to be the second leading cause of death, globally. The South East Asia region had a much higher female age -standardized suicide rate of 11.5 per 100,000 versus the 7.5 per 100,000 rate of the global female average. Women in the low and middle income countries had the highest suicide rate of 9.1 per 100,000, when compared across other income groups [1–3].

Advancing age seems to have a greater divergence between sexes, with decrease in rates of attempted suicides more pronounced in men than women [3–8]. Suicidal attempt to completion ratio is very high (up to 200:1) in younger women compared to older women (4:1), with more direct suicidal communication in younger and

A. Yadiyal
Department of Psychiatry, Father Muller Medical College, Mangalore, India
e-mail: arunag2779@gmail.com

P. S. Chandra (✉)
Department of Psychiatry, National Institute of Mental Health and Neurosciences, Bangalore, India

International Association for Women's Mental Health, Bangalore, India
e-mail: chandra@nimhans.ac.in

more indirect method of communication in older women. Suicide rates in younger women are also more in some Asian countries compared to western countries. Younger women use poisoning as a common method of suicide and have higher rates of substance abuse and depression. In older women, physical illnesses, functional impairment, neuroticism, social isolation and lack of livelihood are unique features. Among older women, suicidal behavior was seen to be of high intent, well planned, more lethal, and less likely to be affected by short-term modelling effect, when compared to their younger counterparts. However greater prevalence of indirect self-destructive behavior like poor adherence to treatment, refusal to eat, self-neglect was seen in older women. The latter also have a unique set of psycho-social stressors like bereavement, chronic physical illnesses, terminal illnesses, spousal loss, untreated or undertreated pain, anxiety related to progression of disease, living alone, fear of dependency or being a burden. Dementia, though, debilitating to elderly, has been thought of as a protective factor, where the execution of suicidal thought becomes difficult [8]. Also, a history of previous suicide attempt, which is one of the prominent risk factors in young women is usually absent in an older cohort as case fatalities are more common (see Table 1) [4–8].

With suicide expected to represent 2.4% of the global disease burden by 2020, it is imperative that focus is shifted towards suicidal behaviors and attempts and not just on mortality statistics arising out of completed suicides. With many countries not reporting suicide attempts, the highly acclaimed suicide data fails substantially to fully represent the major female contribution towards suicidal morbidity. With

Table 1 Differences in suicidal behavior between younger and older women

Variables	Young women	Older women
Suicidal attempts	More	Less
Completed suicides	Less	More
Attempted to completed suicide ratio	Higher	Lower
Suicidal communications	More and detected often	Indirect and missed often
Most common method used	Poisoning	Hanging followed by poisoning
Unique risk factors	(More clinical) Substance use disorders, depressive disorders	(More social) Functional impairment, bereavement, chronic physical illness, terminal illness, spousal loss, pain syndromes, fear of dependency, social isolation
Cognitive style	More flexible	More rigid
Suicidal behavior	Low intent to die, short-term plan, less lethal, highly affected from modelling effect, copycat suicide, direct self-harm more	High intent to die, long planned, highly lethal, indirect self-destruction behavior, poor adherence to treat, refusal to eat, self-neglect
Unique protective factors	Pregnancy, having young children, having a partner	Dementia, less rates of depression

the weight of the disease burden of suicidal behavior clearly skewed towards female gender, more so in younger age groups, it is imperative that research starts focusing on this high-risk group. In the gap between completed suicides and attempted suicide and suicidal behavior lies the hidden potential to tap on preventive strategies to protect this vulnerable socio-demographic cohort from moving along the continuum towards fatal and final outcomes [9–12].

2 Socio-Cultural Threads in the Fabric of Female Suicidality: Would We Do Better here with a Gendered Lens?

As gender is one of the most frequently replicated predictors of suicide, understanding the gender differences in suicidal behavior, and not just suicide, will hopefully lead us to consider current suicide prevention strategies with a gendered lens.

2.1 Difference in Suicidality Between Men and Women

While completed suicides are more in men in most countries, women attempt to take their life two to three times more than men, though this ratio of attempted to completed suicide tends to fall as both genders move to age more [13]. Unlike in men, where older age has a higher risk for suicide, in women it is younger age that appears to confer a higher risk. More differences seem to appear in suicidal behavior in women across cultures and nations, unlike in males, where findings are more stable and similar cross culturally. Differences in cognitive styles related to suicidal behavior also have been described, with women tending to have over-thinking, inclusive thinking, considering feelings of others and being more ready to seek and get help. Men appear to think less, have a more decided attitude, are more plan or action oriented and often refuse help [14]. Also, women tend to have higher rates of suicidal thinking and non-fatal suicidal behavior in addition to higher suicidal attempts. Chosen suicidal methods differ, with women tending to choose less lethal or less violent methods. Poisoning appears to be the commonest method and in case women use a gun, they seldom shoot themselves on the face.

Women have been shown to have different and unique risk and protective factors when compared to men. For example, pregnancy and parenthood appeared to be protective, and post-partum psychiatric disorders, abortions, infertility, death of children, proved to be risk factors unique to female gender. Marriage, found to be a protective factor for men, was not always so for women, and varied across cultures. Forced marriage, early marriage, marriage to an older man and intimate partner violence were found to be risk factors arising out of marriage for women, predominantly from developing countries. Depression, which was one of the most prominent risk factors for suicide, also differs in its manifestation and course across gender. Comorbid psychiatric illnesses like anxiety disorders, eating disorders, body dysmorphic disorder, and physical illnesses were more burdensome in females rather than males. Though 70% of antidepressants use is noted in women, attempted suicides and suicidal behavior are more subjected to under reporting in many countries, especially non-western societies due to stigma associated with suicidality among women [13–23].

2.2   Cultural Patterns with Gender-Specific Subtexts in the Unfolding Saga of Female Suicidality

Diverse cultures with varying dimensions of suicidal behavior in young women are forcing us to shift our focus towards cultural contexts and meanings, which impact each gender differently. Understanding these patterns may help us devise interventions that acknowledge the interface between gender and culture.

The cultural milieu of human behavior has so far been hostile to the female gender, which is evident by the negative impact it has on female suicidal behavior. The rates though high, may still be just the tip of the iceberg, because underreporting of suicidal behavior is rampant in developing countries, owing to various inefficiencies and discrepancies in the civil, legal and social mechanisms in these societies. Suicide rates among women diverge among countries, where in rates are highest in older age groups (>75 years) in Europe, Russia, Korea and China, in the age group of 45–54 years in USA and a much younger age group in South Asia. The method of suicide also varied across cultures, with women in Western countries using over the counter or prescribed medications in overdose, followed by use of firearms. Asian women have been found to use more lethal methods, often without more intent, but rather due to easy accessibility and availability such as consuming pesticides. Self-immolation is also chosen by a sizeable number of women in developing countries, because of prevailing sociocultural norms and higher acceptability. The figures for self-immolation are astonishingly skewed towards females, with it being common in Iran, India, Sri Lanka and other Asian countries. Marriage, seen as a socio-cultural construct, also varies across cultures and genders in its impact on suicidal behavior. Marriage tends to be less protective for females than males across cultures, and even turns into a risk factor for suicidal behavior in younger women in developing countries in South Asia. This seems to be because of the life and marital circumstances, rather than marriage itself, which increases their vulnerability towards suicidal behavior. The most common circumstances include arranged, forced and early marriages, young motherhood, low social status, economic dependency and domestic violence. Intimate partner violence and domestic violence are associated with suicidal risk and behavior in females worldwide, more strikingly so in developing countries of Asia and Middle East, as it is not only socially and culturally condoned but is also acceptable as societal norms in these communities. Studies revealed staggering figures where, 48% of women in Brazil, 61% in Egypt, 64% in India, 11% in Indonesia and 28% in Philippines showed a significant correlation between spousal violence and suicidal behavior [3, 7–10, 24–26]. Recently published systematic reviews have shown strong association between cultural practices like female genital mutilation and adverse mental health outcomes including increased risk of suicide behavior in women [24]. Substance use disorders independently increase risk of suicidal behavior, more so in men and elderly populations. But with increasing substance use disorders in females, globally, and with its association with violence and risk-taking behavior, substance use disorders in both genders needs to be considered as a significant risk factor in female suicidal behavior across cultures [25, 26].

Childhood adversities like physical, emotional and sexual abuse and violence are also associated with suicidal behavior in women. Consistent risk factors that weigh heavily towards female suicidality include intimate partner violence, non-partner physical violence, childhood sexual abuse, being widowed, divorced or separated, and history of partner violence in mother, according to a WHO multi-country study [25]. Sporadic risk factors were also found in some western countries in migrant and minority communities [27]. More common risk factors predominant in western cultures were being widowed, divorced, being single, death of partner, death of child and occasionally abortion and infertility [3]. Pregnancy and childbirth as protective factors may not be applicable uniformly across all countries. In high income countries, suicide is one of the important causes of maternal mortality during pregnancy and related events like abortion and miscarriage, highlighting the cultural variance of suicidal behavior in females [28–30]. Contrary to research findings from developing countries, reports from developed countries like Australia suggest psychiatric illness in young mothers as one of the leading causes of maternal mortality, with most suicides by violent means [30]. WHO, in its report, in 2017, highlights the fact that low-and-middle-income countries account for 78% of world's death by suicide and studies in these cultures point towards family conflict, emotional distress, poverty and illness to be major risk factors for suicidal behavior in women of these cultures [28, 31]. Various studies done in war zones and conflict areas like Pakistan, Afghanistan, Jordan, Thailand-Burma borders have shown that women in these contexts become refugees and are victims of endless traumas including physical and sexual violence, abduction, forced prostitution and forced sale of their children. A range of trauma related psychological aftermath including suicidal behavior have been noted in these women [32]. The socio-cultural milieu of India, though unique, has not been kind towards the female gender, where patriarchy is the main flavor on any day. Culturally colored risk factors in Indian women include stifling patriarchy, archaic stances on sexuality, marriage and female autonomy, sexual and emotional victimization of women, problematic spousal substance abuse, domestic violence, poor physical health and economic impoverishment. Some cultural factors which were found to be protective in Indian women were support from extended family systems, religiosity, resilience, good coping skills and scriptural wisdom in the face of continuing adversities (see Table 2) [32–38].

Table 2 Differences in suicidal behaviour among women in Western and Asian countries

Variables	Western countries	Asian countries
Suicide rate	More in older women	More in young
M:F ratio	High	Low
Risk factors	Commonly studied; clinical risk factors	Unique; culturally colored
Cultural impact on risk factors	Less	More; Negative
Lethality of method used	Low	High
Area	More in urban	More in rural
Reporting bias	Less	More
Stigma associated	Less	More
Socio-economic cost	Less	More
Access to mental health services	Present	Not adequate

3 Cultural Context of Suicidal Behavior in Women of Middle East Countries

With Islam being the fastest growing religion in the world, the higher rates of suicide among young Middle Eastern Muslim females warrants special attention. Though their religion forbids suicide, there is cultural discrimination between sexes, where Muslim females, often of young age, succumb to suicide, usually by violent methods like self -immolation. Many of these women are illiterate, of low socio-economic status, and usually have no desire or intent to die. They choose this gruesome method without much knowledge of consequences, mostly because it is more accepted or available. Many suffer from mental health disorders, the most common being depression, with no access to mental health services. Marriage is more of a risk factor, again, with domestic violence, arranged or forced marriage with much older males, overall oppression in marriage, polygamy practices and secondary designated role in marriage and society as sub-factors. The rights of the men are forced upon, at the cost of liberty of women leading to irrational traditions like honor killing. Restrictions about clothes and movement are also enforced upon women. Infertility, childlessness, abortions, lack of control over one's birthing rights or bodily issues are unique and culturally colored and biased risk factors pushing these women, especially the young ones, towards suicidal behavior [33, 39].

The above descriptions highlight how an understanding of interactions of culture with gender and its roles as both antecedents and explanations of suicidal intent and behavior will definitely help us to focus on culture-sensitive and gender sensitive intervention programs.

4 Components of an Effective Suicide Prevention Program Using Universal, Selected, and Indicated Interventions: Are These Gender and Culture Informed?

Suicide prevention strategies need to be considered among the vital public health goals, taking into account the magnitude of suicide and suicidality and the scope of preventable deaths between them. Though these interventions are limited in developing countries, various preventive approaches, along the lines of Universal, Selective and Indicated interventions have been implemented by developed countries. Universal interventions target whole populations and work towards reducing risk factors across populations. Selective interventions target subgroups of people with risk factors but with no suicidal behavior as yet. Indicated interventions attend exclusively to people who already have exhibited some suicidal behavior like plans, attempts, or to survivors of suicide. For these interventions to become successful, the identified risk factors need to be significant both at individual and population level and should be amenable to modification and fostering acceptability in communities. Acknowledging the diversity and variance of both risk and protective factors across cultures, gender and age is important as it has implications in developing meaningful and relevant prevention strategies (see Table 3) [40–45].

Table 3 Preventive intervention strategies for suicide	**Universal interventions**
	Reducing access to means
	Educating/training of primary care physicians
	Ensuring responsive media portrayal of suicide
	Educating public about mental health and illness
	School based education/awareness programs
	Policy and law changes
	Befriending agencies/crisis centers/national helplines
	Promotion of mental health/media campaigns
	Addressing socio-economic/cultural factors associated with suicidal behavior
	Selective interventions
	Strengthening of screening mechanisms-identify/assess high-risk groups
	Gatekeeper training/consultation/education services
	Support/skills training of at-risk groups
	Focusing on subgroups of at-risk groups
	Indicated interventions
	Treatment and case management of identified cases
	Community outreach programs
	Support/training for family members/survivors of suicide
	Ensuring continuity of care
	Skills building and support to suicide attempters

4.1   Universal Interventions

These interventions aim to reduce risk in the population as a whole, and though difficult, can be highly effective in the long term. Reducing availability of means for suicide is the most widely discussed strategy and has been found to be impactful. Measures like replacing toxic coal gas with non-toxic North Sea gas, cars fitted with catalytic converters to avert carbon monoxide poisoning, restricting availability of firearms, advocating for newer, safer antidepressants like SSRIs, packing of fewer analgesics per pack to reduce paracetamol hepatotoxicity, improving safety at popular sites by erecting suicide barriers on bridges, multi-storey car parks, or skyrises, making psychiatric inpatient units free of hooks, pipes and sharp surfaces, making bed rails collapsible, secure fencing of railway lines or waterways, reducing availability and promoting safe-storage programs for pesticides, have gone a long way in reducing rates of suicide and suicide attempts in areas where it was enforced. Effective local education and training programs for primary care clinicians and general practitioners has led to better detection and management of depression in primary care settings and has also improved referrals to mental health professionals. Joint collaborative committees consisting of the press, clinical and voluntary agencies, local political representatives, non-governmental organizations (NGOs), women support groups and experts in suicidology need to develop consensus statements about media policies in relation to responsible reporting and portrayal of suicide. This strategy needs to be country-specific and culture sensitive to be effective in young women. Psychiatrists also need to continually educate the public about mental illness in general and thereby tackle stigmatization of suicide, specifically, through media campaigns, workshops, articles and leaflets. School based educational programs could do well to teach directly about suicide facts, help recognize psychological distress in themselves and peers and also help screen adolescents at risk of psychiatric disorders with appropriate and timely referrals. Policy and statute changes like imposing a ban on underage drinking, illicit drugs, driving restrictions, and decriminalization of suicide attempts help rein in the rates of suicidal behavior within a population cohort. Befriending agencies, national suicide helplines and crisis centers specifically earmarked for suicide prevention, mainly staffed by volunteers, serves to reach out to the desperate in their weakest moments and helps avert mental suicidal fatality. Promotion of positive health in the public and not just education about mental illnesses helps in building resilience and good coping skills in the masses, which in turn helps to empower them against suicide. Mental health professionals should also lead the way in highlighting to the respective governments and regimes in their areas, the need to modify adverse socio-economic factors, which act as risk factors for suicidal behavior in young women [40–43].

4.2 Selective Interventions

Strategies aimed at addressing at-risk groups and individuals vulnerable to suicidal behavior are valuable in the context of the potential to identify and modify the risk factors found. This requires strengthening of screening mechanisms (through training, better and easy questionnaires, skills training) to identify and assess high-risk groups and take steps to address those particular risk-factors. Gatekeeper training and consultation should be offered to those who serve as first-contact for these high-risk individuals like parents, teachers, school counsellors, primary health care workers, grass root workers, lay mental health workers, religious leaders, school council leaders, youth leaders, women welfare groups and active members of society. Support and skills training should be offered professionally and consistently to families of suicide victims and survivors of suicide attempts to avert a possible future attempt. Also, identification of high-risk occupational groups like farmers, students, women professionals, health care workers and migrants, and addressing their mental needs, forms part of a good selective intervention [43–45].

4.3 Indicated Interventions

These strategies target those who have already exhibited suicidal behavior. As these attempters and survivors form a high-risk group for future suicidal behavior, their treatment and case management need to be done with utmost care to prevent future attempts. Along with good rapport and active collaboration with patients, assessment of factors like preceding life events, motives for the act, personal problems, psychiatric disorders including personality and substance use disorders, family history, current social, domestic and occupational circumstances and previous attempts should be covered. Risk factors, protective factors and factors which suggest high suicidal intent, especially in young women, need special consideration. Pharmacological treatment with newer antidepressants, mood stabilizers (lithium) and neuroleptics (clozapine) is warranted under careful clinical discernment. A range of psychotherapies, to improve problem solving abilities and support the patient, particularly cognitive behavioral therapy, and dialectical therapy, can be effective, if offered over long-term. Provision of emergency cards, crisis center helpline numbers and easing access to emergency psychiatry services, will help in ensuring continuity of care. Also, issuing safety contracts and no-suicide pacts can be thought of at the time of discharge. Community outreach can be impactful with simple telephonic, post or email contact with patients, urging them towards regular follow-up visits. Support, education and training may need to be imparted to family members and survivors of suicide, along with bolstering of coping skills and interpersonal skills for patients during continued follow-up, more so for young women at risk [44–46].

5 Evidence for Effectiveness of Suicide Prevention Interventions: What Does Research Say?

Eighteen suicide prevention experts from 13 European countries have conducted a systematic review to highlight evidence for suicide prevention strategies. The findings include:

- Evidence for restricting access to lethal means has strengthened since 2005.
- School based awareness programs have been significantly effective.
- The anti-suicidal effects of lithium and clozapine are confirmed, although less specific.
- Education of physicians and effective treatment of depression, by pharmacotherapy and psychotherapy, are suitable interventions.

Though these findings have the potential to change public health policies in suicide prevention strategies, the research behind this is not all inclusive. None of the evidence comes from low-and middle-income countries and there is no sex aggregated data available to see which prevention strategies work better for women. Therefore, more research in approaches such as gatekeeper training, regulation of media, helplines, internet-based interventions with specific focus on young women, is definitely warranted [44, 47–49].

All these interventions, though effective, cannot be applied universally across all regions and cultures and fail to focus on vulnerable groups like women. Therefore, it would serve us well to innovate ways to modify these interventions to become more region-specific, culture- sensitive and gender-oriented, as the need of the times demand.

6 From Global to Local: The Path for Prevention Strategies for Suicidal Behavior in Young Women

Worldwide, 70% of suicides occur in low and middle income countries with the South-East Asia region accounting for 39% of global suicides along with higher female age standardized suicide rates. India accounts for 82% of suicides in the South East Asia region and hence patterns in India are applicable across the South-East Asia region [2, 50, 51]. The above mentioned three-pronged intervention strategies may not always be feasible in developing nations with limited mental health resources. Consequently, prevention strategies need to be tailored to the region-specific characteristics of a nation and then implemented in a culture-sensitive approach.

6.1 Nested Suicide Prevention Programs: A Region-Specific and Culture-Sensitive Approach

There is lack of coordinated national suicide prevention programs in most low and middle income countries, except in Sri Lanka, Thailand and Bhutan. Also, most countries of these regions, including India, rely heavily on NGOs for implementation of suicide prevention interventions. For these interventions to be region-specific and culture-sensitive, infrastructure needs to be developed in a decentralized manner. At a national level, financial and political resources will have to be mobilized towards support of NGOs and formation of a multi -partisan committee at community levels. This committee should consist of all stakeholders like policymakers, planners, researchers, health and other service providers, community leaders, religious affiliations, youth representatives, responsible citizens of the community, so that they can devise a country-specific and culturally sensitive plan. This plan needs to be coordinated with relevant health and social agencies, so that it becomes effective and relevant at local levels too [50, 51]. We need to engage in a bottom up rather than a top down approach to prevention.

In order to be feasible in resource strapped developing countries, the interventions need to be risk factor based, low cost, deliverable even by lay mental health workers, micro-sized, and be able to address the felt needs of that community. Some universal interventions feasible here include decreasing availability and accessibility of methods like pesticides and its storage, strengthening of mental health services nationally and district-wise, effective implementation of national and district mental health plans (NMHP, DMHP), promotion and support to NGOs, establishing national chain of crisis centers and suicide helplines, increasing public awareness regarding suicide and de-stigmatization using media campaigns, formulation of guidelines for media for responsible reporting and portrayal of suicides, establishing a good and uniform reporting and monitoring system, and increasing impetus on research on suicidality.

Selective interventions here would include sensitization of primary care physicians and general practitioners in rural areas towards suicide, incorporation of mental health programs in school curriculums and training a cadre of para-mental health professionals to handle crisis at index points.

Indicated interventions can include cost effective use of antidepressants and ECT when essential, in indicated cases, increasing availability and affordability of antidepressants through subsidized dispensaries, easing access to mental health services to suicide attempters and ensuring continuity of care. Propagation of traditionally based and culturally accepted lifestyle modifications like minimalistic living, mindfulness training, meditation, yoga and use of scriptural wisdom, even by lay mental health workers, may help these distressed people adopt good coping skills and build resilience to face future adversities [50–54].

7 Suicide Prevention for Young Women: Can We Envision a New, Yet, Feasible Gender Specific Approach?

For suicide prevention strategies to be appropriate, effective and relevant to women, they need to be culture-sensitive and focus on vulnerable groups at risk (in this case, young women). Preventive efforts can be made more comprehensive by taking into account risk factors and protective factors specific to young women across populations and at individual levels. Preventive strategies should aim to mitigate risk factors and bolster protective factors, which might vary across cultures and nations (see Boxes 1 and 2) [24–26, 55–59].

Box 1 Protective factors for suicide in young women
- Pregnancy (planned, wanted)
- Motherhood
- Very young (<2 years)/dependent children
- Positive family and social support and supportive relationships
- Sense of responsibility to family
- Adequate emotional regulation
- Good social/verbal skills
- Life-satisfaction
- Positive coping/problem solving skills
- More health seeking and treatment-acceptance behavior
- More responsiveness/psychological readiness for psychological interventions
- Use of less lethal means
- Good reality-testing ability
- Religiosity or spirituality

Box 2 Risk factors for suicide in young women
- Psychiatric disorders—depressive disorders, PTSD, eating disorders, anxiety disorders
- Post-partum psychiatric disorders
- Infertility/death of child/child with disabilities
- Perinatal period-abortion and miscarriages
- Domestic violence/intimate partner violence
- Childhood physical/emotional/sexual abuse
- Body image disturbances
- Major surgery like mastectomy, hysterectomy
- Gender disadvantage in society
- Marriage-Socio-cultural factors/living contexts

- Alcohol abuse in spouse
- Unwanted pregnancy/motherhood
- Menstrual cycle associated stressors
- Economic dependency/poverty
- Limited education/financial/vocational opportunities
- Societal and familial pressure on personal issues
- Emotional distress/sensitivity
- Sexism/sexual discrimination/harassment
- Inappropriate media reporting practices
- Criminalization of suicide in some countries.

The cultural diversity in gender patterns in suicidality calls for interventions that are gender and culture specific. However, most suicide prevention interventions including those listed above, are gender neutral. Existing scant evidence indicates that for suicide prevention interventions to be specifically effective for females, it needs to be multipronged, addressing social, economic, political factors and structural inequalities within these factors (see Fig. 1) [60].

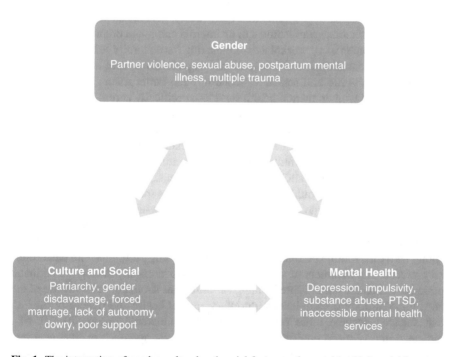

Fig. 1 The interaction of gender, cultural and social factors and mental health in suicide among young women

Universal interventions could include investing in robust public awareness campaigns advocating for gender equality among masses, programs to empower women through educational and economic opportunities, creating women peer support groups, pressing for laws to protect women's rights, laws against female genital mutilation, bolstering existing laws on marital rape, domestic violence, birthing rights and work place benefits, focusing on reducing menace of spousal drinking problems, advocating for compulsory and universal education of girls, abolition of dowry system and child marriages, striving for better representation of women in policy and decision making forums, making access to mental health care easier for women, and supporting NGOs working in areas of women's welfare [46, 60]. As women are significant victims of post disaster situations, disaster intervention programs should work towards gender equity considering the local cultural, social and economic structures of the affected community. Development of support network around women and their care as a family unit would make disaster response strategies more empowering and sensitive towards the needs of women [61].

Selective interventions could include strengthening screening and referrals to mental health services for women in peri-partum conditions, integrating mental health into routine antenatal health care and having appropriate stepped care systems, and developing a chain of mother-baby care units as part of psychiatry in patient services across tertiary care centers. This would also include gender-specific school mental health programs or addressing mental health needs of adolescent girls, reproductive health programs for both genders, gender sensitization programs across all work sectors, establishment of an internal complaint committee and grievance cell for women in all workplaces, advocating for maternity leaves and benefits in all higher educational and occupational organizations, and strengthening of responses to domestic and sexual violence through better managed shelters, one stop centers and women mental health services specifically across the country [59, 60]. By sensitizing health sector workers, mental health policies and services towards violence against women, they can be made to respond appropriately, which may subsequently reduce the health burden associated with violence and suicidal behavior in women [30]. A multi-level program aiming at effective detoxification, followed by rehabilitation and recovery programs in de-addiction wards specially earmarked for women, would be a very desired gender-specific approach as well.

Indicated interventions could include assertive follow-ups and treatment of perinatal women with psychiatric morbidity through accessible psychiatric services, including liaison consultations, which can address suicide in these indicated cases. Along with this, routine perinatal psychosocial screening programs with clear referral protocols and treatment of significant psychiatric morbidity during the perinatal period could be chosen indicated strategies. Clinicians should be made aware of the need for continuity of care between primary, mental health and maternity care, so that suicides become more preventable in this vulnerable group [29, 30, 62]. Indicated interventions could adopt a more empathetic approach in treatment and care of women who attempt suicide, exploring the cultural, social and clinical risk factors in each context, providing continuity of care and outreach through women personnel, and work towards teaching effective coping skills in order to build

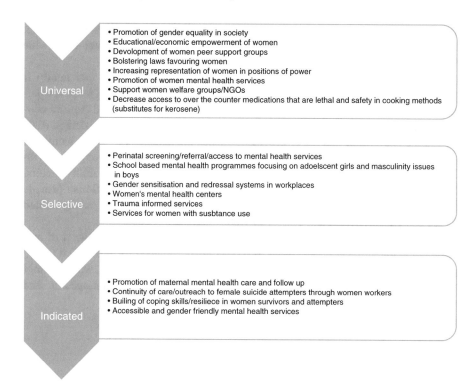

Universal
- Promotion of gender equality in society
- Educational/economic empowerment of women
- Devolopment of women peer support groups
- Bolstering laws favouring women
- Increasing representation of women in positions of power
- Promotion of women mental health services
- Support women welfare groups/NGOs
- Decrease access to over the counter medications that are lethal and safety in cooking methods (substitutes for kerosene)

Selective
- Perinatal screening/referral/access to mental health services
- School based mental health programmes focusing on adoelscent girls and masculinity issues in boys
- Gender sensitisation and redressal systems in workplaces
- Women's mental health centers
- Trauma informed services
- Services for women with susbtance use

Indicated
- Promotion of maternal mental health care and follow up
- Continuity of care/outreach to female suicide attempters through women workers
- Builing of coping skills/resiliece in women survivors and attempters
- Accessible and gender friendly mental health services

Fig. 2 Gender specific interventions for suicide prevention

resilience and to avert suicidal thoughts and behavior in the face of continuing adversities in the future (see Fig. 2) [59–61].

The overall goal would be to bring in a much desired and deserved change in the socio-cultural scene of society as a whole, which should involve the male counterparts as well. Especially in many South Asian and Middle Eastern countries this would include involving men to decrease patriarchy and change traditional masculine roles and power equations.

8 What More Do We Need to Know About Suicide Prevention in Young Women?

Available evidence has shown that no single strategy is found to be better than the rest, advocating need for combinations of strategies at individual and population levels. Insufficient evidence haunts many other acclaimed preventive efforts like gatekeeper training or change in media guidelines. With suicide prevention being a global imperative, future research would do well to fill the voids and discrepancies between expert opinions, legislations, policy changes and available scientific data, to bring about meaningful change on the suicide scene for women worldwide [47–49].

Suicidal behaviors are complex human behaviors which could end fatally if timely preventive interventions are not in place. Young women, as a group, are particularly at risk, taking into account the variability of gender, age and cultural contexts across the spectrum of suicidal behavior. More sex disaggregated data in trials of suicide prevention that try to provide evidence specifically for young women is needed. The inclusion of a question on suicidality in studies related to partner violence or sexual abuse will give a better idea of resilience and vulnerability factors. Psychological autopsy studies related to death of young women will also provide leads. Finally, more biological underpinnings of suicidal behavior, especially related to the postpartum period and other vulnerable states are needed.

A deeper understanding of these complex underpinnings in the context of suicidal behavior in women, will force us to recognize the need for preventive strategies along the lines of universal, selective and indicated interventions, which further needs to be customized to evolve into a women-oriented, region-specific and culture-sensitive approach.

References

1. Bertolote JM, Fleischmann A. A global perspective on the magnitude of suicide mortality. In: Wasserman D, Wasserman C, editors. Oxford textbook of suicidology and suicide prevention. Oxford: Oxford University Press; 2009. p. 91–8.
2. World Health Organization. Suicide in the world: global health estimates. World Health Organization. WHO/MSD/MER/19.3; 2019.
3. Mendez-Bustos P, et al. Life cycle and suicidal behavior among women. Sci World J. 2013;6:1–9.
4. Zeppegno P, Manzetti E, Valsesia R, et al. Differences in suicidal behavior in elderly: a study in two provinces of Northern Italy. Int J Geriatr Psychiatry. 2005;20(8):769–75.
5. De Leo D, Padoani W, Scocco P, et al. Attempted and completed suicides in older subjects: results from WHO/EURO multicenter study of suicide. Int J Geriatr Psychiatry. 2005;20(8):769–75.
6. Skoog I, Aevarsson O, Beskow J, et al. Suicidal feelings in a population sample of non-demented 85-year olds. Am J Psychiatr. 1996;153:1015–20.
7. Abraham VJ, Abraham S, Jacob KS. Suicide in the elderly in the Kaniyambadi block, Tamil Nadu, South India. Int J Geriatr Psychiatry. 2005;10:953–5.
8. Rich C, Young D, Fowler R. San Diego suicide study: young vs old subjects. Arch Gen Psychiatry. 1986;43:577–82.
9. Vijayakumar L. Suicide in women. Indian J Psychiatry. 2015;57:233–8.
10. Beautrais AL. Women and suicidal behavior. Crisis. 2006;27:153–6.
11. Lonnqvist JK. Epidemiology and causes of suicide. In: Gelder M, Andreasen N, Lopez- Ibor JJ, Geddes JR, editors. New Oxford textbook of psychiatry, vol. 1. 2nd ed. Oxford: Oxford University Press; 2009. p. 951–7.
12. Baca-Garcia E, et al. Suicidal behavior in young women. Psychiatr Clin N Am. 2008;31(2):317–31.

13. Garg R, Trivedi JK, Dhyani M. Suicidal behavior in special population: elderly, women and adolescent in special reference to India. Delhi Psychiatry J. 2007;10(2):106–18.
14. Murphy GE. Why women are less likely than men to commit suicide. Compr Psychiatry. 1998;39(4):165–75.
15. Ping Q, Mortensen PB, Agerbo E. Gender differences in risk factors for suicide in Denmark. Br J Psychiatry. 2000;177:546–50.
16. Kolves VK, Allik J, et al. Gender issues in suicide rates, trends and methods among youth aged 15–24 in 15 European countries. J Affect Disord. 2009;113(3):216–26.
17. Chung A. Gender differences in suicide, household production and unemployment. Appl Econ. 2009;41(19):2495–504.
18. Hawton K, Harris L. The changing gender ratio in occurrence of deliberate self-harm across the life cycle. Crisis. 2008;9(1):4–10.
19. Hawton K. Sex and suicide: gender differences in suicidal behavior. Br J Psychiatry. 2000;177:484–5.
20. Edwards MJ, Holder RR. Coping, meaning in life, and suicidal manifestations: examining gender differences. J Clin Psychol. 2001;57(121):1517–34.
21. Mayer P, Ziaian T. Suicide, gender and age variations in India. Are women in Indian society protected from suicide? Crisis. 2002;23:98–103.
22. Webster Rudmin F, Ferrada- Noli M, Skolbekken JA. Questions of culture, age and gender in the epidemiology of suicide. Scand J Psychol. 2003;44:373–81.
23. Canetto SS. Women and suicidal behavior: a cultural analysis. Am J Orthopsychiatry. 2008;78(2):259–66.
24. Abdalla SM, Galea S. Is female genital mutilation/cutting associated with adverse mental health consequences? A systematic review of evidence. BMJ Glob Health. 2019;4(4):e001553.
25. Devries K, et al. Violence against women is strongly associated with suicide attempts: evidence from the WHO multi-country study on women's health and domestic violence against women. Soc Sci Med. 2011;73:79–86.
26. Esang M, Ahmed S. A closer look at substance use and suicide. Am J Psychiatry Resid J. 2018;13(6):6–8.
27. Bhugra D. Suicidal behavior in South Asians in the UK. Crisis. 2002;23(3):108–13.
28. Seponski DM, et al. Family, health and poverty factors impacting suicide attempts in Cambodian Women. Crisis. 2019;40(2):141–5.
29. Khalifeh H, et al. Suicide in perinatal and non-perinatal women in contact with psychiatric services: 15-year findings from a UK national inquiry. Lancet Psychiatry. 2016;3:233–4.
30. Austin MP, et al. Maternal mortality and psychiatric morbidity in the perinatal period: challenges and opportunities for prevention in the Australian setting. MJA. 2007;186:364–7.
31. Cavanaugh CE, et al. Ethnic differences in correlates of suicidal behavior among women seeking help for intimate partner violence. Crisis. 2015;36(4):257–66.
32. Vijayakumar L. Suicide among refugees: a mockery of humanity. Crisis. 2016;37(1):1–4.
33. Rezaeian M. Suicide among young Middle Eastern Muslim females. The perspective of an Iranian Epidemiologist. Crisis. 2010;31(1):36–42.
34. Lasrado RA, et al. Structuring roles and gender identity within families explaining suicidal behavior in South India. Crisis. 2016;37(3):205–11.
35. Parkar SR, Nagarsekar B, Weiss MG. Explaining suicide in an urban slum of Mumbai, India: a sociocultural autopsy. Crisis. 2009;30(4):192–201.
36. Vijayakumar L, John S, Pirkis J, Whiteford H. Suicide in developing countries (2): risk factors. Crisis. 2005;26:112–9.
37. Vijayakumar L. Hindu religion and suicide in India. In: Wasserman D, Wasserman C, editors. Oxford textbook of suicidology and suicide prevention. Oxford: Oxford University Press; 2009. p. 19–26.
38. Maselko J, Patel V. Why women attempt suicide: the role of mental illness and social disadvantage in a community cohort study in India. J Epidemiol Community Health. 2008;62:817–22.

39. Fido A, Zahid MA. Coping with infertility among Kuwaiti women: cultural perspectives. Int J Soc Psychiatry. 2004;50:294–300.
40. Goldsmith SK, Pellmar TC, Kleinarr AM, Barney WE, editors. Reducing suicide: a national imperative. Washington, DC: The National Academies Press; 2002.
41. Hawton K. Prevention and treatment of suicidal behavior: from science to practice. Oxford: Oxford University Press; 2005.
42. Hawton K, Van Heeringen K. The international handbook of suicide and attempted suicide. Chichester: Wiley; 2000.
43. Hawton K, Taylor T. Treatment of suicide attempters and prevention of suicide and attempted suicide. In: Gelder MG, Andreasen NC, Lopez-Ibor JJ JJ, Geddes JR, editors. New Oxford textbook of psychiatry, vol. 1. 2nd ed. Oxford: Oxford University Press; 2009. p. 969–78.
44. Hawton K, Townsend A, Arensman E, et al. Psychosocial and pharmacological treatments of deliberate self-harm. Cochrane Database Syst Rev. 2005;4:CD001764.
45. American Psychiatric Association. Practice guideline for assessment and treatment of patients with suicidal behaviors. Arlington, VA: American Psychiatric Association; 2007.
46. Ahmadi A. Suicide by self-immolation: comprehensive overview, experiences and suggestions. J Burn Care Res. 2007;28:30.
47. Zalsmann G, et al. Suicide prevention strategies revisited: 10 year systematic review. Lancet Psychiatry. 2016;3:646–59.
48. Mann JJ, Apter A, Bertolote J, et al. Suicide prevention strategies: a systematic review. JAMA. 2005;294:2064–74.
49. Turecki G. Preventing suicide: where are we? Lancet Psychiatry. 2016;3:597–8.
50. Vijayakumar L, Pirkis J, Whiteford H. Suicide in developing countries: prevention efforts. Crisis. 2005;26(3):120–4.
51. Vijayakumar L. Challenges and opportunities in suicide prevention in South-East Asia. WHO South-East Asia J Public Health. 2017;6(1):30–3.
52. Radhakrishnan R, Andrade C. Suicide: an Indian perspective. Indian J Psychiatry. 2012;54(4):304–19.
53. Vijayakumar L. Suicide and its prevention: the urgent need in India. Indian J Psychiatry. 2007;49(2):81–4.
54. Chandra PS, Padmavathi D, Anuroopa P, et al. Do newspaper reports of suicides comply with standard suicide reporting guidelines? A study from Bangalore, India. Int J Soc Psychiatry. 2013;60(7):687–94.
55. Qin P, Mortensen PB. The impact of parental status on the risk of completed suicide. Arch Gen Psychiatry. 2003;60:797–802.
56. Oquendo MA, Bongiovi- Garcia ME, Galfalvy H, et al. Sex differences in clinical predictors of suicidal acts after major depression: a prospective study. Am J Psychiatry. 2007;164:134–41.
57. Franko DL, Keel PK. Suicidality in eating disorders: occurrence, correlates and clinical implications. Clin Psychol Rev. 2006;26:769–82.
58. Cougle JR, Resnick H, Kilpatrick DG. PTSD, depression and their comorbidity in relation to suicidality: cross-sectional and prospective analyses of a national probability of women. Depress Anxiety. 2009;26:1151–7.
59. Healey C, Morriss R, Henshaw C, Kinderman P. Self harm in psotpartum depression and referrals to a perinatal mental health team: an audit study. Arch Womens Ment Health. 2013;16(3):237–45.
60. Canetto SS. Prevention of suicidal behavior in females: opportunities and obstacles. In: Wasserman D, Wasserman C, editors. Oxford textbook of suicidology and suicide prevention: a global perspective. Oxford: Oxford University Press; 2009. p. 241–7.
61. Bhadra S. Women in disasters and conflicts in India: intervention in view of the Millenium Development Goals. Int J Disaster Risk Sci. 2017;8:196–207.
62. Lega I, et al. Maternal suicide in Italy. Arch Womens Ment Health. 2020;23:199–206.

Printed in the United States
by Baker & Taylor Publisher Services